T0195336

Musculoskeletal
ULTRASOUND
HOW, WHY AND WHEN

Musculoskeletal
ULTRASOUND
HOW, WHY AND WHEN

Lorelei Waring, DCR (R), PgC AP, MSc Medical Ultrasound, FHEA
Senior Lecturer
Department of Medical Sciences, Institute of Health
University of Cumbria, Lancaster
United Kingdom

Alison Hall, DCR (R), MSc Medical Ultrasound
Consultant Sonographer
School of Primary, Community and Social Care
Keele University, Keele
United Kingdom

Sara Riley, DCR (R), DMU, MHSc Medical Ultrasound
Consultant Sonographer
Leeds Radiology Academy
Leeds Teaching Hospitals NHS Trust, Leeds
United Kingdom

For additional online content visit **ExpertConsult.com**

ELSEVIER

Oxford   2022

Notices

Practitioners and researchers must always rely on their own experience and knowledge in evaluating and using any information, methods, compounds or experiments described herein. Because of rapid advances in the medical sciences, in particular, independent verification of diagnoses and drug dosages should be made. To the fullest extent of the law, no responsibility is assumed by Elsevier, authors, editors or contributors for any injury and/or damage to persons or property as a matter of products liability, negligence or otherwise, or from any use or operation of any methods, products, instructions, or ideas contained in the material herein.

[FOR PRODUCTS CONTAINING ADVERTISING ONLY: Although all advertising material is expected to conform to ethical (medical) standards, inclusion in this publication does not constitute a guarantee or endorsement of the quality or the value of such product or the claims made of it by its manufacturer.]

ISBN: (978-0-7020-8198-9)

Content Strategist: Trinity Hutton
Content Development Specialist: Andrae Akeh
Project Manager: Radjan Lourde Selvanadin
Design: Renee Duenow
Illustration Manager: Narayanan Ramakrishnan
Marketing Manager: Ed Major

Printed in India

Last digit is the print number: 9 8 7 6 5 4 3 2 1

Working together
to grow libraries in
developing countries

www.elsevier.com • www.bookaid.org

CONTENTS

PREFACE

Musculoskeletal ultrasound is an important diagnostic tool used by a range of health professionals in different clinical settings. It is becoming an accepted first-line imaging modality to compliment clinical diagnosis and therapy at point of care and is well established in primary and secondary care with a broad spectrum of use. This includes first-line investigation of choice for many musculoskeletal conditions; a focussed diagnostic and monitoring tool in rheumatology; and an aid to diagnosis, biopsy, and intervention in soft tissue masses and sarcoma assessment.

In comparison to other imaging modalities, ultrasound is operator-dependent and consequently, in the hands of the poorly trained or overconfident practitioner, it has the potential for harm as well as good.

This book is intended as a guide to those practitioners wanting to learn or develop their current practice of musculoskeletal ultrasound but does not claim to be a fully comprehensive resource. It is written by experts in the field from different professional backgrounds including sonographers, physiotherapists, radiologists, and rheumatologists drawing on their experience from many years of practice with practical tips and examples of normal ultrasound appearances and common pathologies.

There are many pitfalls in musculoskeletal ultrasound, which can lead to misdiagnosis or overdiagnosis and may result in poor patient management. These will be discussed in the relevant chapters as they can be due to poor use of the equipment, incorrect technique, or lack of understanding of the range of normal and age-related ultrasound appearances. The book also aims to provide increased awareness to less-experienced practitioners of clinical presentation and management of musculoskeletal conditions.

CONTRIBUTORS

Richard Brindley, BSc (Hons) Diagnostic Radiography
Consultant Sonographer
Radiology
The Royal Wolverhampton New Cross, Wolverhampton
United Kingdom

**Michael Bryant, BSc (Hons) Physiotherapy,
MSc Manual Therapy, PgC MSK Ultrasound**
Consultant MSK Physiotherapist & Sonographer
Integrated Musculoskeletal Service
East Lancashire Hospitals NHS Trust
United Kingdom

**Sophie Cochran, BSc (Hons) Diagnostic Radiography,
MSc Medical Ultrasound**
Clinical Specialist in Medical Ultrasound
Radiology
United Lincolnshire Hospitals Trust, Boston
United Kingdom

Dr Sylvia Connolly, MBChB HONS
Consultant Radiologist
Radiology
St Helens and Knowsley Teaching Hospitals NHS Trust,
    Prescot
Merseyside
United Kingdom

**Nicki Delves, DCR (R), Diploma Medical Ultrasound,
PgC**
Consultant Sonographer
Radiology
Queen Victoria NHS Foundation Hospital, East
    Grinstead
West Sussex
United Kingdom

Clare Drury, DCR (R), PGDip Medical Ultrasound
Clinical Specialist Sonographer
Ultrasound
Hull University Teaching Hospitals NHS Trust, Hull
United Kingdom

**Kirstie Godson, BSc Diagnostic Radiography,
MSc Medical Ultrasound, FHEA**
Academic Lecturer Diagnostic Imaging
Leeds University, Leeds
United Kingdom

Alison Hall, DCR (R), MSc Medical Ultrasound
Consultant Sonographer
School of Primary, Community and Social Care
Keele University, Keele
United Kingdom

Dr Samantha Hider, PhD FRCP MSc BMedSci BM BS
Professor of Rheumatology and Honorary Consultant
    Rheumatologist
School for Primary, Community and Social Care
Keele University, Keele
Staffordshire
United Kingdom

**Andrew Longmead, BSc (Hons) Diagnostic
Radiography, PgD Medical Ultrasound**
Advanced Practitioner Sonographer
Radiology
Chesterfield Royal Hospital NHS Foundation Trust
Chesterfield
United Kingdom

**Mark Maybury, BSc (Hons) Physiotherapy, PgD
Medical Ultrasound (MSK), MSc Neuromusculoskeletal
Health Care**
Research Physiotherapist/Sonographer
IRF, University of Birmingham Laboratories
Queen Elizabeth Hospital University Hospitals
    Birmingham, Birmingham
United Kingdom

Sara Riley, DCR (R), DMU, MHSc Medical Ultrasound
Consultant Sonographer
Leeds Radiology Academy
Leeds Teaching Hospitals NHS Trust, Leeds
United Kingdom

Katie Simm, BSc (Hons) Diagnostic Radiography, MSc Medical Imaging
Advanced Practitioner and Lead Sonographer
St Helens and Knowsley NHS Trust
Radiology
NHS, Merseyside
United Kingdom

Lorelei Waring, DCR(R), PgC AP, MSc Medical Ultrasound, FHEA
Senior Lecturer
Department of Medical Sciences, Institute of Health
University of Cumbria, Lancaster
United Kingdom

ACKNOWLEDGEMENTS

The authors would like to acknowledge the help and support of their families and work colleagues in this venture, with particular recognition of the valuable contributions of Steve Savage and John Leddy. Additional thanks to Tyler Rushton for acting as our model and for his patience throughout.

Image Optimisation and Safety Considerations

Kirstie Godson and Lorelei Waring

CHAPTER OUTLINE

INTRODUCTION

Musculoskeletal (MSK) ultrasound was first introduced in medical imaging in the 1970s[1] and advancements in technology have since enabled a wide scope of practice to develop within this field. Ultrasound is known to be a safe imaging modality with a high sensitivity and specificity for detection of traumatic, inflammatory, and degenerative soft tissue MSK conditions[1]; however, it is operator dependent, and accurate image acquisition and interpretation relies on training and experience of the operator.

It is important to understand the underlying physical principles of ultrasound, the artefacts inherent within the image, and how to operate the equipment in a competent and safe manner.

This chapter will not explain in detail the fundamental physics principles of ultrasound as the reader should have gained a basic understanding of this prior to, or alongside, training for MSK ultrasound.

The learning outcomes of this chapter are to provide the reader with an understanding of the:
- Basic principles and how they influence the ultrasound image.
- Ability to recognise artefacts relevant to MSK ultrasound and how to optimise the image.
- Use of Doppler ultrasound.
- Relevance of safety and medico-legal concerns, record keeping and work-related musculoskeletal disorders.

BASIC PRINCIPLES OF ULTRASOUND

Ultrasound is a high frequency sound wave, operating at frequencies within the range of 2 to 22 MHz.[2] These frequencies are above that which the human ear can hear.

It is produced through a hand-held device termed a transducer or probe by a piezoelectric process. This process involves piezoelectric (PZE) ceramic materials converting electrical energy into mechanical energy and vice versa. An ultrasound transducer housing typically contains 128 to 512 rows of regularly placed PZE elements, often composed of lead zirconate titanate (PZT).[3–5] A voltage is applied across the PZE elements, causing them to expand and contract (resonate) at a specific frequency producing an ultrasound wave which is transmitted into the body. This wave interacts with the body tissues and returns to the transducer which converts the mechanical energy back into electrical energy. This signal is then processed within the machine to produce an ultrasound image which is displayed on a monitor.[3–5]

Some of the physical properties of ultrasound and interactions within the tissues are described in more detail in the following section. They influence the choice of transducer and manipulation of machine settings during the examination; the ultimate aim is to maximise image quality.

Resolution

Spatial resolution describes the ability of the ultrasound system to display fine detail within an image and is determined by a combination of axial, lateral, temporal, and contrast resolution.[5]

- *Axial resolution* is the ability to distinguish between two structures in axis or parallel to the beam (Fig. 1.1). This is determined by wavelength or pulse length. As wavelength is inversely proportional to frequency, the higher the frequency, the shorter the wavelength (shorter pulse length) and the better the axial resolution (Fig. 1.2). However, higher frequency waves are attenuated more readily and therefore have a limited depth penetration.[3–6]

    As MSK structures are often small and superficial, it makes sense to use a high frequency for most examinations.

- *Lateral resolution* is the ability to distinguish between two structures lying side by side or perpendicular to the beam (Fig. 1.3). This is governed by beam width and is optimised by focusing the beam at the level of the structure being examined (Fig. 1.4). The

narrower the beam the better the lateral resolution.[3–6] This is altered during the examination using the focus control.[4,7]

- *Temporal resolution* refers to the ability of an imaging system to accurately distinguish movement of

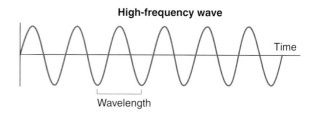

High-frequency wave

Wavelength

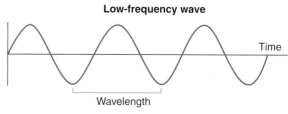

Low-frequency wave

Wavelength

Fig. 1.2 Wavelength and frequency are inversely proportional: the higher the frequency, the shorter the wavelength and the better the axial resolution. (From Powles AEJ, Martin DJ, Wells ITP, Goodwin CR. Physics of ultrasound. Anaesth Intensive Care Med. 2018;19(4):202-205. https://www.sciencedirect.com/science/article/pii/S1472029918300171#fig2)

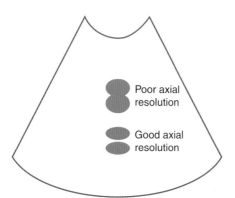

Fig. 1.1 Axial Resolution. The ability to distinguish between two structures along the axis of the beam. (From Gibbs V, Cole D, Sassano A. Ultrasound Physics and Technology. How, Why and When. 1st ed. London: Churchill Livingstone, Elsevier; 2009:40, Fig. 7.3.)

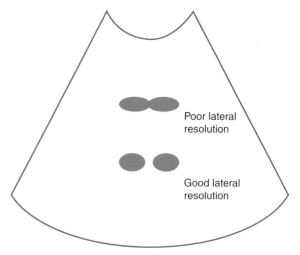

Fig. 1.3 Lateral Resolution. The ability to distinguish between two structures perpendicular to the beam. (From Gibbs V, Cole D, Sassano A. Ultrasound Physics and Technology. How, Why and When. 1st ed. London: Churchill Livingstone, Elsevier; 2009:41, Fig. 7.6.)

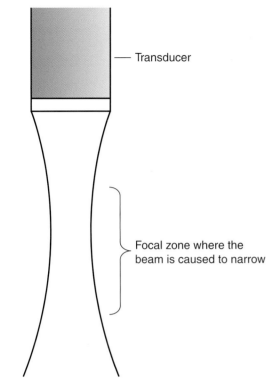

Transducer

Focal zone where the
beam is caused to narrow

Fig. 1.4 Lateral resolution is governed by beam width: the narrower the beam, the better the lateral resolution. (From Gibbs V, Cole D, Sassano A. Ultrasound Physics and Technology. How, Why and When. 1st ed. London: Churchill Livingstone, Elsevier; 2009;25, Fig. 5.5.)

an object over time and is synonymous with frame rate. Frame rate is the rate at which individual images/frames are produced by the system, measured in frames per second.[5] The higher the frame rate, the better the temporal resolution. Frame rate is dependent on several other parameters and can be altered by the operator. The typical range of frame rates utilised in medical ultrasound are between 10 and 30.

- *Contrast resolution* governs the ability of the system to identify closely related structures of similar echo-textures as separate entities. Contrast resolution is influenced by the dynamic range settings, and as MSK ultrasound requires subtle architectural changes to be detected within structures, it is imperative that the dynamic range settings on the equipment are correctly optimised.[5]

Interaction of Ultrasound Within Tissues

The production of an ultrasound image is determined by how the ultrasound wave interacts with structures within the human body.[6]

Attenuation

As the transmitted and returning ultrasound beams traverse through tissue, the intensity and amplitude are reduced, losing energy. This energy loss is dependent on the type of medium the beam is traversing and the frequency of the ultrasound beam.[5,8]

Several processes contribute to attenuation (Fig. 1.5):
- Absorption occurs as energy from the sound wave, as the particles vibrate back and forward, is converted into heat which is transferred to the surrounding tissues. Absorption is greater the higher the frequency.[3]
- Specular reflection occurs when an ultrasound wave interacts with a large smooth interface between tissues with a difference in acoustic impedance. *Acoustic impedance* is the term given to the impedance (resistance) the medium offers to the movement of the sound wave and is determined by the medium's density and compressibility. The "acoustic impedance mismatch" of two mediums determines the proportion of ultrasound that is transmitted and the proportion that is reflected. If the beam interrogates an interface at 90 degrees to the structure, a proportion of the beam is reflected directly back to the transducer and a proportion of the beam will be transmitted deeper into the body (Fig. 1.6A). If the sound beam interrogates the interface with an angle other than 90 degrees, then the angle of incidence (incident beam) will equal the angle of reflection (reflected beam). The steeper the angle of incidence in relation to the interrogated structure, the steeper the angle of reflection, resulting in some of the returning echoes not reaching the transducer and leaving an area of the interrogated structure devoid of information (Fig. 1.6B). This can be identified when imaging the Achilles tendon at the insertion where the tendon fibres are angled away from the direction of the ultrasound beam (Fig. 1.7). The resulting signal void causes an area of reduced echogenicity. This is also known as anisotropy, an artefact which is very important in MSK ultrasound (see 'Artefacts').[8,9]
- Refraction occurs when the ultrasound wave passes from one medium to the next where the speed of sound is different in the two mediums; also, it occurs when the angle of incident beam is not at 90 degrees

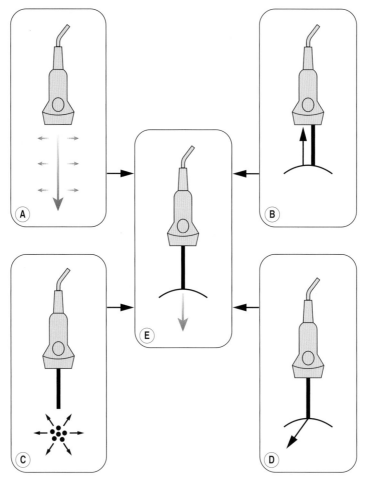

Fig. 1.5 (A) Absorption; **(B)** reflection; **(C)** scatter; and **(D)** refraction all contribute to attenuation of the ultrasound wave **(E)**. (From Powles AEJ, Martin DJ, Wells ITP, Goodwin CR. Physics of ultrasound. Anaesth Intensive Care Med. 2018;19(4):202-205. https://www.sciencedirect.com/science/article/pii/S1472029918300171#fig2 (6))

to the source being interrogated. The ultrasound beam is "bent" from its original direction (Snell's Law) and the received echo is placed in an incorrect location on the ultrasound image[4,5,8]; this can potentially cause misdiagnosis if not recognised (Fig. 1.8).

- Scattering occurs when the size of the medium being interrogated by the ultrasound wave is smaller or equal to the wavelength, resulting in small targets scattering the returning echoes in different directions over a wide range of angles. Known as "Rayleigh" scattering, the returning echoes produce a very weak signal and produce speckle within the image that gives certain MSK structures their typical echotexture (Fig. 1.9).[5]

SUMMARY

Attenuation is due to:
- Absorption
- Specular Reflection
- Refraction
- Scattering

Absorption is the main contributor of attenuation and has an exponential relationship with frequency

Specular Reflection is the angle of incident = angle of reflection

Refraction obeys Snell's Law

Scattering produces most of the echotexture of MSK structures

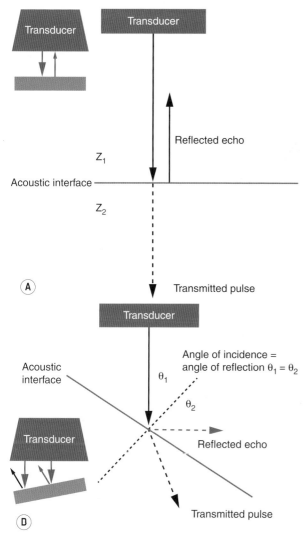

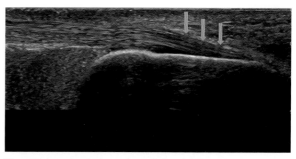

Fig. 1.7 Longitudinal section of the Achilles tendon demonstrating artefactual loss of echogenicity *(blue arrows)* when the incident beam is not perpendicular to the tendon fibers.

Fig. 1.6 (A) The incident beam interrogating a large, smooth structure at 90 degrees with a portion of the sound transmitted and a portion reflected depending on the acoustic impedance of the interface. **(B)** If the ultrasound beam does not interrogate a structure at 90 degrees, the Angle of Reflection = Angle of Incidence and some of the returning echoes do not return to the probe (Refracted echo). (From Dixon AM. Breast Ultrasound. How, Why and When. 1st ed. London: Churchill Livingstone; 2008:23, Figs. 3.3, 3.4.)

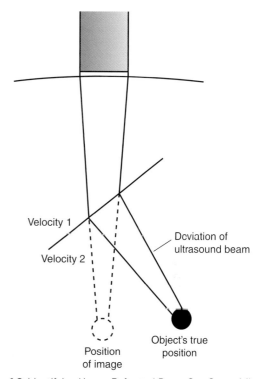

Fig. 1.8 Identifying How a Refracted Beam Can Cause Misregistration of Returning Echoes. (From Gibbs V, Cole D, Sassano A. Ultrasound Physics and Technology. How, Why and When. 1st ed. London: Churchill Livingstone, Elsevier; 2009;48, Fig. 8.8.)

ARTEFACTS

Artefacts are "errors" or misrepresentations within the ultrasound image and are the result of either false assumptions in regards to sound propagation or the presence of irregularities in the investigated tissue.[8,9]

Recognising artefacts is an important aspect of ultrasound practice[9]; and while some artefacts can be used to make a correct diagnosis, others can give false information. The artefacts most commonly encountered in the MSK ultrasound field include:

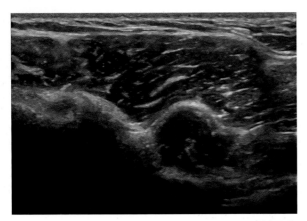

Fig. 1.9 Image of Muscle Architecture Governed by the Principle of Scattering.

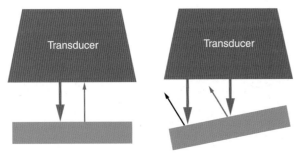

Fig. 1.10 Anisotropy occurs when the ultrasound beam is not perpendicular to the structure being imaged *(right image)* and, due to the steeper angle of reflection, not all the returning echoes reach the transducer *(black arrow)*.

Anisotropy

Anisotropy occurs when the ultrasound beam is not perpendicular to the structure being imaged[10] and is specific to imaging muscles, tendons, ligaments, and to a lesser degree, nerves. The resultant image demonstrates an area of reduced echogenicity within the structure as not all the returning echoes reach the transducer (Fig. 1.10). In tendons and muscle, areas of reduced echogenicity may be suggestive of tendinopathy or tears (see Chapter 2); therefore, this artefact has the potential to cause misdiagnosis. This scenario is commonly encountered in the shoulder when interrogating the long head of biceps tendon at an incorrect angle (Figs. 1.11A and 1.12A). In order to remove the artefact, the operator needs to alter the angle of insonation to bring the structure perpendicular to the transducer (Figs. 1.11B

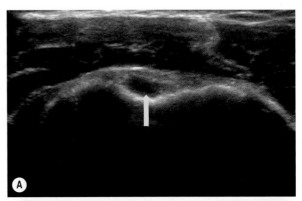

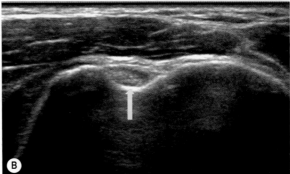

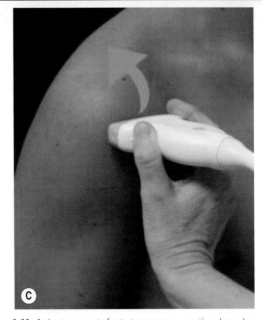

Fig. 1.11 Anisotropy artefact, transverse section long head of biceps tendon *(yellow arrows)*. **(A)** Incorrect insonation of tendon fibers. **(B)** Correct insonation of tendon fibers. Note in image A the artefactual echo-poor appearance of the tendon which can mimic pathological appearances. Tilting the probe **(C)** confirms normal appearances.

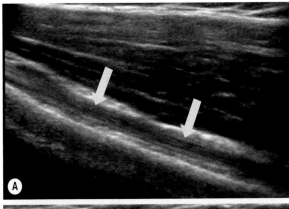

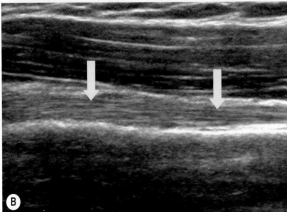

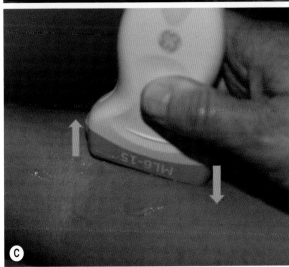

and 1.12B). This manipulation of the transducer is commonly termed "tilting" (Fig. 1.11C), "rocking," or "heel/toeing" (Fig. 1.12C) the transducer.[9,11,12] Utilising beam steering or cross beam imaging facilities (discussed in next section) if available may also help to reduce this artefact.[12]

Posterior Acoustic Enhancement

Posterior acoustic enhancement (otherwise known as through transmission) refers to the increased echoes deep to structures that easily transmit sound.

This is commonly seen with fluid-filled structures as fluid attenuates the sound less than the surrounding tissue. The time gain compensation is the same throughout the image and overcompensates through the fluid-filled structure, causing deeper tissues to be brighter[5,6,12] (Fig. 1.13). Although this artefact is often associated with fluid in cysts, bursae, and ganglions,[12] it should not be used to confirm that a structure is purely fluid-filled or benign as it can also be seen posterior to some low attenuation, solid lesions with a high fluid content, such as peripheral nerve sheath tumors and malignant cystic sarcomas.[13]

Posterior Acoustic Shadowing

This artefact is an area devoid of information ("a shadow") posterior to a structure that strongly reflects, refracts, or absorbs ultrasound.[5] This is demonstrated posterior to a bony structure[8] such as the coracoid process (Fig. 1.14A), limiting evaluation of structures deep

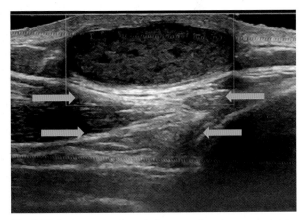

Fig. 1.12 Anisotropy artefact, longitudinal section long head of biceps tendon *(yellow arrows)*. **(A)** Incorrect insonation of tendon fibers. **(B)** Correct insonation of tendon fibers. Note in image A the artefactual echo-poor appearance of the tendon which may mimic pathological appearances. Heal/toeing the probe **(C)** confirms normal appearances.

Fig. 1.13 An example of posterior acoustic enhancement posterior to a epidermoid cyst. Note the increased echogenicity of the tissues deep to the cyst *(arrows)* when compared to the surrounding tissues.

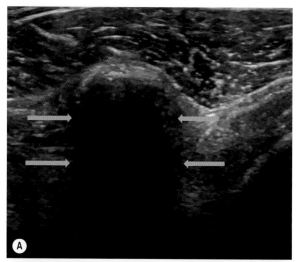

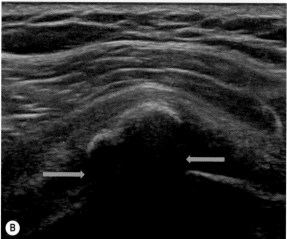

Fig. 1.14 Posterior Acoustic Shadowing. An area devoid of information posterior to the structure is identified *(blue arrows)*. This is demonstrated posterior to bony structure such as the coracoid process **(A)**, which limits evaluation of structures deep to the bone, and **(B)** mature calcification within tendons.

to the bone surface, and behind mature calcification within tendons[8] (Fig. 1.14B) where it is a helpful feature to confirm pathology.

Edge Enhancement Artefact

This artefact is evident when interrogating a curved structure which has a different acoustic impedance to its surrounding structures. The phenomenon occurs due to both reflection and refraction and results in parallel "hypoechoic" regions adjacent to the edges of

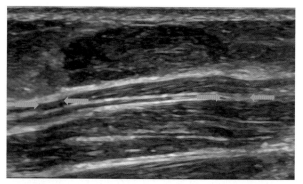

Fig. 1.15 Edge enhancement occurs due to both reflection and refraction and results in parallel "hypoechoic" regions adjacent to the edges of the structure *(blue arrows)*.

the structure[5] (Fig. 1.15). This can limit visualisation in the immediate area, but it can be useful to assist in the identification of the proximal and distal tendon ends of torn tendons such as the Achilles tendon.[8] To try to reduce this artefact the operator can change the angle of the beam either manually or electronically.[8]

Reverberation Artefact

This artefact occurs when there is a strong reflector situated parallel to the beam. Multiple reflections are repeated at depth behind the reflector at the same distance apart as the distance between the transducer and the reflector.[4,5] An example of this artefact is seen in Fig. 1.16 behind a needle used for injection or aspiration of fluid.[8] The needle is the strong reflector and the artefact helps in this case with location of the shaft of the needle (Fig. 1.16).

Beam Width Artefact

This occurs due to the shape of the ultrasound beam (Fig. 1.17). The beam exits the transducer at a pre determined width. It narrows at the focal point (discussed later), then diverges, resulting in the beam width being wider at depth. If a strong reflector is positioned in the beam path which is outside of the margins of the transducer, the ultrasound system will display the echoes as coming from within the main beam path resulting in overlapping of information (Fig. 1.18). In MSK ultrasound this may be seen when false echoes from adjacent soft tissue structures are displayed within a fluid-filled bursa or cyst.[3,5] The artefact can be removed by narrowing the beam in the

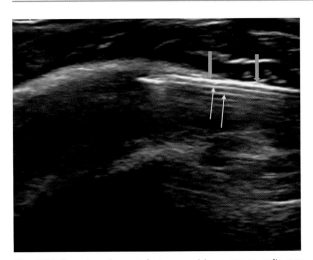

Fig. 1.16 Reverberation artefact caused by a strong reflector situated parallel to the beam such as a needle *(blue arrows)*. Multiple reflections are repeated at depth behind the reflector at the same distance apart *(yellow arrows)*.

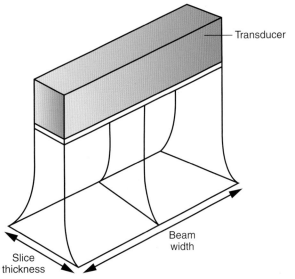

Fig. 1.17 Ultrasound Beam Shape Demonstrating Beam Width and Slice Thickness. (From Gibbs V, Cole D, Sassano A. Ultrasound Physics and Technology. How, Why and When. 1st ed. London: Churchill Livingstone, Elsevier; 2009;58, Fig. 9.17.)

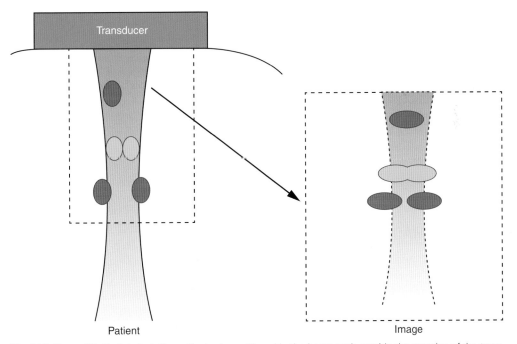

Fig. 1.18 Beam Width Artefact. The reflector is positioned in the beam path outside the margins of the transducer, and the ultrasound system will display the echoes as if they are coming from within the main beam path, resulting in false echoes. (From Dixon AM. Breast Ultrasound. How, Why and When. 1st ed. London: Churchill Livingstone; 2008:28.)

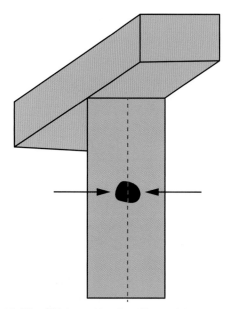

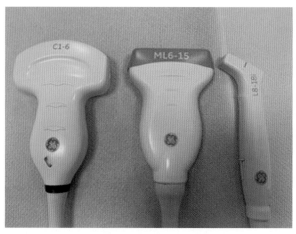

Fig. 1.20 The Typical Probes Utilised for Musculoskeletal Work. **(A)** Curvilinear. **(B)** Linear array. **(C)** Hockey stick. (Courtesy GE Medical Logic, Chicago, IL.)

Fig. 1.19 Slice Thickness Artefact. Tissue *(black arrows)* situated in front or behind a cystic structure *(black dot)* will be represented in the resultant image, creating spurious echoes. (From Dixon AM. Breast Ultrasound. How, Why and When. 1st ed. London: Churchill Livingstone; 2008:29, Fig. 3.17.)

region of interest, which is achieved by changing the position of the focus.[3,5,11]

It is important that beam width is not confused with slice thickness (Fig. 1.17). Slice thickness artefact may occur when imaging cystic structures that are smaller than the thickness of the probe. The tissues which are situated in front or behind this area can be represented in the resultant image, creating spurious echoes (Fig. 1.19). Slice thickness is infrequently encountered and is an inherent property of the beam and cannot be manipulated.[5]

EQUIPMENT AND IMAGE OPTIMISATION

An ultrasound machine should be "fit for purpose"[14] to accommodate the range of examinations performed, manage the current and predicted workload, and allow for any future developments in the service. It is tempting to go for the cheapest option; however, this is often at the expense of image quality, transducer options, durability, and manufacturer support.

Even with good quality equipment, only by "driving the machine" well can you expect a quality examination.[1,15,16]

Transducer selection should be the first consideration, and a suggested range of transducers for MSK examinations would include:

- High frequency linear array,[1,10,12] typically operating in the frequency range of 6 to 15 MHz. This provides high spatial resolution which enables the operator to identify and differentiate fine detail at the expense of depth. It provides a rectangle field of view producing good skin-to-probe contact.
- Hockey stick linear array, 15 to 18 MHz. This transducer has a small, rectangular footprint making it an excellent choice for interrogating the fingers or small joints of the wrist and ankle. It also provides excellent spatial resolution but at the expense of depth and a small field of view.[13]
- Low frequency curvilinear, 2- to 6-MHz transducer, allows increased penetration, and having a curved footprint provides a large field of view, but this is at the expense of spatial resolution.[17] It is useful when imaging a large deep-seated tumor or collection/abscess/hematoma (Fig. 1.20).

Examination pre-sets are programmed into the system by the manufacturers prior to purchase. They provide standardised settings[4,17] for different examinations and can be selected once the correct transducer has been chosen. For example, when using an 18-MHz transducer to examine the hand tendons, a superficial MSK pre-set would be appropriate. These pre-sets may need altering by the manufacturer's application specialist in the support period after purchase to make sure they are optimised to suit the service. The pre-set can also be linked to appropriate annotation for the examination to save time during the scan. It is possible, for instance, to create an individual pre-set e.g., "shoulder" to include labels for all the areas imaged.

After choosing the correct transducer and initial pre-set, the most utilised controls during the examination are explained in more detail below. It is important to understand when and why these are altered.

Depth

Depth defines how deep the image is in centimeters and should be set to ensure the region under investigation occupies approximately two-thirds of the field of view. This should be the first parameter altered to ensure that the structures under investigation are fully visualised within the image whilst irrelevant information is excluded. Appropriate use of the depth control improves image quality[10] because reducing the depth also increases the number of frames created per second[4] as the pulse of ultrasound has less distance to travel. This results in higher frame rates, improving both spatial and temporal resolution.[4,5]

Focus

When the depth has been optimally set, the focus should be adjusted according to the area under investigation. The focus is usually indicated on the screen by small arrows along the side of the image, and it corresponds to the narrowest part of the beam (Fig. 1.21).[4] As discussed earlier, lateral resolution is governed by the width of the beam and is optimal in a narrow, nondivergent beam.[4,5,17] If the focus is set too superficially in the image, poor image resolution will be evident in the far field due to divergence of the beam distal to the focal zone. For this reason, the focus should be set at the same level as or just behind the region under investigation.[17]

Multiple focal zones can be utilised which can be advantageous in MSK ultrasound as it facilitates improved image resolution at multiple depths (Fig. 1.22), but this may depend on specific systems. The disadvantage of using multiple focal zones is the frame rate will be reduced, resulting in a slower refresher rate, lagging of the moving image, and reduced temporal resolution; however, in MSK ultrasound this is not as much of an issue as in abdominal or obstetric ultrasound when there is more movement of the structures being examined.

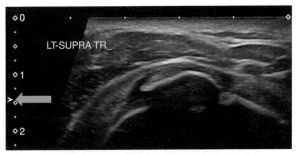

Fig. 1.21 Focus. Focus should be adjusted to ensure it is at the level of or just behind the area of interest. The level of the focus is often indicated by a small arrow to the side of the image *(blue arrow)*.

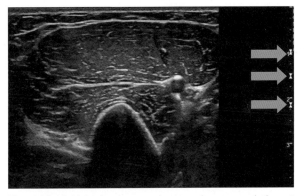

Fig. 1.22 Multiple focal zones improve image resolution at multiple depths, which is advantageous when imaging larger areas in the musculoskeletal field. The three focal zones are indicated on the right side of the image *(blue arrows)*.

With new technology, recent advances in software allows the whole of the image to be focused at all depths with no intervention required by the operator.

Frequency

Modern-day transducers are termed broad-band[17] or multi-frequency. This means that the individual transducer operates at multiple frequencies enabling the operator to change the frequency by adjusting a control on a touch screen or a "toggle switch," rather than having to switch to another transducer. Imaging at higher frequencies[10,13,17] improves axial resolution and image quality due to the shorter wavelengths (pulse length) (Fig. 1.23), but this is at the expense of depth penetration.[4,5] Therefore, any change in frequency will result in a trade-off between resolution and penetration.[4,10] When the depth and focus are set correctly, the frequency can be altered

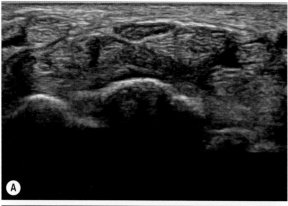

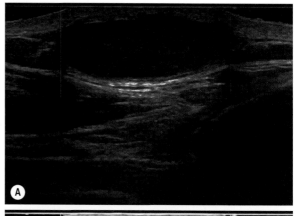

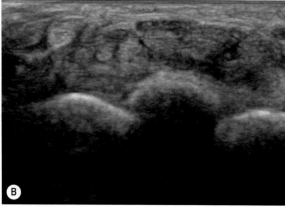

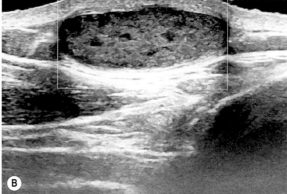

Fig. 1.23 Frequency. Images of the volar aspect of the wrist demonstrating superior resolution when scanning at **(A)** high frequency (17 MHz), compared with the poor resolution seen in **(B)** when scanning at a lower frequency (9 MHz).

Fig. 1.24 Overall Gain. (A) Decreasing the gain too much results in an image which is too dark, and **(B)** increasing the gain too much results in an image which is too bright, resulting in suboptimal imaging.

if necessary to optimise resolution or to ensure the ultrasound beam is able to penetrate to the deepest structure being imaged. Penetration is not often an issue when undertaking MSK examinations, so the highest possible frequency should be utilised to maximise resolution. Other settings, such as overall gain and time gain compensation (TGC), should be adjusted[17] to increase amplitude of the signal (brightness) before reducing the frequency or changing to a lower frequency transducer.

Overall Gain

Overall gain increases or decreases the amplitude of the returning echoes[5] across the whole image, so altering this setting adjusts the brightness of the entire area under investigation without increasing the power or strength of the transmitted sound wave. Overall gain should only be adjusted when the previously discussed parameters have been optimally set and must be adjusted carefully as inappropriate gain settings can affect contrast resolution. Decreasing the gain too much results in an image which is too dark and increasing the gain too much results in a "noisy" image which is too bright. This can make it difficult to visualise detail in the structures or pick out pathology from the background noise (Fig. 1.24).

Time Gain Compensation (TGC)

Attenuation does not always affect the whole of the image equally. TCG compensates for this as it allows the operator to increase or decrease the amplitude of the returning echoes at different depths, creating uniformity in the brightness of the image.[4,5] As MSK

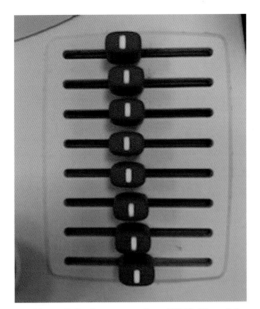

Fig. 1.25 Time Gain Compensation (TGC). The slider scale allows the operator to increase or decrease the amplitude of the returning echoes at different depths. (Courtesy GE Medical Logic, Chicago, IL.)

imaging involves imaging mainly superficial structures, this is not a parameter that is utilised often, but prior to commencing an examination it is important to ensure all the TGC sliders are centred (vertical)[5] (Fig. 1.25). This ensures the image is a true representation of the area being interrogated. Altering the TGC may be useful when imaging large deep muscles or when imaging behind a fluid-filled structure, such as a bursa, to reduce posterior enhancement or inversely to enable better visualisation of the echotexture of an attenuating lesion deep in the image.[5]

Power

Adjusting the power on the ultrasound machine alters the voltage applied to the PZE crystal, which subsequently adjusts amplitude or strength of the emitted beam.[4,5] It is usually displayed as a percentage, where 100% is the maximum safe level. Power determines the rate at which ultrasound energy flows,[18] so increasing the power increases the amplitude of the wave and ultimately the amount of energy the patient receives.[4,5,18,19] In theory, this also increases the potential risk of thermal and non-thermal bioeffects (see Ultrasound Safety section). Ultrasound examinations should be performed using the lowest output power setting possible.[15] It is not normally necessary to alter the power during an examination as the other settings we have already discussed accommodate the changes required.

Dynamic Range (DR)

The DR control allows the operator to determine how the returning echoes are displayed on the image in regard to the number of different shades of grey.[4,5,15] Increasing the DR will display a higher number of shades, resulting in lack of contrast and an overall smoother image. A narrow or reduced DR will display fewer shades and will produce an image with more contrast. The pre-set DR is often satisfactory,[4] and it is rarely necessary to alter this parameter; however, it is possible to adjust these settings to the satisfaction of the operator during the examination.

Trapezoid/Wide View

This increases the footprint of the linear transducer by steering the beam at the edges, producing a wider footprint, rather like that produced by a curvilinear transducer. This function allows clearer evaluation of structures that are greater than the footprint of a linear transducer (Fig. 1.26).[5]

The disadvantages are a reduced frame rate and poor lateral resolution in the region of the steered beam.

The following functions are not available on all equipment, but their application should be considered if available.

Compound Imaging/Beam Steering

This is an advanced function which utilises electronic beam steering to obtain sonographic information of an

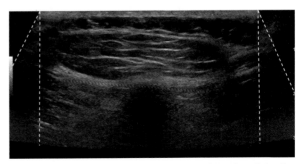

Fig. 1.26 Trapezoid imaging increases the footprint of the linear transducer by steering the beam at the edges producing a wider footprint (yellow lines).

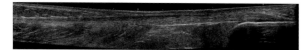

Fig. 1.27 Panoramic Image Demonstrating the Full Length of the Achilles Tendon.

object from several different scan angles.[5] The angle of the beam is altered by adding delays to the transmit and receive times. These overlapping scans are then combined and averaged to produce a single image. This technique improves image resolution by improving visualisation of image borders and reducing noise (speckle) and can also reduce anisotropy artefacts.[20]

Panoramic/Extended Field of View

This facility allows multiple frames to be acquired by dynamically imaging in real-time whilst moving the transducer over an extended area. This function "stitches together" multiple frames into an extended view image.[5,13] This is advantageous in MSK ultrasound[13] as it allows imaging and measurement of large structures or lesions which are greater than the footprint of the transducer, such as the Achilles tendon or large lipomata (Fig. 1.27). It can also be useful when assessing subtle findings, for instance when looking for a soft tissue mass by making a sweep to include both sides for comparison.

It takes a lot of practice to perfect the technique, however, especially when scanning a curved or irregular surface, and there may be a margin of error when performing measurements.

DOPPLER ULTRASOUND

Colour and power Doppler imaging is routinely utilised within MSK ultrasound[1,13,16,17] to identify the presence or confirm the absence of blood flow within a structure or lesion. The identification of blood flow can help when assessing an inflammatory process[17] such as inflammatory arthritis, and it can be valuable when assessing soft tissue masses as the presence or absence of flow and the vessel morphology[13] can help with the differential diagnosis. Spectral Doppler may also be indicated on occasion to sample the blood flow within a vascularised lesion. An example would be when assessing a vascular malformation[21] to check whether the vessels within the lesion contain venous or arterialised flow.

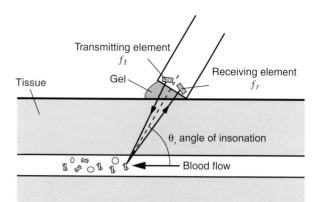

Fig. 1.28 Doppler Principle. The transmitted frequency (f_t) and received frequency (F_r) determine the Doppler shift. The angle of insonation (θ) provides the final parameter for the Doppler equation. (From https://www.slideshare.net/shaffar75/principles-of-doppler-ultrasound [slide 7].)

The Doppler principle describes the change in frequency of a sound wave due to a reflector (blood) moving towards or away from the emitting source (transducer).[5,6,22] If the reflector is moving towards the source, the received frequency will be higher than the emitted frequency (positive Doppler shift); and if the reflector is moving away from the source, the received frequency will be lower (negative Doppler shift) and this determines the colour of the blood flow demonstrated during scanning (blue or red)[6,7] (Fig. 1.28).

Correct parameter adjustment is paramount when utilising Doppler techniques to maximise diagnostic accuracy.

Pulsed Repetition Frequency (PRF)

PRF is the Doppler sampling frequency of the transducer measured in kilo Hertz (KHz), and it determines the maximum Doppler shifts obtainable.[4,6,7] Optimal PRF settings are vital and will vary depending on the flow velocity in the vessel examined. If it is set too low, "aliasing" occurs[4]; if set too high, slow flow will not be detected.

- A high PRF should be used for high velocity vessels such as arterial work in order to filter out artefact
- A low PRF should be set when assessing low velocity flow, which is the aim in most MSK examinations

The PRF will be set by manufacturers in the specific presets but the level should be refined by operators, especially when examining joints for inflammatory disease or soft tissue lesions for hyperemic changes when the detection of low velocity flow is vital.

Wall Filter

Movement of vessel walls and the surrounding tissues generate their own low-level Doppler shifts,[23] often termed motion artefacts. The wall filter eliminates these artefacts; however, the system cannot determine which low-frequency Doppler shifts originate from slow moving blood and which originate from motion artefacts. Consequently, both will be removed when the filters are high. Hence, to detect low velocity flow, the wall filter needs to be set to low.

These two controls (PRF and wall filter) are linked and altering one will automatically alter the other: increasing or decreasing the PRF will elicit the same effect on the wall filter.[22] They determine the sensitivity of colour and power Doppler by filtering out unnecessary signal.[22] Low PRF will use less filters and detect vessels of low velocity, such as those in synovitis.

Doppler Gain

Doppler gain determines the sensitivity of the system to flow.[22] Low gain settings minimise noise, blooming, and motion artefacts but may result in minimal neovascularisation being missed. Gain settings set too high result in random noise or blooming, which may result in an over estimation of the degree of vascularity.

As mentioned, in MSK ultrasound, the main modes used for detecting and assessing blood flow are colour, power, and spectral Doppler: these techniques provide slightly different information on blood flow.

Colour Doppler (CD)

CD provides a map of directional flow superimposed on a B mode image. Blood flow is colour coded depending on its direction. Flow towards the transducer is red (positive Doppler shift) and away from the transducer is blue (negative Doppler shift).[6,7,16,22] This CD information is represented in a colour scale box on the side of the ultrasound image and operators need to understand the significance of the colours orientation when evaluating the image. To optimise the use of CD in MSK, when placing the colour box over the region of interest, make sure it is as small as possible whilst ensuring all relevant structures are included.[4,6,22] This improves Doppler sensitivity and the colour scale, PRF, and wall filter will also need to be low to pick up low flow velocities[4] (Fig. 1.29).

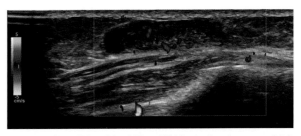

Fig. 1.29 Identifying Blood Flow Within an Arteriovenous Malformation in the Upper Arm Utilizing Color Doppler.

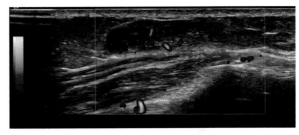

Fig. 1.30 Identifying Blood Flow Within an Arteriovenous Malformation in the Upper Arm Utilizing Power Doppler.

Power Doppler (PD)

PD provides information on the presence of blood flow; however, it does not give directional information.[16,22] It represents the energy/back-scattered energy of the blood and is identified as being more sensitive than CD[16] (Fig. 1.30). As with CD, the PD box should just include the relevant area, and, to ensure low velocities are observed, the PRF and wall filter need to be low.

When utilising either Doppler techniques within MSK ultrasound it is imperative that probe pressure is kept to a minimum as this could compress small blood vessels resulting in a failure to identify the presence of low velocity flow.[16,17]

ULTRASOUND SAFETY

Ultrasound is recognised as a safe diagnostic imaging modality, and to date there have been no reported adverse effects in patients. However, it is the responsibility of the practitioner not the manufacturer to ensure safe practice when operating the equipment, and the operator must appreciate the principles of ultrasound safety to ensure standards are maintained.

TABLE 1.1   Factors Affecting the Thermal Index and Mechanical Index During Examinations
• Length of exposure time • Utilisation of any of the Doppler modes • Output power • Utilisation of advancing technology • Incorrect parameter settings

TABLE 1.2   Work-Related Musculoskeletal Disorders (WRMSD)
• Ensure correct posture is maintained at all times • Do not put undue strain or tension on your dominant scanning arm • Prevent over stretching • Take regular breaks • Have mixed lists • If WRMSD symptoms are evident, perform a risk assessment and speak to your line manager

The safety indices on the ultrasound machine are presented as two output display standards (ODS) which are displayed on the monitor as TI (thermal index) and MI (mechanical index)[4,6,15,18]:

• Thermal index indicates the relative risk of a temperature rise in the tissues being insonated.[4,5,6,18]
• Mechanical index indicates the relative risk of a nonthermal effect such as cavitation.[4,5,6,18]

The British Medical Ultrasound Society (BMUS), Royal College of Radiologists (RCR), Society of Radiographers (SoR), and the Food and Drug Administration (FDA) are governing bodies that provide guidance on appropriate TI and MI values.[6,15,19] Several factors can affect these parameters (Table 1.1).

It is recommended that the ALARA (as low as reasonably achievable) principle is adhered to[4,5,14,15,19] and this can be achieved by:

• Monitoring the length of time of the examination and keeping this to a minimum.
• Keeping the transducer in "freeze" mode when not in use.
• Keeping the power output to as low as possible, utilising the overall gain initially.

OTHER SAFETY CONSIDERATIONS

Referring Request

All MSK referrals should be vetted to ensure the referral is appropriate and has been raised by a recognised and appropriately qualified professional.[15]

Quality Assurance (QA)

Ultrasound departments are required to undertake routine QA testing to ensure there is no degradation of the equipment or image. Failure to undertake regular QA could result in physical damage to the patient or operator and potential misinterpretation of the image, leading to an incorrect diagnosis.[5,6,15]

Work Related Musculoskeletal Disorders (WRMSD)

Many ultrasound practitioners have experienced or will experience WRMSD at some point in their career.[6,14,15,24] Extensive research has been undertaken into the cause and effect of such disorders on both the individual and the organisation,[15,24,25] and several strategies have been identified to help operators reduce the risk of WRMSD (Table 1.2). WRMSD is problematic in MSK as many of the joint examinations require the operator to perform fine movements of the hand and wrist putting strain on the joints.[6,14,25] In the following chapters the authors will give recommendations for patient positioning which can help to reduce the strain on the operator. Other factors to consider are using an ergonomic seat when sitting for the examination and having mixed lists if possible, to introduce changes in posture, e.g., shoulder followed by soft tissue lump followed by ankle, etc.

Record Keeping and Medico-Legal Factors

Lastly, we should address the importance of image recording and report writing as safety considerations.

Every ultrasound practitioner with the appropriate training in a well-supported workplace should be capable of good practice. However, it is becoming more common for practitioners of ultrasound to be required to defend themselves following claims of medical negligence. A selection of well-annotated, good quality images should be taken as a record of the scan.[15,26] This will allow the expert witness in a medico-legal investigation to assess the quality of the examination performed. Review of recorded images (now widely available in all sectors via digital and internet-based platforms) also helps when formulating a report and for comparison with future examinations.

The report is the main form of communication to the referring clinician and therefore could be considered as the most important part of the examination.[15,26] It is also an important medico-legal document and should be carefully constructed. There are examples of reports within the following chapters and references are given for further reading recommendations.

MULTIPLE CHOICE QUESTIONS

1. Axial resolution is the ability to:
   a) distinguish between two structures lying side by side or perpendicular to the beam
   b) distinguish between two structures in axis or parallel to the beam
   c) accurately distinguish movement of an object over time

2. Which processes contribute to attenuation?
   a) Scattering, specular reflection, refraction, and absorption
   b) Wavelength, absorption, reflection, and depth
   c) Frequency, reflection, refraction, and motion

3. Anisotropy occurs when the ultrasound beam is not perpendicular to the structure being imaged and it:
   a) can affect any tissue in the human body
   b) can cause areas of tendons to appear artefactually echo poor
   c) can cause areas of tendons to appear artefactually echo bright

4. PRF is the Doppler sampling frequency of the transducer.
   a) PRF is not important when undertaking MSK examinations.
   b) A high PRF should be set when assessing low velocity flow, which is the aim in most MSK examinations.
   c) A low PRF should be set when assessing low velocity flow, which is the aim in most MSK examinations.

5. It is recommended that the ALARA principle is adhered to during an ultrasound examination and this can be achieved by:
   a) minimizing scan time and power output
   b) minimizing scan time and using multiple focal zones
   c) minimizing scan time and using higher power outputs

REFERENCES

1. Czymy Z. Standards for musculoskeletal ultrasound. J Ultrason. 2017;17(70):182–187.
2. Abu-Zidan FM, Hefny AF, Corr P. Clinical ultrasound physics. J Emerg Trauma Shock. 2011;4(4):501–503.
3. Dixon AM. Principles of diagnostic medical ultrasound. In: Breast Ultrasound, How, Why and When. 1st ed. London: Churchill Livingston, Elsevier; 2008:23–29.
4. Gibbs V, Cole D, Sassano A. Ultrasound Physics and Technology. How, Why and When. 1st ed. London: Churchill Livingstone, Elsevier; 2009:13–62, 95–97.
5. Hoskins PR, Martin K, Thrush A, eds. Diagnostic Ultrasound. Physics and Equipment. 3rd ed. Boca Raton, FL: CRC Press; 2019:7–32, 78–81, 105–124, 305–315.
6. Thrush A, Hartshorne T. Vascular Ultrasound. How, Why and When. 3rd ed. London: Churchill Livingstone, Elsevier; 2010:9–14, 18–19, 23–47, 84–86.
7. Bates J. Abdominal Ultrasound. How, Why and When. 3rd ed. London: Churchill Livingstone, Elsevier; 2011:2–7.
8. Krishnan S. Artefacts in musculoskeletal ultrasound. Indian J Rheumatol. 2018;13:S9–16.
9. Matthieu J, Rutten CM, Jager GJ, Blickman JC. US of the rotator cuff: pitfalls, limitations and artifacts. Radiographics. 2006;26:589–604.
10. Taljanovic MS, Melville DM, Gimber LH, et al. High-resolution US of rheumatologic diseases. Radiographics. 2015;35(7):2026–2048.
11. Rafaildis V. Delianidou A, Sferopoulos N, Torounidis I. Ultrasonographic imaging of the biceps tendon rupture at the myotendinous junction. European Federation of Societies for Ultrasound in Medicine and Biology. 2016.
12. Krishan S. Artefacts in musculoskeletal ultrasound. Indian J Rheumatol. 2018;13(5):9–16.
13. Teh J. Ultrasound of soft tissue masses of the hand. J Ultrason. 2012;12(51):382–401.

14. Bates J. Abdominal Ultrasound. How, Why and When. London: Elsevier, Churchill Livingstone; 2011:12–13.

15. BMUS: British Medical Ultrasound Society Musculoskeletal Ultrasound. Accessed December 28, 2019. https://www.bmus.org/musculoskeletal-ultrasound/.

16. Taljanovic MS, Melville DM, Scalcione LR, Gimber LH, Lorenz EJ, Witte RS. Artefacts in musculoskeletal ultrasonography. Semin Musculoskelet Radiol. 2014;18:3–11.

17. Serafin-Krol M, Maliborski A. Diagnostic errors in musculoskeletal ultrasound imaging and how to avoid them. J Ultrason. 2017;17(70):188–196.

18. Ter HG, Duck FA, eds. The Safe Use of Ultrasound in Medical Diagnosis. London: BMUS/BIR; 2000.

19. Maeda K. Diagnostic ultrasound safety ultrasound safety indices. J Health Med Inform. 2014;5(3):1000160.

20. Lin DC, Nazarian LN, O'Kane PL, McShane JM, Parker L, Merritt CRB. Advantages of realtime spatial compound sonography of the musculoskeletal system versus conventional ultrasound. Am J Roentgenol. 2002;179:1629–1631.

21. Samadi K, Salazar GM. Role of imaging in the diagnosis of vascular malformations. Cardiovasc Diagn Ther. 2019;9(Suppl. 1):S143–151.

22. Terslev L, Diamantopoulos AP, Døhn UM, Schmidt WA, Torp-Pedersen S. Settings and artefacts relevant for Doppler ultrasound in large vessel vasculitis. Arthritis Res Ther. 2017;19(1):167. Available at: https://doi.org/10.1186/s13075-017-1374-1.

23. Evans DH, Jensen JA, Nielsen MB. Ultrasonic colour Doppler imaging. Interface Focus. 2011;1(4):490–502.

24. The Society & College of Radiographers. Work related musculoskeletal disorders (Sonographers). 3rd ed. London: SCoR; 2019:3–10.

25. Monnington SC, Dodd-Huges K, Milnes E, Ahmad Y. Risk management of musculoskeletal disorders in sonography work. Health and Safety Executive. Corporate Science, Engineering and Analysis Directorate; 2012. Available at: https://www.hse.gov.uk/HEALTHSERVICES/management-of-musculoskeletal-disorders-in-sonography-work.pdf

26. The Royal College of Radiologists, The Society and College of Radiographers. Standards for the Provision of an ultrasound service. London: The Royal College of Radiologists; 2014. Available at: http://www.sor.org/sites/default/files/document-versions/bfcr1417_standards_ultrasound.pdf

Overview of General Musculoskeletal Principles

Mark Maybury and Michael A. Bryant

LEARNING OBJECTIVES

This chapter provides the reader with an appreciation of:
- Anatomical terminology used in musculoskeletal (MSK) medicine
- The ultrasound appearance of MSK tissue and associated pathological changes in these tissues
- The terminology and models of tendinopathy behind tendon changes
- History taking, and its relevance for MSK conditions

INTRODUCTION

Ultrasound is the investigation of choice for many musculoskeletal (MSK) conditions.[1] Numerous professions from various backgrounds are using MSK ultrasound[2]; its value on patient care and patient experience has been demonstrated in point of care ultrasound (POCUS).[3–5] Nevertheless, a cautionary note has been struck with respect to governance and education as mistakes made by inadequately trained operators could jeopardise patients' wellbeing.[6] It is well established that scan results alone without clinical integration or interpretation can be misleading, as changes established on imaged structures do not necessarily correlate to the cause of symptoms. Therefore, the onus is on those performing scans to appreciate not only the science and instrumentation of ultrasound, but also MSK medicine so that they can provide clinically useful information and enhance patient management.

STANDARD ANATOMICAL CONVENTION AND ACCEPTED ULTRASOUND NOMENCLATURE

Understanding anatomical terminology is an important consideration when describing the position of structures and movement of limbs relative to the body. This is important for accurately communicating findings to those requesting ultrasound examinations.

The "anatomical position" is the theoretical reference standard which describes all limb positions and relative motions enabling communication of anatomy in a clear, unambiguous way (Fig. 2.1). In reality, it is rare that patients/people adopt this position as postures and movements are complex.

The Cardinal Planes and Axes of Movement

Ultrasound is a dynamic imaging modality, and familiarity with the three cardinal planes and their associated

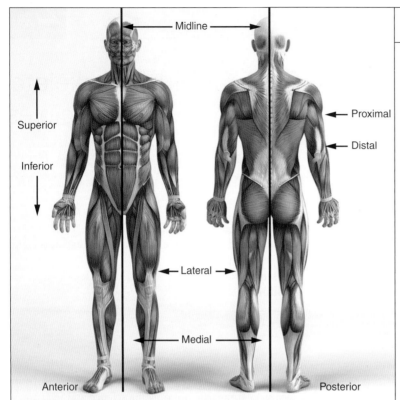

	Descriptive term relative to the anatomical position

	Anterior – in front
	Posterior – behind/rear
	Superior – above (see cephalic)
	Inferior – below (see caudal)
	   • Cephalic – towards the head
	   • Caudal – towards the tail
	Lateral – away from midline
	Medial – towards midline
	Distal – away from the root of the limb
	Proximal – towards the root of the limb
	Superficial – close to the body surface
	Deep – away from the body surface

Fig. 2.1 The Anatomical Position. (Image from https://3dmusclelab.com/anatomical-position and adapted to demonstrate midline position and related terminology.)

axes of movement is fundamental when examining the dynamic integrity of a structure, e.g., ankle ligaments or impingement syndrome of the shoulder. The relationship between the cardinal planes and axes of motion are summarised in Fig. 2.2.

It is worth noting that there are some additional terms describing motion occurring around joints that are used:

1. Forearm—Rotation occurring in the radiocapitellar and distal radioulnar joints enabling the palm of the hand to face up or down is termed supination and pronation, respectively.
2. Ankle—Flexion and extension produced by motion at the ankle is referred to as plantar and dorsiflexion.
3. Foot—Inversion and eversion of the foot is a combined motion of the subtalar and midfoot joints and are biplanar movements.

ULTRASOUND APPEARANCE OF COMMON MUSCULOSKELETAL TISSUES

Joints

These skeletal articulations are classified as fibrous, cartilaginous, and synovial.

Fibrous joints (syndesmotic) utilise strong fibrous ligaments to join two bones together, e.g., the distal radioulnar and inferior tibiofibular joints. These joints can be injured following a traumatic event, e.g., a fall on an outstretched arm/hand or following an ankle sprain (Fig. 2.3).

Cartilaginous joints permit a small amount of motion, subclassified into primary (for example, ribs and first sternocostal joint) and secondary (for example, the pubic symphysis) joints.

Synovial joints permit a high degree of mobility as their surface is covered in articular cartilage providing them with an almost friction-free surface. The joints are

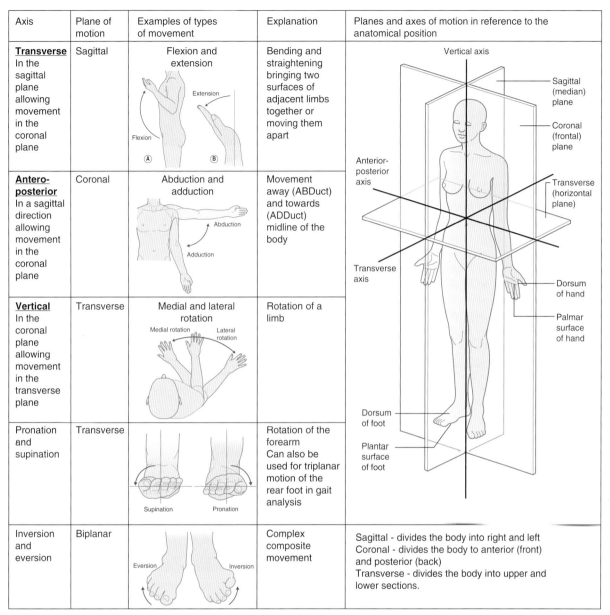

Axis	Plane of motion	Examples of types of movement	Explanation	Planes and axes of motion in reference to the anatomical position
Transverse In the sagittal plane allowing movement in the coronal plane	Sagittal	Flexion and extension	Bending and straightening bringing two surfaces of adjacent limbs together or moving them apart	
Antero-posterior In a sagittal direction allowing movement in the coronal plane	Coronal	Abduction and adduction	Movement away (ABDuct) and towards (ADDuct) midline of the body	
Vertical In the coronal plane allowing movement in the transverse plane	Transverse	Medial and lateral rotation	Rotation of a limb	
Pronation and supination	Transverse		Rotation of the forearm Can also be used for triplanar motion of the rear foot in gait analysis	
Inversion and eversion	Biplanar		Complex composite movement	Sagittal - divides the body into right and left Coronal - divides the body to anterior (front) and posterior (back) Transverse - divides the body into upper and lower sections.

Fig. 2.2 Planes and Axes of Motion and Commonly Occurring Movements That Occur About These Axes. (Adapted from Soames R, Palastanga N. Anatomy and Human Movement: Structure and Function. 7th ed. Elsevier Ltd; Edinburgh; 2019.)

covered by a dense fibrous capsule lined by a specialised synovial membrane that secretes a viscoelastic fluid which both cushions and nourishes the joint. In its normal state, the synovial layer is indistinguishable from the fibrous joint capsule, but this differs considerably from the pathological state where the synovium becomes clearly visible. These are the most frequently scanned joints in MSK ultrasound practice (Fig. 2.4). The relevance of these structures to pathological states will be developed in the rheumatology section (see Chapter 10).

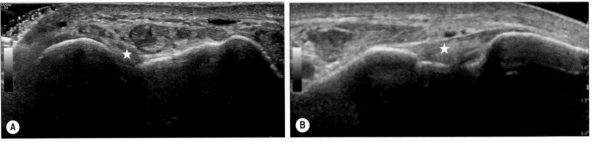

Fig. 2.3 Syndesmotic Joints. (A) Distal radioulnar joint of the wrist and **(B)** inferior tibiofibular joint of the ankle. Note the dense fibrous ligamentous attachment *(white star)* which connect the bones together representing the syndesmosis, very stable joints not prone to injury.

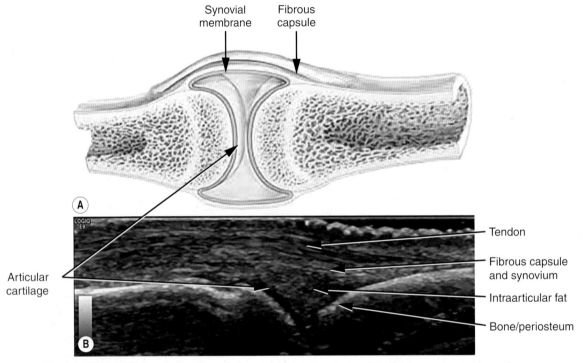

Fig. 2.4 (A) Simplified example of a typical synovial joint. The shape of the joint may change depending on its location. **(B)** A corresponding ultrasound image of the dorsal aspect of a metacarpophalangeal joint.

Synovial joints differ in size and shape depending on their position and these factors help determine the range of motion and function. They are classified as plane, saddle, hinge, ball and socket, condyloid, and ellipsoid (Fig. 2.5).

Bone

Ultrasound is not the imaging modality of choice for bone, although this premise has been recently challenged by those working in rural/remote point of care settings with limited access to X-ray equipment.[7]

Bone is covered by periosteum, and cortical bone and periosteum are normally indistinguishable on ultrasound, appearing as a single thin bright line[8] (Fig. 2.6).

The periosteum is a fibrous, dual-layered, highly vascular membrane that controls bone homeostasis, with vascular connections to adjacent muscles. When bone is injured, the periosteal changes are identified on

Type of joint	Description	Ultrasound image
Plane	Ends of the joint allow twisting and gliding movement, i.e., acromioclavicular joint	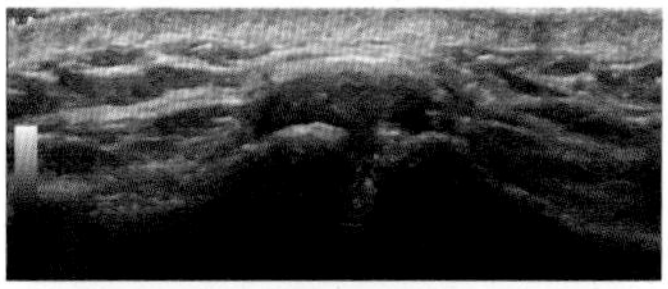 Acromioclavicular joint transverse
Saddle	Two joint surfaces are concavoconvex allowing movement in two perpendicular axes, i.e., carpometacarpal joint of the thumb	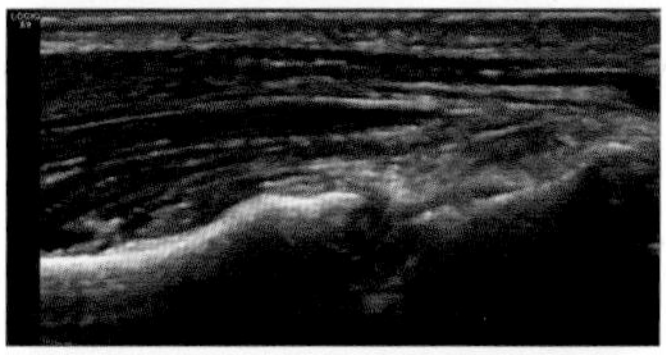 Carpometacarpal joint thumb longitudinal
Hinge	Allows movement about one axis and is supported by strong ligaments, i.e., elbow joint. The knee is another example but is thought to be a modified hinge joint as it allows for some movement about a vertical axis, endowed by the intraarticular menisci	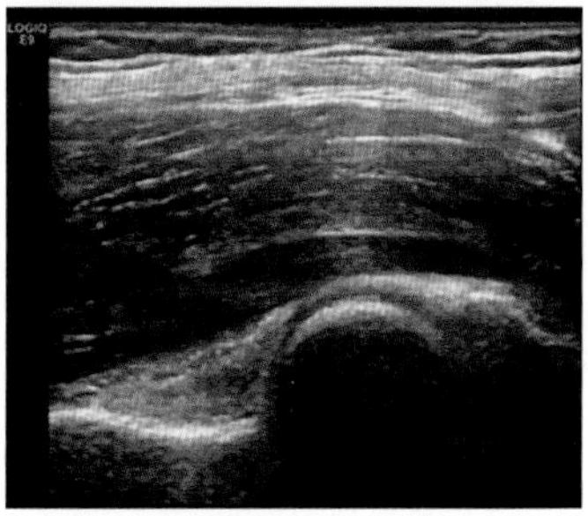 Elbow anterior longitudinal
Ball and socket joint	These are the most mobile joints allowing movement in three axes, i.e., shoulder and hip	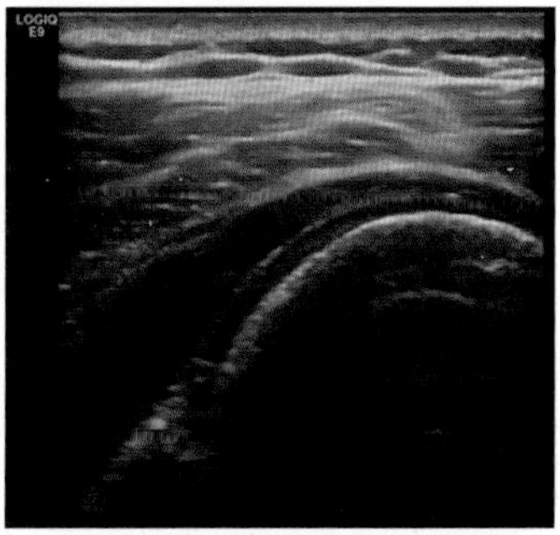 Glenohumeral joint posterior aspect longitudinal
Condyloid	This is a modified ball and socket joint with 3 axes of motion, 2 active and 1 passive, i.e., MCP joint	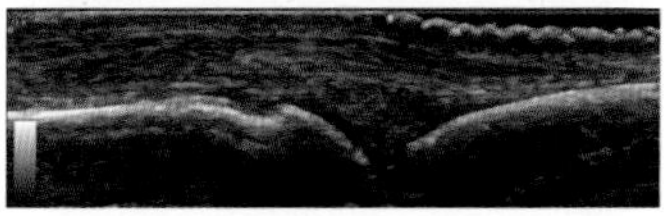 Metacarpophalangeal (MCP) joint hand longitudinal
Ellipsoid	Modified ball and socket joint with 2 axes of motion, i.e., radiocarpal joint	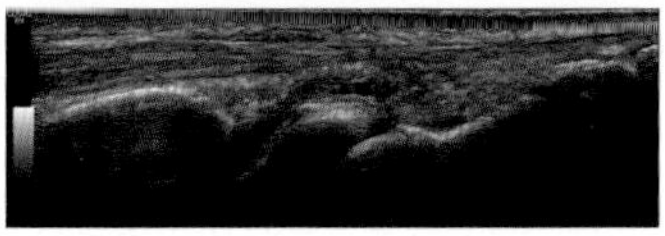 Radiocarpal joint (radio-lunate-capitate) longitudinal

Fig. 2.5 Examples of different types of joints that sonographers will encounter, with typical ultrasound appearances in one plane of view and examples of locations. (Adapted from Soames R, Palastanga N. Anatomy and Human Movement: Structure and Function. 7th ed. Elsevier Ltd; Edinburgh; 2019.)

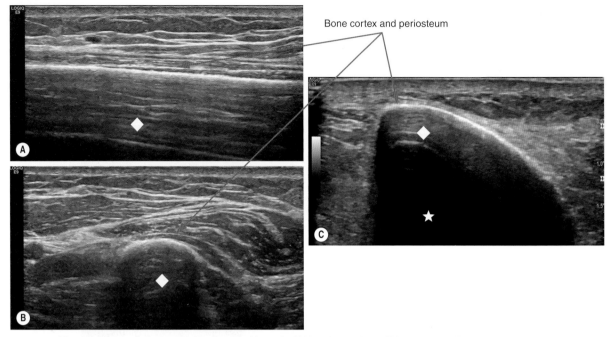

Bone cortex and periosteum

Fig. 2.6 Ultrasound appearance of cortical bone in **(A)** longitudinal and **(B)** transverse. The continuous bright line represents the cortical bone and periosteum that are indistinguishable on ultrasound. Note the reverberation artefacts under the bone *(white diamonds)* and the posterior acoustic shadowing in **(C)** *(white star)*, all characteristic artefacts of bony tissue.

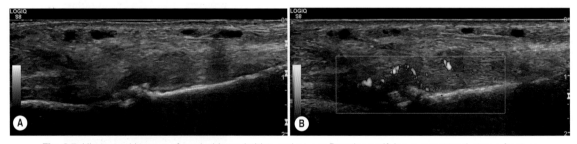

Fig. 2.7 Ultrasound images of cortical irregularities and power Doppler typifying a metatarsal stress fracture in a patient who presented 1 week after treatment for plantar fasciitis with lateral foot pains. **(A)** Demonstrates a cortical/periosteal reaction—note the irregularity in an otherwise smooth cortex/periosteal line. **(B)** Power Doppler images showing increased vascularity overlying the cortical irregularity. (From Leddy J, Maybury M. Ultrasound imaging. In: Watson T, Nussbaum E, eds. Electrophysical Agents. 13th ed. London: Elsevier; 2019:383.)

ultrasound[9] long before calcification reaction occurs on X-ray.[8]

Bony fractures have a classic sonographic appearance as a defect in the cortex extending over the bony surface. Depressions in the cortex can also represent compression fractures, though in these cases erosive causes should also be considered. Stress fractures may also be detected by observing lifting of the periosteum,

haematoma, increased vascularity, and thickening of the cortex[10] (Fig. 2.7).

Care must be taken when subtle defects are seen as small localised breaks in the cortex may represent nutrient canals allowing vessels to pass into the bone.

Bony exostoses and osteophytes can also be visualised as smooth outlined, well-defined lesions continuous with the cortex (Fig. 2.8).

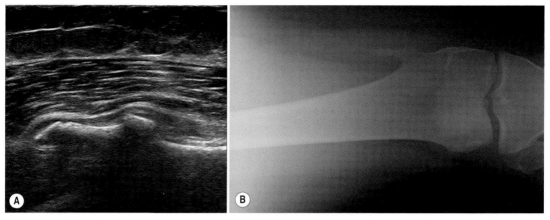

Fig. 2.8 Bony Exostosis at the Metaphysis of the Femur. (A) Ultrasound image. **(B)** Corresponding X-ray. The patient reported left knee pain following a road traffic collision after her knee hit the dashboard.

Muscles, Muscle Tendon Junction, and Enthesis

Skeletal muscle makes up 25% to 35% of total body mass. Its form is governed by fibre orientation and attachment to the respective tendons: (1) flat, (2) parallel (fusiform), and (3) oblique (pennate).

Pennate muscles have three patterns with respect to their tendon attachments: unipennate (attaches to one side of the tendon), bipennate (attaches to both sides of the tendon), and multipennate (several intermediate short tendon-like structures) (Fig. 2.9).

In common with tendons, muscle has a highly organised hierarchical structure composed of cylindrical muscle fibres held together by endomysium and grouped together in bundles to form fascicles. These fascicles in turn are grouped together to form a muscle and are covered by the epimysium. The strong, dense fibrous collagen network that holds the fascicles in position, called the perimysium, eventually forms the tendon, which becomes a separate entity at the myotendinous junction. Muscle has a typical ultrasound appearance, and in longitudinal section (LS) appears as hypoechoic (myofibrils), with obliquely orientated hyperechoic parallel lines (perimysium). In transverse section (TS) the muscle has a "starry sky" appearance; the bright perimysium septa is seen as dots contrasted against the dark myofibrils (Fig. 2.10).

Muscle Injury

Historically, muscle injuries were classified by the causative/mechanical force, anatomical location, and whether it was an internal (stretching) or external (direct trauma) event.[11] These injuries were graded on a three-point scale: (1) mild, (2) moderate, and (3) severe.

As ultrasound scanning became more accessible, a variety of ultrasound grading systems were proposed which emulated the clinical grade, although based on ultrasound appearance and description (hyper/hypo/anechoic).[12] However, the key issue with all grading systems is the prognostic information obtained both clinically and through imaging is generally poor,[11] with poor prediction of return to play in sport (RTP). This has led to the development of more sophisticated muscle grading scales, and one such example is the British Athletics muscle injury classification.[13] This is a five-point scale ranging from 0, representing an injury undetectable by imaging suggesting microtrauma to muscle tissue, to 4, representing the worst injury involving the muscle and tendon. Each point on this scale is further subclassified to denote the anatomical region (muscle, musculotendinous junction, and tendon) that is affected.

The images in Fig. 2.11A and B show examples of a low-grade muscle injury and a high-grade avulsion injury.

Tendons

The function of a tendon is to transmit the force of muscle contraction to the adjacent bone at the insertion or enthesis. Tendons have many forms from strong, round, cordlike structures to flattened bands with thin/sheets (aponeuroses). When a tendon is subjected to friction, it may develop a sesamoid bone, which act as

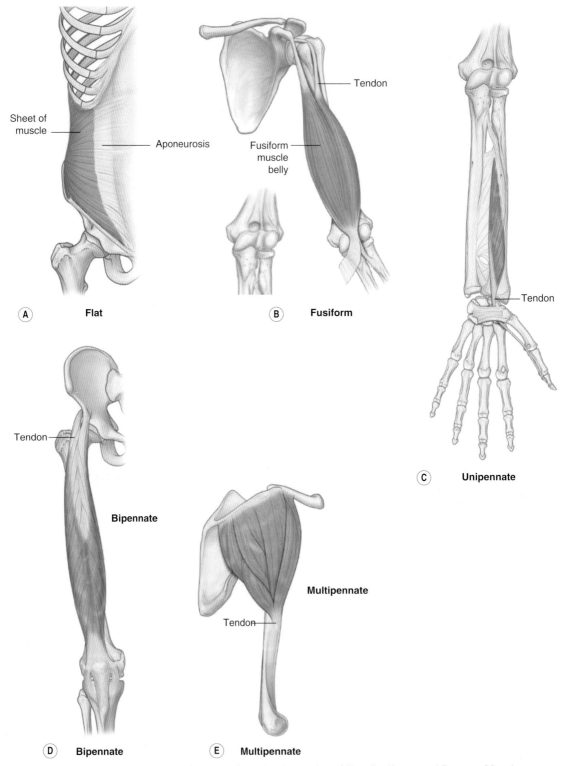

Sheet of muscle

Aponeurosis

(A)   **Flat**

Tendon

Fusiform muscle belly

(B)   **Fusiform**

Tendon

(C)   **Unipennate**

Tendon

Bipennate

(D)   **Bipennate**

Multipennate

Tendon

(E)   **Multipennate**

Fig. 2.9 Examples of Muscle Structure Showing Examples of Flat, Fusiform, and Pennate Muscles.

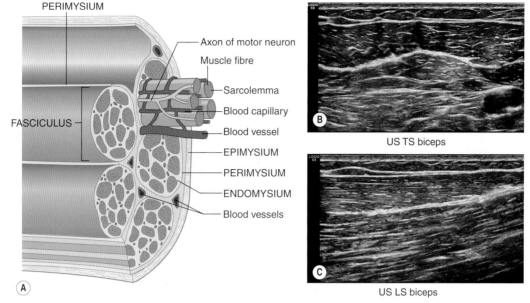

Fig. 2.10 **(A)** Schematic diagram of muscle structure. **(B)** Transverse section (TS) demonstrating the "starry sky" appearance. **(C)** Longitudinal section (LS) of the muscle. *US,* Ultrasound. (From Soames R, Palastanga N. Anatomy and Human Movement: Structure and Function. 7th ed. Elsevier Ltd; Edinburgh; 2019.)

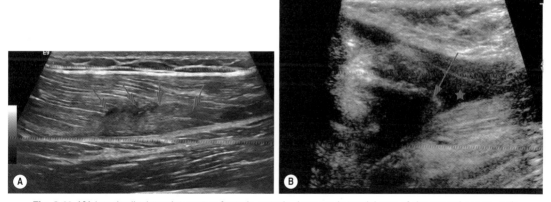

Fig. 2.11 **(A)** Longitudinal section rectus femoris muscle. Low grade partial tear of the central aponeurosis of rectus femoris, affecting only a small proportion of the muscle fibres with very little fibre retraction *(arrows).* **(B)** Longitudinal section right adductor muscles. High grade complete avulsion of the adductor longus origin, retraction, and bunching of the avulsed tendon *(arrow)* and resolving haematoma *(*).* The deeper fiberes of adductor brevis and magnus are intact.

pulleys to produce mechanical advantage for muscle contraction, thus magnifying the force of contraction, e.g., the patella within the quadriceps tendon/ligamentum patella complex.

Tendon structure. Tendon structure is complex and composed of type I collagen and elastin. Long strands of type I collagen form tendon fibrils which are enveloped by extracellular matrix (ECM) and are supplied by sparse neurovascular bundles and tenocytes. The fibres are further organised into fascicles and then into primary-secondary-tertiary bundles, each being surrounded internally by an endotenon and grouped together to form the

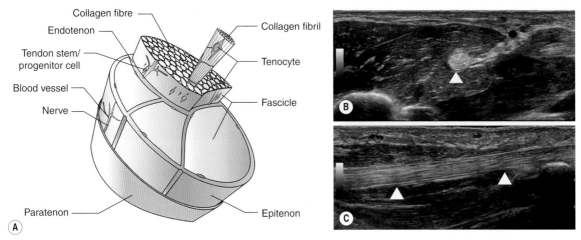

Fig. 2.12 Tendon Structure. **(A)** Schematic representation of a tendon. **(B)** Transverse and **(C)** longitudinal sections demonstrating typical sonographic appearances of a tendon *(arrowheads)*. (From Docheva et al. Biologics for tendon repair. Adv Drug Deliv Rev. 2015;84:222-239.)

tendon. The tendon is partially covered by a paratenon or enveloped by a tendon sheath.

Typically, tendons possess characteristically similar sonographic appearances, in that they appear as thin, uniformly linear structures composed of alternating hyperechoic and hypoechoic uniform bands in LS. This reflects their organised internal architecture and fibrillar patterning. In TS, they appear as rounded, slightly elliptical structures with a stippled appearance (Fig. 2.12).

Terminology of tendon dysfunction. Assessment of "tendinopathy" has become one of the most common requests on MSK ultrasound referrals and continues to promote discussion. Historically, in the literature and in clinical practice, most tendon pathology was referred to as "tendinitis" (inflammation of the tendon). Following studies that failed to show inflammatory processes, this changed to "tendinopathy" (clinically thickened without imaging) and "tendinosis" (thickened with hypervascularity on imaging).

The term "tendinosis" has been further challenged[14] in recent research as a misnomer because imaging findings are nonspecific and can relate to normal physiological adaptations to ageing, repair, and regeneration. Opinion suggests it is difficult to predict symptomatic versus asymptomatic tendon changes based on imaging findings alone.[15,16]

Recently, the International Consensus (ICON) 2019 statement[14] on clinical tendon terminology was published. The conclusion based on the findings of a panel of tendon experts was that the preferred term for tendon-related pain is "tendinopathy" and that this term should be used when communicating findings relating to tendons. The ICON 2019 statement recommends a number of other terminology changes when communicating tendon findings, and suggests that tendon-related pain should be termed *tendinopathy* and that imaging is not always necessary for this diagnosis. It also advises standardising nomenclature used by clinicians when communicating pathology in tendons and associated structures by recommending the avoidance of multiple terminologies frequently used by clinicians to describe one pathology, which can confusing to some. The ICON 2019[14] statement suggests the following proposals:

- Longstanding lateral and medial elbow pain = Lateral or medial elbow tendinopathy
- Longstanding patella tendon pain = Patella tendinopathy
- Longstanding Achilles pain = Achilles tendinopathy
- Longstanding Peroneal (fibularis) pain = Peroneal tendinopathy

These conditions are frequently induced, related to, and exacerbated by mechanical load/overload, resulting in pain and loss of function in the affected limb. These conditions can also be associated with tears within the structure, but the ICON 2019[14] statement suggests that if imaged, defects contained within the structure under investigation should be demonstrable (macro-tears) without the need for magnification (micro-tears). The group that produced the ICON 2019[14] statement anticipate that changes in terminology would become widespread and adopted over time.

Tendon models of injury. Tendons have evolved to perform movements at varying loads and frequencies without injury. When the tendon's capacity is exceeded, through excessive compressive or tensile loading, it breaks down.

Numerous patho-aetiological models have been proposed:
1. The inflammatory model
2. The collagen disruption/tear model
3. The tendon cell response model
4. The tendon continuum model (Fig. 2.13).

The tendon continuum model[17] has become the widely accepted model of tendon pathology and suggests that the key factors in the development of tendinopathy are repeated energy storage/release and excessive compressive forces, primarily occurring at tendon/bone entheses. Currently, the volume, intensity, and frequency of load required to cause overuse tendinopathy is unknown. Current opinion suggests that it is a multifactorial problem with age, sex, genetics, biomechanics, body composition, and circulating level of cytokines playing a role in the development of tendinopathy. The continuum model is used to guide treatment and outcome, placing the patient on a tendon change spectrum ranging from reactive tendinopathy (reversible tendon changes) to degenerative tendinopathy (irreversible tendon changes). The goal of therapy is to move the patient towards a normal tendon by load management (increasing or decreasing load). A very degenerate tendon can achieve a high functional level with careful management. However, in this case, the tendon will always look abnormal on ultrasound and will be clinically thickened. It is important to understand that even in chronically degenerate tendons there will be some "normal" tendon fibres contained within the degenerative structure, and these can be prone to tendinopathy, which gives rise to acute-on-chronic presentations. An understanding of the tendon continuum helps the ultrasound practitioner provide a detailed survey of the tendon to inform the clinical decision-making process (Fig. 2.14).

Pathological appearance of tendons. Tendon disorders share some similar ultrasound characteristics wherever their location:
1. Thickened (swollen)
2. Hypoechoic (oedematous)
3. Loss of fibrillar pattern giving rise to a disorganised internal structure
4. Colour or power Doppler reveals varying degrees of hypervascularity (depending on location)

Inflammatory model	Acute tendon injury heals with the standard inflammatory response of cell proliferation, maturation, and scar formation. A classic inflammatory response to overload in tendinopathy is not observed; whilst increases in inflammatory cytokines have been reported, it does not support that inflammation is the primary driver.
Collagen disruption/tear model	The oldest model used to explain tendon response to injury which has been challenged in recent years because the postulated collagen tearing and remodeling, does not occur as a result of normal loading (microtrauma).
Tendon cell response model	Proposes that tendon injury is caused by an abnormal adaptive response to tendon loading, and instead of normal collagen synthesis, an abnormal response occurs leading to a separation of collagen fibres with concomitant capillary proliferation. This leads to mechanically "silent" areas within the tendon which are unresponsive to load. This is hypothesised to play a role in degenerative tendinopathy. It is the lack of tendon cell response that may explain limited reversibility of degenerative tendinopathy.
Pathology continuum model	A three-stage continuum of tendinopathy consisting of reactive, disrepair, and degeneration phases. The addition or removal of tendon load being responsible for moving forward or backward along the tendon continuum. In the reactive tendinopathy phase, there is a non-inflammatory proliferation in extracellular matrix resulting in a thickening of the tendon. In the disrepair phase, repair is attempted, resulting in increased cells and proteoglycan (collagen) production. In the degenerative phase there are continued changes in the extracellular matrix alongside areas of cell death infiltrated with new blood vessels, resulting in considerable heterogeneity with degenerative tendon tissue interspersed with normal tendon.

Fig. 2.13 Summary of Tendon Models of Degeneration.

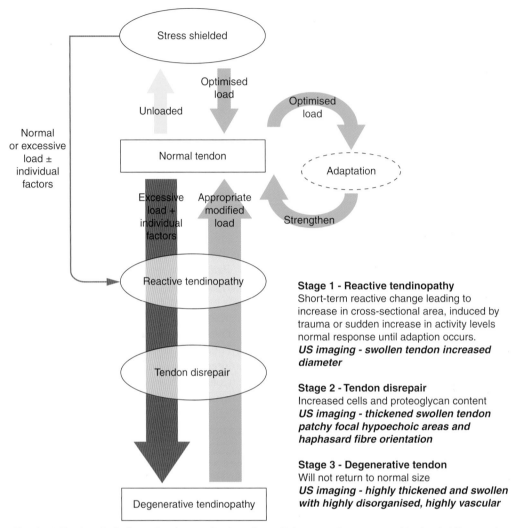

Fig. 2.14 Tendon Pathology Continuum Explanations. Relates to changes noted in the Achilles tendon but can be adapted for other tendons. *US*, Ultrasound. (From Cook JL, Purdam CR. Is tendon pathology a continuum? A pathology model to explain the clinical presentation of load-induced tendinopathy. Br J Sports Med. 2009;43(6):409-416.)

Stage 1 - Reactive tendinopathy
Short-term reactive change leading to increase in cross-sectional area, induced by trauma or sudden increase in activity levels normal response until adaption occurs.
US imaging - swollen tendon increased diameter

Stage 2 - Tendon disrepair
Increased cells and proteoglycan content
US imaging - thickened swollen tendon patchy focal hypoechoic areas and haphasard fibre orientation

Stage 3 - Degenerative tendon
Will not return to normal size
US imaging - highly thickened and swollen with highly disorganised, highly vascular

5. If ruptured, complete loss of internal architecture discontinuity and bunching of the fibres at the site of retraction (Fig. 2.15)

Detailed examples will be shown in the respective chapters.

Entheses

Entheses are specialised regions of muscle-tendon-bone units allowing for the attachment of tendons, ligaments, and joint capsules to bones. They can be categorised as fibrous or fibrocartilaginous.[18] Fibrous entheses are located where the tendon inserts directly on to periosteal bone, and fibrocartilages entheses are located in regions without periosteum such as epiphyses or apophyses.[19]

Their anatomical structure is complex, which in part explains the number of different pathologies that can affect them.[20,21] The extraarticular enthesis

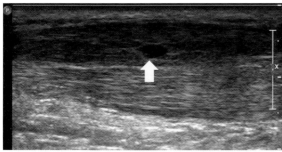

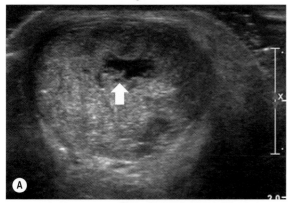

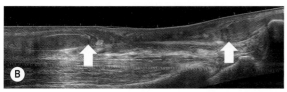

Fig. 2.15 Examples of Degenerative Changes That Can Occur in Tendons (Achilles Tendon Shown). (A) Longitudinal and transverse grey scale changes highlighting the swollen, disorganised loss of internal architecture and fibrillar pattern and a macroscopic intrasubstance tear *(white arrow).* **(B)** Extended field of view of a complete rupture of the Achilles tendon. Note the bulging of the retracted ends *(white arrows)* on the tendon, both proximal and distal.

of the Achilles tendon is presented in Fig. 2.16 demonstrating the complexity of the tendon bone unit, with the addition of an intervening bursa. This tendon-bursa-bone arrangement is typical of other entheses, such as the distal biceps insertion onto the radial tuberosity.

Typically, the normal ultrasound appearances of entheses are smooth and free of any enthesophytes or cortical irregularities, with regular internal pattern/fibrillar structure of the tendon.

Pathological appearance of entheses. Pathological appearances of entheses on ultrasound include cortical irregularities with concomitant changes in the overlying tendon such as microcalcifications, disorganised fibrillar patterning of the overlying tendon, and if a bursa is present, concomitant bursitis.[20,21] Any pathological condition that affects the enthesis, such as trauma, degenerative, inflammatory, endocrine, or metabolic, has been termed "enthesopathy," but in view of changes suggested by ICON 2019, the term "insertional tendinopathy" may need to be used to reflect current clinical opinions.[14]

Nerves

Considered as an advanced skill in MSK ultrasound, nerves can be technically challenging but rewarding structures to image, particularly when attempting to problem solve complex MSK problems.

Anatomically, nerves lie close to blood vessels so from a practical perspective, if a nerve is difficult to see, finding the vessels will aid its detection. This is important when first starting to scan nerves and when looking for small nerve branches.

Nerves are best visualised in TS where they appear as a collection of tiny, low echo balls within bright capsules, resembling a "bunch of grapes," "pepper pot top," or "honeycomb" appearance (Fig. 2.17).

Pathological Appearance of Nerves

Peripheral nerves are susceptible to compression produced by:

- Trauma
- Tumour
- Systemic conditions, e.g., diabetes and inflammatory arthritis
- Internal constraints, e.g., fibrous bands
- External loads

Typically, an abnormal nerve appears thickened with degradation of its internal architecture at, or just proximal to, the site of compression due to the build-up of oedema (Fig. 2.18). It can also demonstrate hypervascularity when examined with power Doppler.

Low grade blunt trauma to a nerve may produce similar appearance to that of compression. High grade blunt trauma and/or penetrating injuries can dissect nerves, resulting in discontinuity of the fascicles.

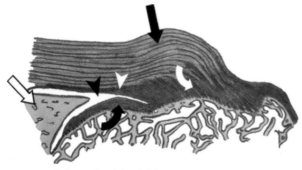

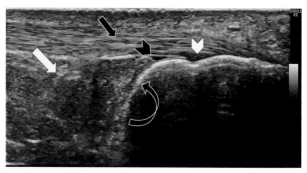

Schematic of the Achilles tendon insertion
which is an extraarticular enthesis

US image of Achilles tendon insertion

Fig. 2.16 Example of a Typical Extraarticular Enthesis from the Achilles Tendon. *Black arrow,* Achilles tendon; *black arrowhead,* synovial lined retrocalcaneal bursa separating fibrocartilaginous surfaces of the calcaneum and tendon; *black curved arrow,* superior tubercle of the calcaneum; *white arrow,* Kager's fat pad; *white arrowhead,* deep layer of the tendon lined with sesamoid fibrocartilage; *white curved arrow,* fibrocartilaginous enthesis. (Adapted from Tadros AS, Huang BK, Pathria MN. Muscle-tendon-enthesis unit. Semin Musculoskelet Radiol. 2018;22(3):263-274.)

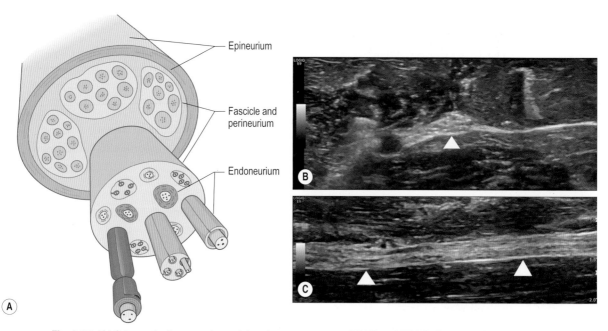

Fig. 2.17 (A) Schematic diagram of a peripheral nerve structure. **(B)** TS and **(C)** LS ultrasound images of the ulna nerve mid-forearm, demonstrating a typical ultrasound appearance. The tip of the *white triangle* points to the nerve. Note the dark regions within the nerve denoting the fascicles and the brighter perineurium and epineurium. *LS,* Longitudinal section; *TS,* transverse section. (A, from Soames R, Palastanga N. Anatomy and Human Movement: Structure and Function. 7th ed. Edinburgh; Elsevier; 2019.)

Differentiating Tendon and Nerves

Tendons and nerves share similar visible internal architecture—both possess a similar pattern and differentiation between the two may be challenging to the novice. Essentially, a tendon comprises of "solid" fibrils and a nerve is comprised of fluid-filled tubes, both "bundled" together. Nerve fascicles are larger and appear more widely spaced, whereas the tendon collagen fibres exhibit a finer fibrillar architecture (Fig. 2.19). Tendons and nerves are both affected by anisotropy, however, due to the larger nerve fascicles, nerves suffer with anisotropy to a lesser degree than tendons. In practical terms, when scanned in transverse, tendons will "darken" as the transducer is rocked forwards and backwards, whereas nerves stay relatively unchanged. This makes differentiation between the two slightly easier.

Fat

This versatile and often neglected tissue has a variety of functions including insulation, food storage, and shock absorbency. In areas where shock absorbency is important, fat is organised into specialised pads with a different sonographic appearance to subcutaneous fat (Fig. 2.20).

These pads are found in the following areas:
- Plantar heel and metatarsal heads

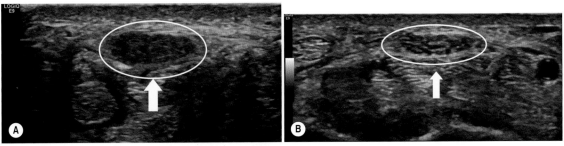

Fig. 2.18 Changes in Median Nerve on the Flexor Aspect of the Wrist Due to Internal Constraints. **(A)** Median nerve at the level of the carpal tunnel, demonstrating oedematous changes and loss of fascicular patterning compared with the normal fascicular pattern in **(B)**.

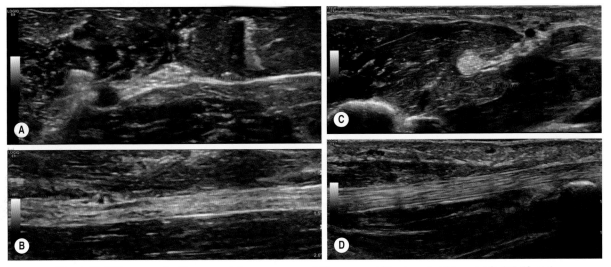

Fig. 2.19 Differences in Ultrasound Appearances of Nerves and Tendons in TS and LS. (A) TS and **(B)** LS nerve. **(C)** TS and **(D)** LS tendon. *LS,* Longitudinal section; *TS,* transverse section.

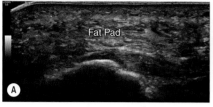
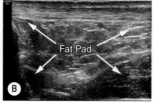
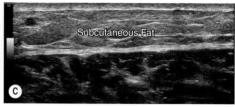

Plantar heel Fat pad   Hoffa's Fat pad anterior knee   Subcutaneous Fat

Fig. 2.20 **Examples of Different Appearances of Fatty Tissue. (A)** Plantar heel. Note the increased density of fibrous tissue giving a more structured appearance than in C. **(B)** Patella tendon and Hoffa's fat pad with a looser fibrous appearance. **(C)** Subcutaneous fat. Note how the fat lobules are held in less echogenic fibrous connective tissue than either A or B.

- Palm aspect of hand
- Buttocks
- Deep to Achilles and patellar tendons

Recognition of these structures is important because they can be a source of pain, particularly near the patella and metatarsals. They are also susceptible to iatrogenic damage (steroid atrophy) by poorly placed steroid injection.

Ligaments

These variably sized, dense, discrete, bands of strong collagenous tissue span joints attaching bone to bone. Ligaments have an adequate blood supply provided by the epi-ligament to maintain homeostasis—the two tissues are indistinguishable and blend with the periosteum of the bone. Each ligament complex is tailored to the joint that they protect,[22,23] and function to stabilise and restrict joint motion.[19,22] Biomechanically, ligaments have an inherent ability to stretch and un-stretch during load relaxation cycles, helping to prevent ligament damage during movement.[23]

On ultrasound, ligaments appear as bright structures due to their tightly bound collagen content, or dark structures due to their frequent deep and oblique orientation. A hockey stick transducer is particularly useful when scanning ligaments, particularly around the ankle as the bony contours often limit the degree of transducer manipulation, limiting the view of the ligament (Fig. 2.21).

Bursae

Bursae are loose, sac-like extraarticular structures providing a potential space between different types of skeletal tissue such as soft tissues and bony areas.[19]

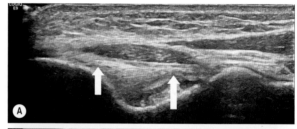
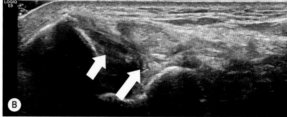

Fig. 2.21 (A) Ulnar collateral ligament of the elbow and **(B)** middle deltoid ligament of the ankle.

Their prime function is to protect, reduce friction, and improve movement between adjacent structures.

Bursae can be divided into two broad categories: native and nonnative types. Native bursae (Fig. 2.22) are generally associated anatomically with a synovial joint and are lined with synovial tissue (Fig. 2.23).

Nonnative bursae are adaptations formed because of friction. They lack a synovial layer and develop from potential spaces allowing extravasation of fluid, serum protein, and hyaluronic acid though increased tissue permeability.[24] Nonnative bursae can commonly be found on the plantar aspect of the heel or metatarsals and superficial to the distal Achilles tendon.

In their normal, nonpathological state, bursae can be difficult to see on ultrasound, except for the subacromial

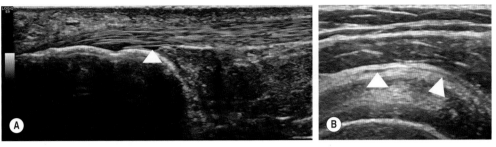

Fig. 2.22 Examples of Native Bursae Found in the Body. **(A)** Retrocalcaneal bursa. **(B)** Subacromial subdeltoid bursa *(white triangles).*

Shoulder	Subacromial-subdeltoid, Subcoracoid
Elbow	Olecranon, Bicipitoradial
Hip	Iliopsoas, Trochanteric, Ischiogluteal
Knee	Suprapatellar, Prepatellar and Infrapatellar (superficial and deep), Gastrocnemio-semimembranosus, Pes anserine, Semimembranosus
Ankle/foot	Retrocalcaneal, Intermetatarsal

Fig. 2.23 Positions of Native Bursae Possessing a Synovial Lining. (From Ruangchaijatuporn T, Gaetke-Udager K, Jacobson JA, Yablon CM, Morag Y. Ultrasound evaluation of bursae: anatomy and pathological appearances. Skeletal Radiol. 2017;46(4):445-462.)

bursa in the shoulder, which is the largest and most easily seen. However, some normal bursae may contain a very small quantity of anechoic fluid which makes them easier to identify, i.e., the retro-calcaneal bursa at the ankle and the deep infrapatellar bursa at the knee. Care must be taken not to mistake or misinterpret these as pathological findings. Symptomatic bursae become fluid-filled, appearing hypoechoic or anechoic on ultrasound. They may be hypervascular, with a thickened wall and may demonstrate a mixed echogenic appearance due to synovial proliferation.

Bursal distension alone is a nonspecific finding and as such, is insufficient to differentiate aetiology of a condition. It may be related to a myriad of aetiologies including trauma, or inflammatory or proliferative disorders.[24] Integrating ultrasound findings, patient history, physical examination, and laboratory tests are critical in order to arrive at a differential diagnosis.[24]

HISTORY TAKING

Obtaining a succinct history is an art-form rather than a science and is a skill that takes time to develop. For those unfamiliar with history taking, once mastered, it delivers a better understanding of MSK conditions and pain behavior.

Taking a brief history during the ultrasound examination performs a number of functions:
1. May supplement the clinical information contained on the request card
2. Confirms the correct structure and side to be scanned
3. Quickly builds a rapport with the patient
4. Gains additional information on how the condition affects the patient's life
5. Improves the patient's experience and journey

Below is a short list of questions that could be asked during an ultrasound examination.[25]
1. **How did the problem start?**
   a. Was this a sudden or slow onset pointing to a traumatic event (minutes/seconds), or due to repetitive activities (days/weeks/months) (eliciting mechanism of injury)?
   b. Was it due to occupation (work) or recreation (hobbies)—is this problem affecting either or both?
2. **How long has the problem been present for?**
   a. Is this problem acute, subacute, or chronic? This helps work out the healing timescale—an important consideration as MSK conditions, e.g., ruptured distal biceps, need surgery within 6 weeks.
3. **Where did the pain start and where is it now?**
   a. A relevant question if lumbar or cervical radiculopathy is suspected. Pain may start centrally, i.e., neck or back, and radiate to a limb, leading a referring agent to ask for a shoulder or knee scan, although these

sites are not the source of the problem. Bursitis can have strong referral patterns, i.e., subacromial-subdeltoid bursa.

4. **Does the pain disturb your sleep?**
   a. Generally, inflammatory conditions cause sleep disturbances and produce constant pain. Mechanical conditions broadly produce pain on movement but not necessarily sleep disturbances.

6. **Is it getting better or worse?**

7. **Have you had this before?**
   a. Useful question to ask as it can explain acute-on-chronic presentations, i.e., chronically thickened Achilles with acute tendinopathy.

8. **Which movements cause pain?**
   a. Mechanical conditions produce intermittent pains in some part of the movement cycle, and if a patient is pain free at rest but in pain during a particular movement, it may help to scan the suspected structure during movement if this is possible.

9. **What does the pain feel like?**
   a. Different tissues produce different sensations of pain: (1) nerve, a burning, pins and needles sensation; (2) bone, a local deep and boring sensation; (3) vascular, diffuse, achy, and poorly localised, and can refer; and (4) muscle, ligaments, and joint capsule, a dull, achy, hard to localise sensation which can refer.

SUMMARY

It is important to use correct anatomical terminology to locate and describe the position of an MSK lesion when communicating scan findings to other professionals. Knowing planes of motion helps with dynamic scanning.

Synovial joints are the most commonly scanned joints in MSK ultrasound practice.

Ultrasound detects periosteal changes after bony injury, before calcification reaction can be demonstrated on X-ray.

Tendons and nerves share similar characteristics, i.e., fibrillar patterning, but nerves, due to the larger fibres, have a coarse appearance.

Tendinopathy is the preferred term for persistent tendon pain and loss of function related to mechanical loading—please avoid tendinosis/tendinitis.

Entheses have a complex structure which a number of different pathologies can affect.

Bursae can be native and/or non-native, and it is normal to have a small amount of physiological fluid associated with native bursae.

History taking, though a skill in itself, is useful in order to supplement the examination and region requested.

REFERENCES

1. Sconfienza LM, Albano D, Allen G, et al. Clinical indications for musculoskeletal ultrasound updated in 2017 by European Society of Musculoskeletal Radiology (ESSR) consensus. Eur Radiol. 2018;28(12):5338–5351.

2. Klauser AS, Tagliafico A, Allen GM, et al. Clinical indications for musculoskeletal ultrasound: a Delphi-based consensus paper of the European Society of Musculoskeletal Radiology. Eur Radiol. 2012;22(5):1140–1148.

3. Wheeler P. What do patients think about diagnostic ultrasound? A pilot study to investigate patient-perceived benefits with the use of musculoskeletal diagnostic ultrasound in an outpatient clinic setting. Int Musculoskelet Med. 2010;32(2):68–71.

4. Sahbudin I, Bell J, Kaur K, Raza K, Filer A. Observing real-time images during ultrasound-guided procedures improves patients' experience. Rheumatology 2016, 55(3): 585-6

5. Lumsden G, Lucas-Garner K, Sutherland S, Dodenhoff R. Physiotherapists utilizing diagnostic ultrasound in shoulder clinics. How useful do patients find immediate feedback from the scan as part of the management of their problem? Musculoskeletal Care. 2018;16(1):209–213.

6. Edwards H. Let's all jump on the ultrasound bandwagon. Ultrasound. 2010;18:4–7.

7. Champagne N, Eadie L, Regan L, Wilson P. The effectiveness of ultrasound in the detection of fractures in adults with suspected upper or lower limb injury: a systematic review and subgroup meta-analysis. BMC Emerg Med. 2019;19(1):17. doi:10.1186/s12873-019-0226-5.

8. Moraux A, Gitto S, Bianchi S. Ultrasound features of the normal and pathologic periosteum. J Ultrasound Med. 2018;38(3):775–784.

9. Docheva D, Müller SA, Majewski M, Evans CH. Biologics for tendon repair. Adv Drug Deliv Rev. 2015;84:222–239.

10. Rao A, Pimpalwar Y, Sahdev R, Sinha S, Yadu N. Diagnostic ultrasound: an effective tool for early

detection of stress fractures of Tibia. J Arch Mil Med. 2017;5(2):e57343.

11. Hamilton B, Valle X, Rodas G, et al. Classification and grading of muscle injuries: a narrative review. Br J Sports Med. 2015;49(5):306.

12. Grassi A, Quaglia A, Canata GL, Zaffagnini S. An update on the grading of muscle injuries: a narrative review from clinical to comprehensive systems. Joints. 2016;4(1):39–46.

13. Pollock N, James SL, Lee JC, Chakraverty R. British athletics muscle injury classification: a new grading system. Br J Sports Med. 2014;48(18):1347–1351.

14. Scott A, Squier K, Alfredson H, et al. ICON 2019: International Scientific Tendinopathy Symposium Consensus: clinical terminology. Br J Sports Med. 2020;54(5):260–262.

15. Moosmayer S, Smith HJ, Tariq R, Larmo A. Prevalence and characteristics of asymptomatic tears of the rotator cuff: an ultrasonographic and clinical study. J Bone Joint Surg. 2009;91(2):196–200.

16. McCreesh K, Lewis J. Continuum model of tendon pathology - where are we now? Int J Exp Pathol. 2013;94(4):242–247.

17. Cook JL, Purdam CR. Is tendon pathology a continuum? A pathology model to explain the clinical presentation of load-induced tendinopathy. Br J Sports Med. 2009;43(6):409–416.

18. Benjamin M, Toumi H, Ralphs JR, Bydder G, Best TM, Milz S. Where tendons and ligaments meet bone: attachment sites (entheses) in relation to exercise and/or mechanical load. J Anat. 2006;208:471–490.

19. Soames R, Palastanga N. Anatomy and Human Movement: Structure and Function. 7th ed. Edinburgh: Elsevier Ltd; 2019.

20. Tadros AS, Huang BK, Pathria MN. Muscle-tendon-enthesis unit. Semin Musculoskelet Radiol. 2018;22(3):263–274.

21. Benjamin M, Moriggl B, Brenner E, Emery P, McGonagle D, Redman S. The "enthesis organ" concept: Why enthesopathies may not present as focal insertional disorders. Arthritis Rheum. 2004;50(10):3306–3313.

22. Frank CB. Ligament structure, physiology and function. J Musculoskelet Neuronal Interact. 2004;4(2):199–201.

23. Bray RC, Salo PT, Lo IK, Ackerman P, Rattner JB, Hart DA. Normal ligament structure, physiology and function. Sports Med Arthrosc Rev. 2005;13(3):127–135.

24. Ruangchaijatuporn T, Gaetke-Udager K, Jacobson JA, Yablon CM, Morag Y. Ultrasound evaluation of bursae: anatomy and pathological appearances. Skeletal Radiol. 2017;46(4):445–462.

25. Magee DJ, Orthopedic Physical Assessment. 6th ed. St Louis, Missouri: Elsevier Saunders; 2014.

Ultrasound of the Shoulder

Lorelei Waring, Clare Drury, and Mark Maybury

CHAPTER OUTLINE

LEARNING OBJECTIVES

This chapter aims to provide the reader with the relevant knowledge of:
- Shoulder anatomy
- Imaging technique and normal ultrasound appearances
- Pathological appearances and clinical presentations
- Management options

INTRODUCTION

Shoulder pain is common in the general population and is a frequent reason for referral to musculoskeletal services. This is attributed to the fact that the shoulder is the most mobile joint of the body and thus the most unstable, rendering it susceptible to injury.[1–4]

Many centres now utilise ultrasound as the first-line imaging investigation for the painful shoulder,[5–7] and although there are many benefits to ultrasound, the most documented limitation is its operator dependency.[7,8] The practitioner must have a sound knowledge of the anatomy and physiology of the shoulder, know how to employ the standardised ultrasound technique, and have an appreciation of the normal and pathological ultrasound appearances, as well as an understanding of the management options available to the patient.

ANATOMY OF THE SHOULDER JOINT

The shoulder is composed of four articulations: the glenohumeral joint (GHJ), acromioclavicular joint (ACJ), sternoclavicular joint (SCJ), and scapulothoracic unit. The two joints which are routinely included in a shoulder ultrasound examination are the GHJ and ACJ.

The GHJ is a synovial ball and socket joint between the head of the humerus and the glenoid fossa of the scapula. The head of the humerus is much larger than the shallow glenoid fossa despite the presence of a fibrocartilage labrum which encircles and deepens the glenoid. The joint is therefore capable of a wide range of movement, but this is at the expense of stability.[4]

The ACJ (between the clavicle and acromion of the scapula) is a plane synovial joint allowing gliding movement. As it attaches the scapula to the thorax, it enables additional movement of the scapula and assists in shoulder abduction and flexion (Fig. 3.1).

Static and dynamic stabilisers control movement and stability of the shoulder, and these are susceptible to repetitive injury and trauma.[9]

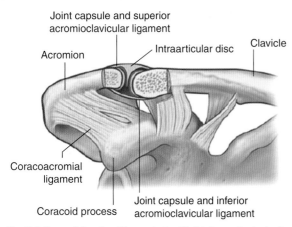

Fig. 3.1 Frontal Section Through the Right Acromioclavicular Joint Showing the Intraarticular Disc and Capsular Attachments. (From Soames R, Palastange N. Anatomy and Human Movement Structure and Function. 7th ed. London: Elsevier; 2019.)

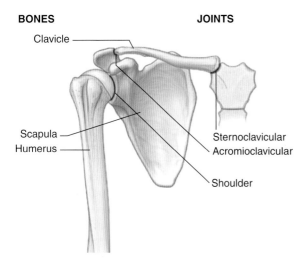

Fig. 3.2 Static Stabilisers. The acromioclavicular, shoulder (glenohumeral) and sternoclavicular joints. (From Soames R, Palastange N. Anatomy and Human Movement Structure and Function. 7th ed. London: Elsevier; 2019.)

The static stabilisers include the glenoid labrum, the GHJ, ACJ, and SCJ (Fig. 3.2) as well as the glenohumeral, coracohumeral, coracoclavicular, and acromioclavicular ligaments (Fig. 3.3).[4]

The dynamic stabilisers include the four muscles of the rotator cuff, as well as the biceps brachii, coracobrachialis, and deltoid muscles and the scapulothoracic unit (serratus anterior, trapezius, latissimus dorsi, rhomboids, pectoralis major, and minor and levator scapula) (Fig. 3.4).

The scapula itself has important bony landmarks that can help to locate other musculoskeletal structures during clinical and ultrasound examination. The acromion is the expanded lateral end of the spine of the scapula. It projects forwards at right angles making its anterior edge easily palpable (Fig. 3.5).

The coracoid process is a hook-like projection with a broad base located on the anterior aspect of the scapula (see Fig. 3.5).

On the posterior aspect of the shoulder blade, the palpable spine of the scapula separates the supraspinous fossa and the infraspinous fossa. These fossae communicate via the spinoglenoid notch which is located between the lateral end of the spine and neck of the scapula (see Fig. 3.5).[4]

> ### ◎ TOP TIP
>
> Be "hands on."
> Palpating bony landmarks such as the acromion, coracoid, and spine of the scapula (on willing volunteers) will help you to build up a clearer picture of the anatomy of the shoulder and will allow you to appreciate the position of the tendons and muscles associated with these landmarks. Having this clearer understanding of the anatomy will improve your confidence when scanning.

Shoulder Joint Capsule

The GHJ has a thick, fibrous capsule that forms a loose sleeve between the humeral head and the scapula. It is strengthened anteriorly by the three glenohumeral ligaments and superoposteriorly by the coracohumeral ligament (see Fig. 3.3).

There are two natural openings within the joint capsule. The first is located at the upper aspect of the bicipital (intertubercular) groove between the greater and lesser tuberosities of the humerus through which the long head of biceps tendon passes. The second opening is located on the anterior aspect of the capsule between the superior and middle glenohumeral ligaments, and this communicates with the subscapular bursa deep to the subscapularis tendon. These openings allow communication between the joint cavity and the corresponding anatomical structures.[4]

Subacromial-Subdeltoid (SASD) Bursa

The subacromial bursa is a synovial cavity and, in most individuals, it communicates with the subdeltoid

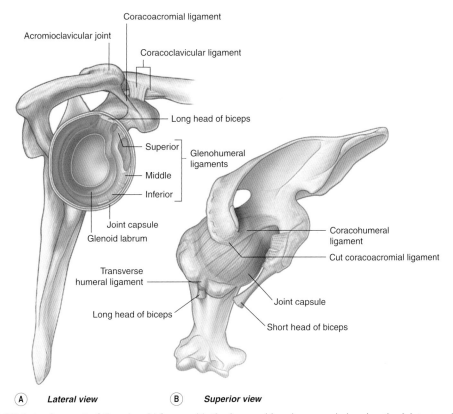

A **Lateral view**   B **Superior view**

Fig. 3.3 (A) Lateral aspect of the glenoid fossa with the humeral head removed showing the joint capsule and glenohumeral ligaments; **(B)** anterolateral aspect of the shoulder joint showing the transverse humeral, coracohumoral, coracoacromial, and coracoclavicular ligaments. (From Soames R, Palastange N. Anatomy and Human Movement Structure and Function. 7th ed. London: Elsevier; 2019.)

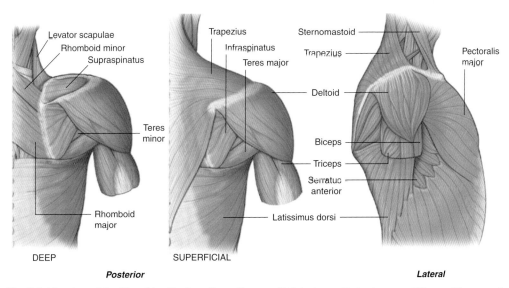

Fig. 3.4 Muscles of the Shoulder Region. (From Soames R, Palastange N. Anatomy and Human Movement Structure and Function. 7th ed. London: Elsevier; 2019.)

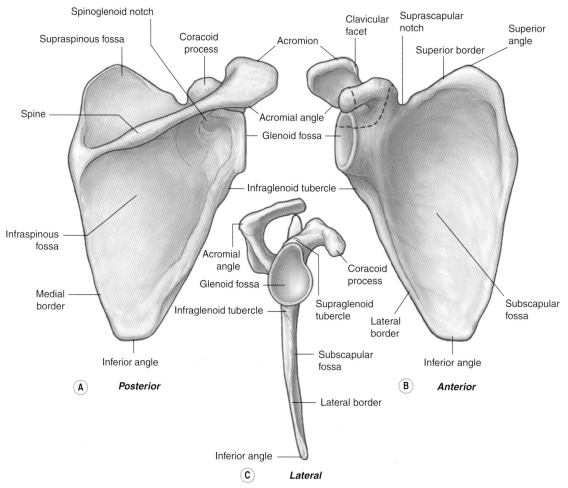

Fig. 3.5 Posterior **(A)**, anterior **(B)**, and lateral **(C)** aspects of the right scapula. (From Soames R, Palastange N. Anatomy and Human Movement Structure and Function. 7th ed. London: Elsevier; 2019.)

bursa forming the SASD bursa. This bursa separates the coracoacromial arch and the deltoid muscle from the underlying rotator cuff tendons. It allows smooth movement between these structures, minimising friction (Fig. 3.6).[4]

Rotator Cuff

The tendons of the subscapularis (SSC), supraspinatus (SST), infraspinatus (IST), and teres minor (TM) muscles are the stabilising structures most closely related to the shoulder joint as they cover the joint capsule and merge with it at their humeral insertions. As such, they act as extensible ligaments and are very important in maintaining joint integrity (Fig. 3.7). They are known

collectively as the rotator cuff tendons and are the main structures evaluated in shoulder ultrasound.

Recent developments show that the anatomy of the rotator cuff is more complex than originally believed, and although this next section describes the tendons separately, they are blended structures. A recent discovery is the rotator cable (RCa), a strong fibrous suspensory structure, which originates from the deep layer of the coracohumeral ligament, extending perpendicularly along the SST and IST tendon fibres (Fig. 3.8). It is thought to protect an avascular crescentic-shaped area in the tendons (rotator crescent) at the insertion of the SST/IST tendons, which is prone to damage and becomes thinner in elderly patients. The RCa can be seen

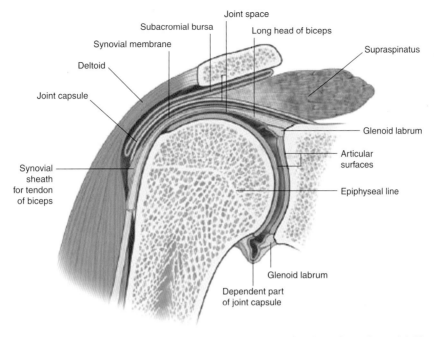

Fig. 3.6 Coronal Section of the Shoulder Joint Showing the Reflection of the Synovial Membrane Around the Long Head of Biceps. (From Soames R, Palastange N. Anatomy and Human Movement Structure and Function. 7th ed. London: Elsevier; 2019.)

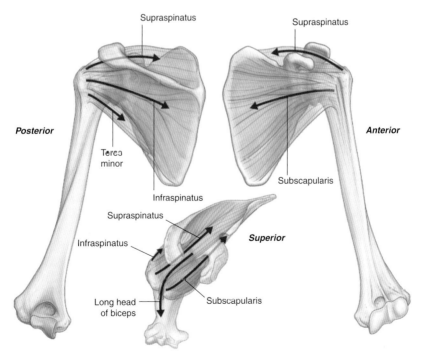

Fig. 3.7 Posterior, anterior, and superior aspects of the scapula and humerus showing the action of the rotator cuff muscles in stabilising the shoulder joint. Collectively, interplay between the musculotendinous rotator cuff reduces sliding and shearing movements during movement of the humeral head on the glenoid. (From Soames R, Palastange N. Anatomy and Human Movement Structure and Function. 7th ed. London: Elsevier; 2019.)

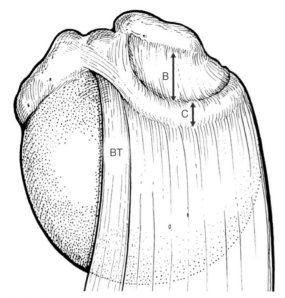

Fig. 3.8 The rotator cable *(C)* is a thick fibrous reinforcement which shields the rotator crescent *(B)* from mechanical stress. *BT,* Biceps tendon. (From Burkhart et al. The rotator crescent and rotator cable: an anatomic description of the shoulder's "suspension bridge." Arthroscopy. 1993;9(6):611-616. Copyright © 1993, Elsevier.)

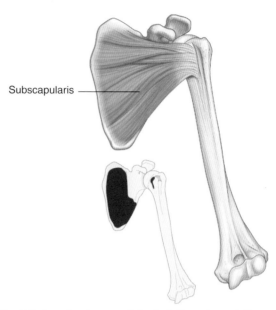

Fig. 3.9 Anterior Aspect of the Left Scapula and Humerus Showing the Position and Attachments of Subscapularis. (From Soames R, Palastange N. Anatomy and Human Movement Structure and Function. 7th ed. London: Elsevier; 2019.)

on ultrasound especially in younger patients but is better demonstrated on magnetic resonance imaging (MRI).[10,11]

Subscapularis

The SSC muscle arises from the medial two-thirds of the subscapular fossa on the costal surface of the scapula. It is a multipennate muscle and its fibres run medially to form a broad, thick tendon that inserts on to the lesser tuberosity of the humerus (Fig. 3.9). The main action of this muscle is internal rotation of the arm at the shoulder.[4]

Supraspinatus

The SST muscle originates from the medial two-thirds of the supraspinous fossa on the posterior aspect of the scapula and courses laterally below the trapezius muscle, acromion, and coracoacromial ligament, over the top of the shoulder. The tendon inserts onto the upper facet of the greater tuberosity of the humerus (Fig. 3.10). The SST muscle initiates abduction of the arm but is only responsible for the first 20 degrees of abduction; after this, the deltoid takes over.[4]

Infraspinatus

The IST muscle originates from the medial two-thirds of the infraspinous fossa and converges to form a narrow tendon which inserts on to the middle facet of the greater tuberosity of the humerus (Fig. 3.11).

It is an external rotator of the arm at the shoulder.[4]

Teres minor

The TM muscle originates from the upper two-thirds of the lateral border of the scapula, running laterally to form a narrow tendon which inserts on to the lower facet of the greater tuberosity of the humerus (see Fig. 3.11).

This muscle is an external rotator of the arm at the shoulder but also acts as an adductor.[4]

Long Head of Biceps Brachii (LHB)

Although not part of the rotator cuff, the LHB tendon is an important structure in shoulder ultrasound. It plays an important role in stabilising the shoulder during elbow flexion and forearm supination. The tendon originates on the supraglenoid tubercle of the scapula and is enclosed within a synovial sheath. It enters the bicipital

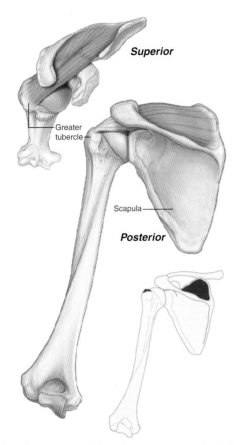

Fig. 3.10 Posterior and Superior Aspects of the Left Scapula and Humerus Showing the Position and Attachments of Supraspinatus. (From Soames R, Palastange N. Anatomy and Human Movement Structure and Function. 7th ed. London: Elsevier; 2019.)

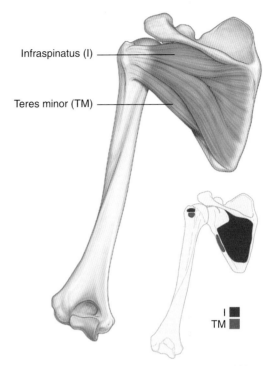

Fig. 3.11 Posterior Aspect of the Left Scapula and Humerus Showing the Position and Attachments of Infraspinatus *(I)* and Teres Minor *(TM)*. (From Soames R, Palastange N. Anatomy and Human Movement Structure and Function. 7th ed. London: Elsevier; 2019.)

groove of the humerus by passing deep to what is commonly called the "transverse humeral ligament" (THL). This is now felt to be a conjoint ligamentous structure, sometimes termed the "biceps sling" or "pulley," and is made up of fibres from the coracohumeral and superior glenohumeral ligaments, reinforced by fibres of the SSC and SST tendons (Fig. 3.12).

The biceps brachii muscle has a second short tendinous head which originates on the apex of the coracoid process[4] (see Fig. 3.12).

Pectoralis Major Tendon

The pectoralis major tendon acts as an important landmark when assessing the full extent of the LHB tendon with ultrasound as the anterior lamina of this tendon inserts on to the humerus at the same level of the myotendinous junction of the LHB tendon[4] (Fig. 3.13).

Deltoid Muscle

The deltoid muscle lies superficial to the rotator cuff muscles and is separated from them by the SASD bursa. It affords the shoulder its rounded shape. It has an extensive origin and inserts on to the deltoid tuberosity on the lateral aspect of the shaft of the humerus[4] (Fig. 3.14).

◎ **TOP TIP**

Know your anatomy!

Knowing the origins, insertions, and functions of the rotator cuff tendons and the other relevant structures and being able to appreciate their anatomical positions within the shoulder will enable you to approach your scanning with more confidence.

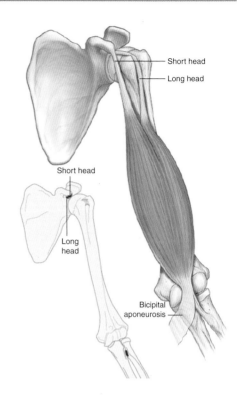

Fig. 3.12 Anterior Aspect of the Left Arm and Forearm Showing the Position and Attachments of Biceps Brachii. (From Soames R, Palastange N. Anatomy and Human Movement Structure and Function. 7th ed. London: Elsevier; 2019.)

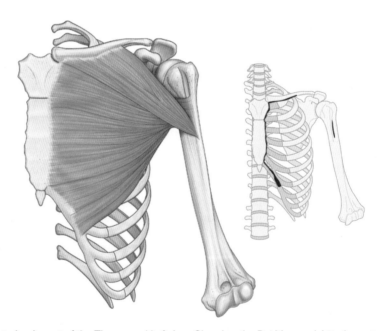

Fig. 3.13 Anterior Aspect of the Thorax and Left Arm Showing the Position and Attachments of Pectoralis Major. (From Soames R, Palastange N. Anatomy and Human Movement Structure and Function. 7th ed. London: Elsevier; 2019.)

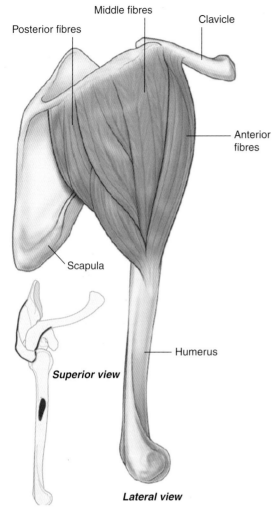

Fig. 3.14 Lateral Aspect of the Right Clavicle and Scapula Showing the Position and Attachments of Deltoid. (From Soames R, Palastange N. Anatomy and Human Movement Structure and Function. 7th ed. London: Elsevier; 2019.)

ULTRASOUND TECHNIQUE AND NORMAL APPEARANCES

There are various patient positions advocated for shoulder ultrasound examinations, including scanning the patient from behind or from in front. The decision is often based on which approach is most comfortable for the individual practitioner. It is recommended that the patient is asked to sit on a rise and fall chair without a back or with lumbar support to facilitate the necessary arm movements,[4] but it is advisable to avoid chairs on wheels for safety reasons.

It can be difficult to elicit the origin of symptoms in the shoulder clinically, and it has therefore become standard practice to perform a global ultrasound assessment of the shoulder regardless of the clinical differential diagnosis. The European Society of Skeletal Radiologists (ESSR) and British Medical Ultrasound Society (BMUS) guidelines suggest that as a minimum the following structures are imaged[12,13]:

- Long head of biceps tendon
- Rotator interval
- Subscapularis tendon
- Supraspinatus tendon
- Infraspinatus tendon
- Any visible bursae around the shoulder
- Posterior glenohumeral joint
- Acromioclavicular joint

The order in which these structures are examined varies between individual centres and practitioners. The technique highlighted in the ESSR shoulder guidelines is widely accepted as good practice.[12]

When annotating images, it is important to remember that very few anatomical structures within the body lie in the true anatomical planes, and it is commonly accepted that when ultrasound images are annotated as "longitudinal" or "transverse" or "axial" and "coronal," this refers to the section of the structure under investigation not the anatomical position of the probe. For the purposes of the images in this chapter, the long axis of the tendon will be termed longitudinal (LS) and the short axis of the tendon will be termed transverse (TS).

Long Head of Biceps (LHB) Tendon

The patient's arm is relaxed down by their side with slight internal rotation of the shoulder. The elbow is flexed at 90 degrees and tucked into the side with the palm of the hand facing towards the ceiling (Fig. 3.15). The probe is placed in the transverse plane at the level of the bicipital groove to image the LHB in TS (see Fig. 3.15).

The LHB tendon will be identified within the bicipital groove as a hyperechoic oval-shaped structure with the lesser tuberosity medially and the greater tuberosity laterally (see Fig. 3.15). The biceps sling or THL can be seen traversing the tuberosities (see Fig. 3.15). Maneuvering the probe superiorly facilitates examination of the proximal LHB tendon. Moving inferiorly, the myotendinous junction is reached when the tendon dives

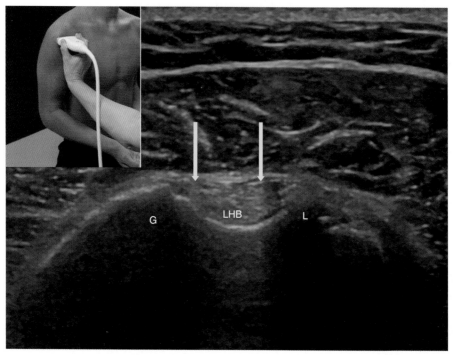

Fig. 3.15 Transverse Image of long head of biceps tendon (LHBT). Inset: Patient position for imaging the LHB tendon in the TS plane. *G,* Greater tuberosity; *L,* lesser tuberosity; *LHB,* long head of biceps tendon; *yellow arrows,* biceps sling (transverse humeral ligament).

deep to the pectoralis major tendon, which can be seen on ultrasound in its longitudinal plane as a linear fibrillar structure[14] (Fig. 3.16).

The probe is then turned through 90 degrees to image the LHB tendon in LS (Fig. 3.17), where it appears as a striated hyperechoic fibrillar structure of uniform thickness (see Fig. 3.17) which is noted to widen at its myotendinous junction (MTJ) (Fig. 3.18).

Tilting the probe in TS and 'heel toeing' the probe in LS is required to ensure the beam remains perpendicular to the tendon fibres thus avoiding anisotropy, which can mimic tendinopathy and rupture (see Chapter 1).

The much shorter tendon of the short head of biceps can be seen in LS by directing the transducer medially in an oblique orientation to the coracoid process—this tendon does not usually lie within the normal shoulder protocol, but may be imaged if pathology is suspected.

Subscapularis (SSC) Tendon

With the elbow still flexed at 90 degrees and the palm facing towards the ceiling, the patient's arm is rotated

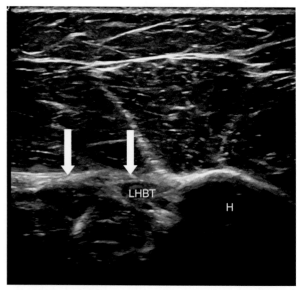

Fig. 3.16 Transverse Image of Distal LHBT at the Level of the MTJ. *H,* Humerus; *white arrows,* pectoralis major tendon.

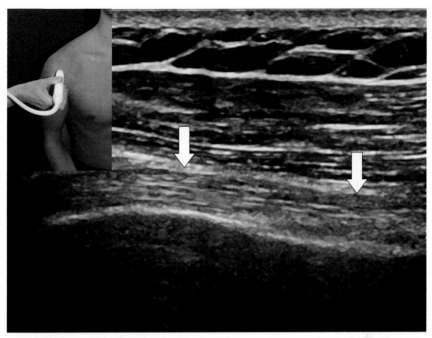

Fig. 3.17 Longitudinal Image of LHBT. Inset: Patient and probe position for imaging the LHBT in the transverse plane. *White arrows,* Long head of biceps tendon.

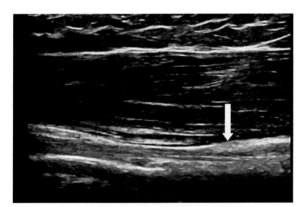

Fig. 3.18 Longitudinal Image of LHBT at the MTJ. Note the widening distally as the biceps muscle belly appears *(white arrow)* and the subtle change in echogenicity.

externally with the elbow tucked into the side (Fig. 3.19). This allows access to the SSC tendon as it emerges from underneath the coracoid process. With the probe in a transverse plane the tendon is imaged in LS (see Fig. 3.19).

The probe is moved medially and laterally, superiorly and inferiorly to ensure the tendon is imaged in its entirety from myotendinous junction to insertion on the lesser tuberosity as it is a broad tendon. In LS, this tendon has a convex superficial surface with a striated, fibrillar architecture and is uniformly echogenic as it tapers to its insertion[15] (see Fig. 3.19).

By maintaining the patient's arm position and rotating the probe through 90 degrees, a TS view of the SSC tendon is obtained (Fig. 3.20).

The SSC muscle is multipennate and is made up of 4 to 8 muscle/tendon bundles. In this plane, the individual echogenic "tendon bundles" are most apparent towards the medial aspect, at the MTJ, where the hypoechoic muscle fibres are seen between the "tendon bundles." These appearances should not be mistaken for tears or tendinopathy[15,16] (see Fig. 3.20). Again, the tendon is imaged in its entirety by moving the transducer from the MTJ, laterally to the lesser tuberosity.

Rotator Cuff Interval (RI)

The RI describes the appearance of the proximal LHB tendon positioned between the SSC and SST tendons. The superior glenohumeral and coracohumeral ligaments are also seen in this view.

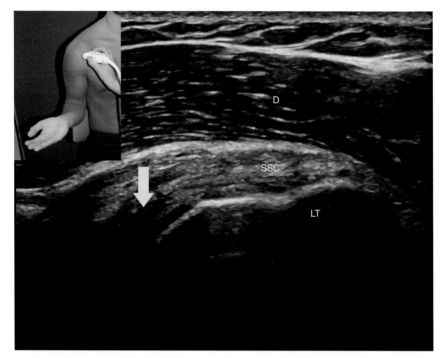

Fig. 3.19 Longitudinal Image SSC. Inset: Patient and probe position for imaging the subscapularis tendon in the LS plane. *D,* Overlying deltoid muscle; *LT,* lesser tuberosity of the humeral head; *SSC,* subscapularis tendon; *yellow arrow,* myotendinous junction (note hypoechoic changes here).

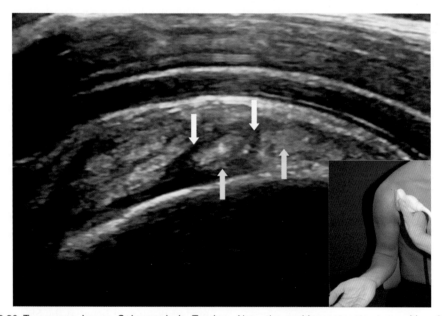

Fig. 3.20 Transverse Image Subscapularis Tendon. Note the multipennate structure with echopoor "clefts" *(white arrows)* interspacing the tendon bundles *(yellow arrows).* Inset: Patient and probe position for imaging the subscapularis tendon in the transverse plane.

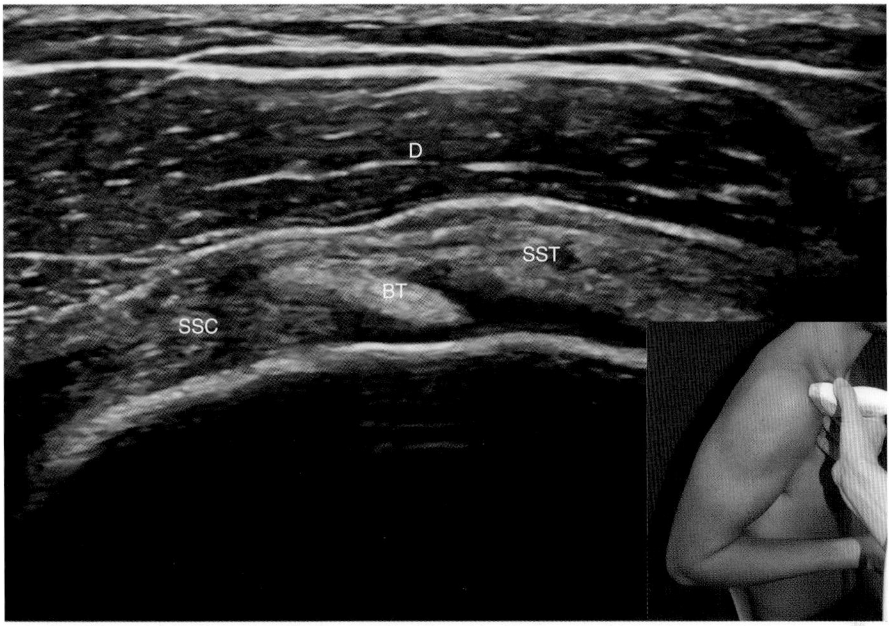

Fig. 3.21 Rotator Cuff Interval. The oval echogenic long head of biceps *(BT)* located between the rounded anterior leading edge of the supraspinatus tendon *(SST)* laterally and the upper aspect of the subscapularis tendon *(SSC)* medially. The deltoid muscle *(D)* is noted overlying the rotator cuff tendons. Inset: Patient and probe position for imaging the rotator interval tendon in the transverse plane.

With the patient's elbow still in flexion, the arm is returned to the neutral position and with the elbow tucked in to the side, the elbow is eased backwards until the medial aspect of the hand rests at the patient's side (Fig. 3.21). In this position the distal SST tendon emerges from under the acromion. As the humerus is only minimally internally rotated, the LHB assumes a more medial position but is still clearly identified. It is important to appreciate that the SST tendon takes an oblique course as it reaches its insertion and its true long axis lie can be described as being on virtually the same plane as a line drawn between the ear and tip of the shoulder[6] (Fig. 3.22). For this reason, the transducer is placed in an oblique transverse plane to image the interval in TS (see Fig 3.21 and Fig. 3.22, *yellow line*).

The resultant ultrasound image reveals the oval echogenic LHB between the rounded anterior leading edge of the SST tendon laterally and the upper aspect of the SSC tendon medially[15] (see Fig. 3.21). Rotator cuff tears often originate at the anterior leading edge of the SST tendon, so undertaking a thorough interrogation of this area is critical.[6] It can also help detect small tears of the superior fibres of SSC where they merge with the "biceps sling."

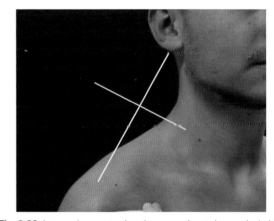

Fig. 3.22 Image demonstrating the approximate long axis *(white line)* and short axis *(yellow line)* lie of the supraspinatus tendon. This indicates the probe positioning required to image the SST tendon in true TS (yellow line) and LS (white arrow) axis.

Supraspinatus (SST) Tendon

To facilitate optimal imaging of the whole SST tendon, the arm is then moved more posteriorly with the elbow close to the patient's side and the palm of the hand placed on the posterior aspect of the ipsilateral hip/lower back. This pulls

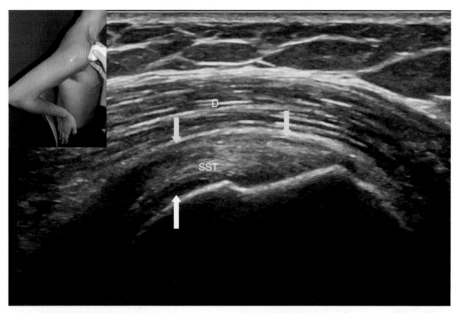

Fig. 3.23 Longitudinal Image Supraspinatus Tendon. Note the convex superior surface. The normal subacromial-subdeltoid bursa *(yellow arrows)* appears as a thin hypoechoic band between the supraspinatus tendon *(SST)* and the deltoid muscle *(D)*. The articular cartilage is also demonstrable *(white arrow)*. Inset: Patient and probe position for imaging the supraspinatus tendon in longitudinal plane.

the proximal aspect of the tendon from under the acromion. This view is commonly known as the modified crass position or hand in back pocket position (Fig. 3.23). The transducer is placed in an oblique sagittal plane to image the tendon in LS (see Fig. 3.23 and Fig. 3.22, *white line*).

Using the highly echogenic LHB in true LS as a starting point, the probe is then moved laterally without changing its orientation and the medial aspect of the SST tendon comes into view. It appears as a uniformly hyperechoic structure with a convex superior surface which tapers smoothly to its insertion on the greater tuberosity, also known as the tendon footprint[15] (see Fig. 3.23). The RCa may be noted as a hyperechoic, fibrillar structure 1 to 1.5 cm distal to the crescent area of the SST tendon tracking in a perpendicular axis to the tendon fibres[10] (Fig. 3.24). As the probe is moved across the tendon footprint, the cartilage overlying the humeral head can also be demonstrated (see Fig. 3.23). The normal SASD bursa appears as a thin hypoechoic band between the SST tendon and the deltoid muscle (see Fig. 3.23). The tendon should be imaged in its entirety, which may require moving superiorly as well as laterally following the curved surface of the shoulder.

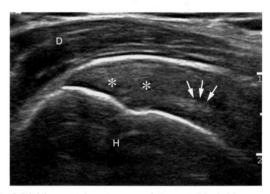

Fig. 3.24 Ultrasound appearance of rotator cable *(white arrows)* and of the crescent area *(asterisks)*. D, Deltoid; H, humerus. (From Sconfienza LM, Orlandi D, Fabbro E, et al. Ultrasound assessment of the rotator cuff cable: comparison between young and elderly asymptomatic volunteers and interobserver reproducibility. Ultrasound Med Biol. 2012;38(1):35-41.)

To image the SST in TS, the arm position is maintained and the transducer is turned through 90 degrees (Fig. 3.25).

A useful starting landmark is the LHB, which is seen in TS at the RI adjacent to the anterior leading edge of

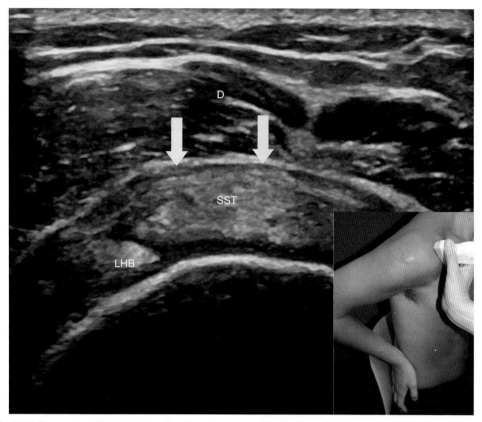

Fig. 3.25 Transverse Supraspinatus Tendon Demonstrating Uniform Thickness from the Biceps Tendon Landmark. Note the change in position of the long head of biceps tendon *(LHB)* when compared to Fig. 3.21 due to the increased internal rotation of the humerus. The SASD bursa *(yellow arrows)* is again noted separating the supraspinatus tendon *(SST)* and the deltoid muscle *(D)*. Inset: Patient and probe position for imaging the supraspinatus tendon in the TS plane.

the SST tendon (see Fig. 3.25). As the transducer is moved posteriorly (for a distance of approximately 2 cm) the rest of the SST tendon can be evaluated. Thorough examination of the entire tendon requires making greater excursions with the transducer in an anteroposterior direction but also in a slight cranial to caudal direction following the natural curved contour of the shoulder. The tendon should be uniformly echogenic and it is important to note that the normal tendon gradually thins out in its anterior aspect (not to be mistaken as tendon rupture) whilst posteriorly, it blends with the IST tendon[15] (see Fig. 3.26). The RCa is noted as a hyperechoic fibrillar structure deep to the SST tendon tracking perpendicular relative to the tendon fibres[10] (Fig. 3.26).

> ◎ **TOP TIP**
>
> Utilising the LHB tendon as a landmark is a useful way of reorientating oneself as it is easily recognisable and also aids in ensuring accurate transducer positioning.

An alternative arm position for imaging the SST tendon is the crass position where the patient's arm is placed further behind their back with the dorsal aspect of the hand over the opposite hip/lower back. The elbow is kept close to the body with no space between the arm and the lateral chest wall[16] (Fig. 3.27). This increased internal rotation brings the greater tuberosity and the SST tendon into a more anterior position,

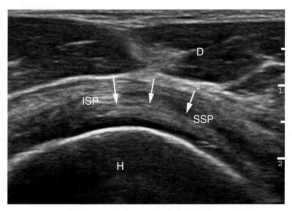

Fig. 3.26 Short axis view of the supraspinatus tendon demonstrating the rotator cable *(arrows)* at the junction of supraspinatus *(SSP)* and infraspinatus *(ISP)* tendons. *D*, Deltoid; *H*, humerus. (From Sconfienza LM, Orlandi D, Fabbro E, et al. Ultrasound assessment of the rotator cuff cable: comparison between young and elderly asymptomatic volunteers and interobserver reproducibility. Ultrasound Med Biol. 2012;38(1):35-41.)

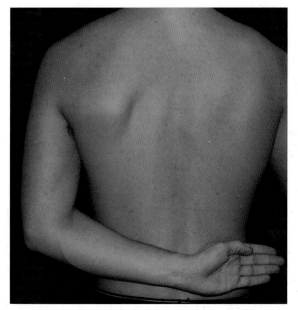

Fig. 3.27 Crass Position for Imaging the Supraspinatus Tendon.

ensuring that more of the tendon is exposed from beneath the acromion. The tendon adopts an almost vertical (sagittal) anatomical position and it is important that the transducer position is altered accordingly as a truer sagittal and transverse approach is required.

There are some limitations associated with the crass position. These include:

- Patients may find this position difficult to achieve and maintain.
- The increased internal rotation of the shoulder shifts the LHB tendon and anterior leading edge of the SST tendon into a more medial position which in some patients may make these structures disappear out of view.
- Additional stress and tension are placed on the SST tendon, and it has been suggested that this can lead to over estimation of the size of tendon tears.[6,13,17]

However, this position can help detect very small tears as it can separate the torn tendon ends, aiding diagnosis.[18]

◎ TOP TIP

When imaging patients with a significantly reduced range of movement, any degree of arm manipulation may be difficult. In these cases, allowing the patient to hang their arm down by their side and asking them to turn their palm posteriorly can elicit a degree of internal rotation of the shoulder and allow for some supraspinatus tendon visualisation.

Infraspinatus and Teres Minor Tendons and Posterior Glenohumeral Joint

The patient's arm is placed across the anterior chest with the hand rested on the contralateral shoulder (Fig. 3.28). The transducer is placed in an oblique transverse plane below the spine of the scapula (Fig. 3.29). The IST muscle belly is located in long axis and the probe is moved laterally to follow the muscle to its tendinous attachment. On ultrasound, the LS IST tendon appears as a uniformly hyperechoic tendon which tapers smoothly to its insertion on the greater tuberosity[15] (see Fig. 3.29). By sliding the transducer inferiorly, the LS view of the much thinner TM tendon is obtained. This tendon has similar ultrasound appearances to the IST tendon but can be distinguished from the former due to its slightly more lateral myotendinous junction (Fig. 3.30). These tendons and their muscle bellies can be imaged in TS by rotating the probe through 90 degrees (Fig. 3.31).

Returning to the long axis view of the IST tendon, the probe is shifted medially (Fig. 3.32) until the posterior GHJ (PGHJ) is visualised deep to the IST tendon/muscle. Depending on patient build, the depth, frequency, and focal position may need to be adjusted. The echogenic

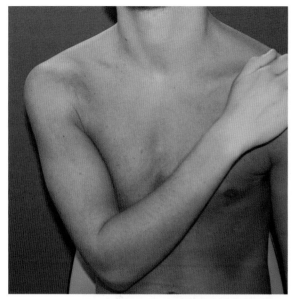

Fig. 3.28 Patient Arm Position for Imaging the Infraspinatus Tendon, Teres Minor Tendon, and Posterior Glenohumeral Joint.

labrum can be seen within the posterior joint capsule adjacent to the glenoid. The posterior joint recess is one of the sites where effusion may be identified in addition to signs of osteophytosis in osteoarthritis (OA) and synovitis[15] (see Fig. 3.32). More medially, the spinoglenoid notch is imaged as a recess containing the suprascapular neurovascular bundle (see Fig. 3.32).

In this position the IST muscle can be compared to the overlying deltoid muscle and by sliding the probe superiorly over the spine of the scapular, the SST muscle can be compared to the overlying trapezius muscle to assess for fatty infiltration/atrophy.

Acromioclavicular Joint (ACJ)

The probe is placed in the coronal plane on the superior aspect of the shoulder across the ACJ (Fig. 3.33). This can be easily palpated in most patients, enabling accurate probe placement. The joint margins and acromioclavicular ligament (ACL) can be clearly imaged (see Fig. 3.33), and the probe should be swept anteriorly and posteriorly over this joint for full evaluation.

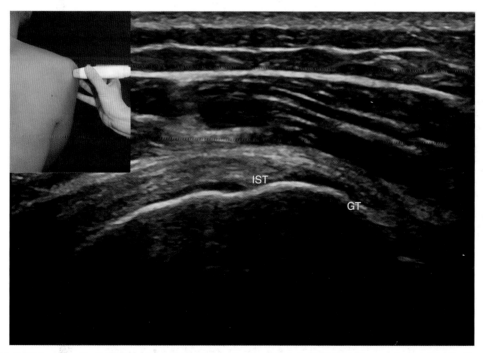

Fig. 3.29 Longitudinal (LS) Section of the Infraspinatus Tendon *(IST)* Inserting on to the Middle Facet of the Greater Tuberosity of the Humeral Head *(GT)*. Inset: Patient and probe position for imaging the infraspinatus tendon in the LS plane. Note the probe is moved slightly inferiorly from this position to image the teres minor tendon.

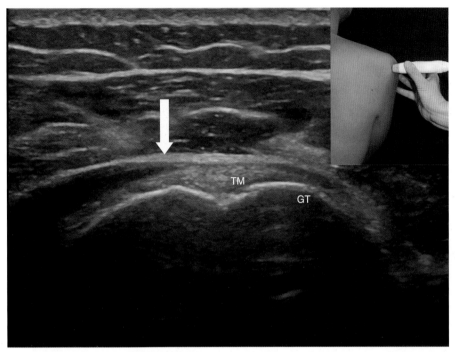

Fig. 3.30 Longitudinal Section of the Teres Minor Tendon *(TM)* Inserting onto the Inferior Facet of the Greater Tuberosity *(GT)*. Note the shorter tendon and more proximal myotendinous junction *(white arrow)*.

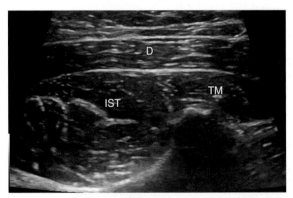

Fig. 3.31 Transverse Image of Infraspinatus Tendon *(IST)* and Teres Minor *(TM)* Muscles. *D,* Deltoid.

❗ PITFALL

Anisotropy is particularly prevalent when imaging the shoulder as the rotator cuff tendons follow the curved shape of the humeral head. Probe maneuvers such as heel toeing and tilting are an essential element of the technique for scanning shoulders.

Dynamic assessment techniques can be utilised when imaging the shoulder with ultrasound. These include[12,19]:

- Assessing LHB tendon in transverse plane for subluxation during external rotation. Subluxation is diagnosed if the tendon is seen to temporarily "pop out" of the bicipital groove.
- "Impingement" is a clinical diagnosis but dynamic imaging can demonstrate bunching of the SASD bursa and/or SST tendon against the acromion or coracoacromial ligament during abduction. The transducer is placed in the coronal plane with its medial edge at the lateral margin of the acromion (Fig. 3.34). The patient abducts their arm whilst in internal rotation (see Fig 3.34). The SST and the bursa can be seen passing deep to the acromion (Fig. 3.35). The coracoacromial ligament is imaged by maintaining the lateral edge of the transducer on the acromion and rotating the medial edge of the probe inferiorly towards the coracoid process (Fig. 3.36). The ligament is visualised in long axis as a thin linear fibrillar structure traversing the two bony landmarks (Fig. 3.37). Turning the

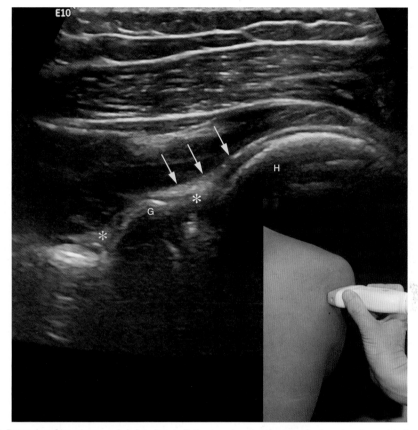

Fig. 3.32 Posterior Glenohumeral Joint. Inset: Patient and probe position for imaging the posterior glenohumeral joint in the longitudinal plane. *G,* Glenoid; *H,* humeral head; *white asterisk,* posterior labrum; *yellow asterisk,* spinoglenoid notch (SGN); *yellow arrows,* joint capsule.

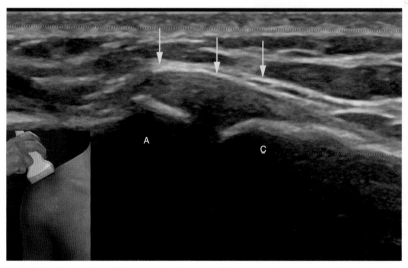

Fig. 3.33 Acromioclavicular Joint. Note the clear joint margin between the acromion *(A)* and clavicle *(C)* and joint capsule/superior ACL *(yellow arrows).* Inset: Patient and probe position for imaging the acromioclavicular joint.

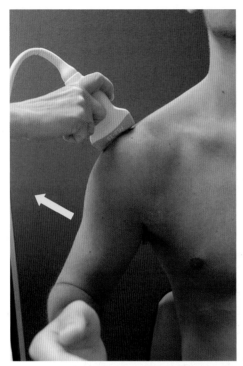

Fig. 3.34 Patient and Probe Position for Performing a Dynamic "Impingement" Test. The *yellow arrow* indicates the direction of the dynamic abduction of the arm.

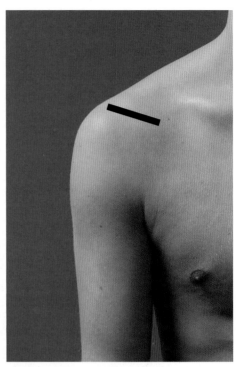

Fig. 3.36 Probe position *(black line)* for imaging the coracoacromial ligament.

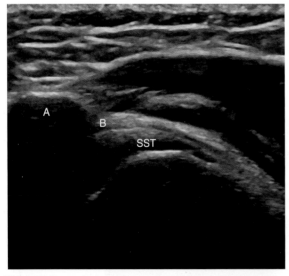

Fig. 3.35 Dynamic assessment demonstrates the supraspinatus tendon *(SST)* and subacromial-subdeltoid bursa *(B)* sliding under the acromion *(A)* as the patient abducts their arm.

transducer through 90 degrees allows this ligament to be imaged in its short axis.

- PGHJ recess: to assess for a glenohumeral joint effusion. The probe is positioned as if imaging the PGHJ (see Fig. 3.32) and the patient's arm is internally and externally rotated. An effusion would be most evident during external rotation.

> **◎ TOP TIP**
>
> Contralateral scanning is essential as it will assist in determining the clinical significance of certain changes related to the patients' age and the activities they undertake. Images of the contralateral shoulder should be archived and it should also be documented in the report that comparison has been made. Of course, this is of less value if both shoulders are symptomatic.

THE PATHOLOGICAL SHOULDER

Painful shoulders are known to cause significant disruption to patients' lives and whereas some shoulder problems

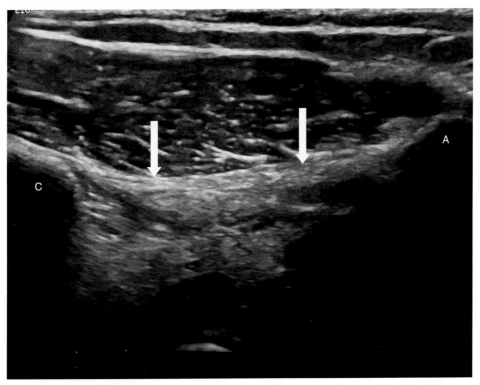

Fig. 3.37 Coracoacromial ligament *(white arrows)* noted traversing between the acromion *(A)* and the coracoid process *(C)*.

are the result of trauma, others have a more insidious onset. Prior to referral for an ultrasound, all patients should have undergone some form of clinical assessment. However, there are over 120 clinical tests for the shoulder, reflecting the difficulties clinicians face when assessing the cause of symptoms. From a practical perspective the clinical examination attempts to differentiate between shoulder lesions arising from either the contractile structures (rotator cuff tendons) or the passive structures (ACJ, SCJ, GHJ).[20,21] It is recognised that tendons fail due to vascular insufficiency and cumulative damage; however, this mechanism is complex, and a variety of intrinsic and extrinsic factors contribute to the pathogenesis of rotator cuff pathology, not impingement alone. Many researchers are now suggesting that more appropriate terminology for the patient presenting with nontraumatic pain around shoulder should be considered, with the term subacromial pain syndrome being suggested as a more accurate expression.[3,19,20]

Whether it is termed subacromial impingement or subacromial pain syndrome, it is widely cited as a major contributor to nontraumatic shoulder pain, and this pain is usually elicited during or after lifting the arm. This concept concerns the progressive cuff damage that may occur due to interaction between the rotator cuff and coracoacromial arch (the anterior acromion, coracoacromial ligament, and ACJ). The distal anterior aspect of the SST tendon is especially susceptible to damage due to vascular insufficiency in this region. This is a continuum of pathology progressing from bursitis to tendinopathy and fibrosis of the cuff tendons and finally to rotator cuff tears. Calcific tendinopathy and LHB tendon pathology are also considered part of this manifestation.[3,15,19]

Symptoms can occur anywhere between an arc of 45 to 120 degrees abduction (Fig. 3.38) and produces an intermittent catch of pain clinically known as a painful arc. Neer's, Hawkins Kennedy, and Jobe's tests (Fig. 3.39) are frequently used to assess for "impingement" as they focus on reducing the subacromial space and are considered positive if the pain is reproduced.[22]

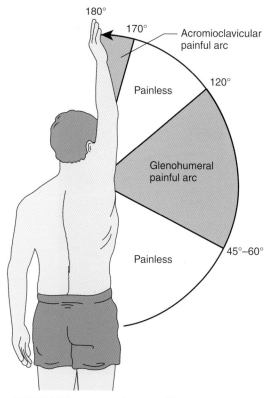

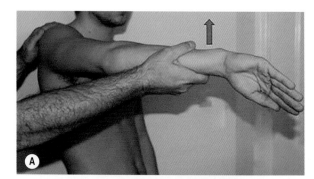

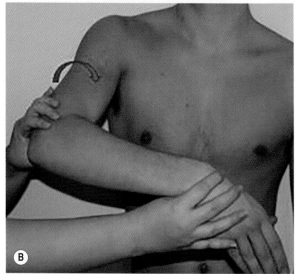

Fig. 3.38 Painful arc occurs between 60 and 120 degrees suggesting subacromial impingement syndrome. Impingement occurring towards the end of abduction range "high-arc" is more suggestive of acromioclavicular joint pathology. (From Magee DJ. Orthopedic Physical Assessment. 6th ed. London: Elsevier; 2014:273, which has been modified from Hawkins RJ, Hobeika PE. Impingement syndrome in the athletic shoulder. Clin Sports Med. 1983;2(20):391.)

A second point of impingement can also occur towards end of range and is frequently associated with ACJ degeneration as the joint approximates and compresses towards end of range[23] (see Fig. 3.38).

Common Pathological Appearances

Accurate and appropriate use of ultrasound can play a crucial role in determining the best management strategy for the patient. Assessing the stage of rotator cuff disease is considered the main role of ultrasound as this may help to direct management.[6,22]

When undertaking the scan, it is important to appreciate that restricted patient movements can determine a variety of joint conditions and may help the practitioner to decide on a differential diagnosis. For example, patients

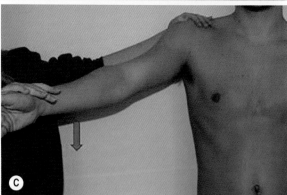

Fig. 3.39 (A) Neer's impingement sign. Patient's arm internally rotated, then examiner passively moves patient's arm until a vertical overhead position is achieved. **(B)** Hawkins Kennedy test. The patient's elbow and shoulder are flexed and the examiner internally rotates the shoulder, reducing the subacromial space. **(C)** Jobe's test. The patient's arm is abducted. The examiner then attempts to forcibly lower the arm whilst the patient resists.

presenting with painful restriction in movement, particularly external rotation, may be suffering from adhesive capsulitis (AC) commonly referred to as "frozen shoulder." AC can result from trauma or may be idiopathic in origin and it is described as an inflammatory contracture of the shoulder joint capsule, although the pathoanatomy is poorly understood. The early "freezing" and acute, severe pain may be due to inflammation, which then reduces in the later stages, when restriction in movement becomes the predominant feature and the pain is not as pronounced.[24] AC is considered a clinical diagnosis as there is a lack of specific ultrasound diagnostic criteria; however, recent research suggests that coracohumeral ligament thickening and increased hypervascular soft tissue in rotator interval are features that are indicative of the initial stages of the condition, but these features should be considered in the clinical context.[25]

Bursitis

The term "bursitis" refers to an inflammatory condition of any of the bursae around the shoulder, usually the SASD bursa. It is commonly caused by overuse/dysfunction and it develops over time, but direct trauma to the shoulder following a fall can also precipitate the problem.[26,27]

The patient presents with constant, often severe shoulder pain. All active and passive movements of the shoulder may be limited by pain, and the pain may be evident at rest. Patients often suffer from pain at night and may struggle to sleep on the affected shoulder. A painful arc may be present, and resisted tests produce discomfort. Due to the proximity of the rotator cuff to the SASD bursa, it can be difficult to distinguish between chronic bursitis and rotator cuff tendinopathy.

On ultrasound, SASD bursitis presents as focal or diffuse thickening of the synovial lining of the bursa (Fig. 3.40) which may be hyperemic on Doppler. As the synovial lining secretes fluid, in some cases there may also be fluid distension of the bursa[7,28] (Fig. 3.41).

A measurement of over 2 mm has been suggested as abnormal for the SASD bursa; however, normal thickness varies between individuals and may be dependent on their profession/sport, so this may not always be an appropriate way to assess the bursa. Comparison to the opposite shoulder (if asymptomatic) is essential prior to making the diagnosis of "bursitis" and a difference of 2 mm or more between the two sides can then be considered as abnormal. Bursitis is most commonly observed overlying the SST tendon and anterior to the LHB tendon. Fluid

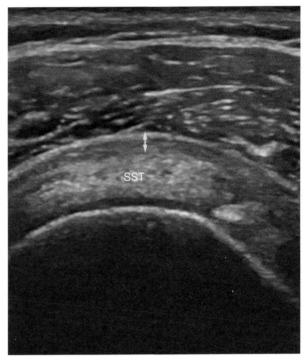

Fig. 3.40 Mild subacromial-subdeltoid bursitis overlying the supraspinatus tendon *(SST)* with synovial thickening *(arrow)* but no fluid.

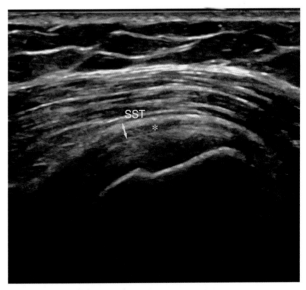

Fig. 3.41 Mild subacromial-subdeltoid bursitis overlying the supraspinatus tendon *(SST)* with synovial thickening *(arrow)* and evidence of fluid distension *(*).*

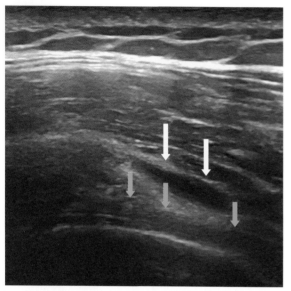

Fig. 3.42 Subacromial-subdeltoid (SASD) bursal fluid *(white arrows)* noted anterior to the proximal long head of biceps (LHB) tendon *(blue arrows)*.

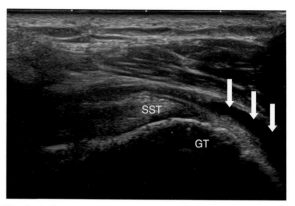

Fig. 3.43 Subacromial-subdeltoid (SASD) inferior recess fluid *(arrows). GT,* Greater tuberosity; *SST,* distal supraspinatus tendon insertion.

within the bursa can be distinguished from fluid within the LHB tendon sheath in two ways:
- Bursal fluid is seen anterior to the proximal aspect of the tendon, whereas tendon sheath fluid often extends more distally.
- Bursal fluid is only demonstrated anterior to the tendon, whereas tendon sheath fluid surrounds the tendon[27,29] (Fig. 3.42).

> ◎ **TOP TIP**
>
> Ensure you examine the dependent aspect of the bursa to avoid missing small quantities of fluid within the inferior margin of the bursa. When imaging the supraspinatus tendon in the long axis, guide the probe distally off the insertion of the tendon to image the inferior recess of the bursa (Fig. 3.43)

Excessive fluid noted within the bursa with no evidence of synovial thickening may be a sign of a rotator cuff tear. However, if a large amount of fluid is present within the bursa with associated synovial proliferation (with or without evidence of hyperemia on Doppler assessment) (Fig. 3.44), other causes should be considered[28]:
- Inflammatory conditions such as rheumatoid arthritis
- Infection

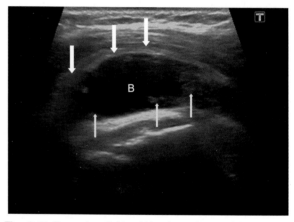

Fig. 3.44 Excessive fluid within the subacromial-subdeltoid (SASD) bursa *(B)* with thickened bursal wall *(white arrows)* and synovial proliferation *(yellow arrows)*.

- Haemorrhage (this is unlikely without a history of trauma)
- Hydroxyapatite crystal deposition (usually associated with sudden onset severe pain)

Bunching of the bursa against the lateral border of the acromion on dynamic abduction can help to support the diagnosis of impingement but this should be reported in context with the clinical presentation and the ease with which the patient is able to perform the maneuver.

Rotator Cuff (RC) Pathology

RC pathologies including tendinopathy, partial thickness tears, and complete tears, are more prevalent with age

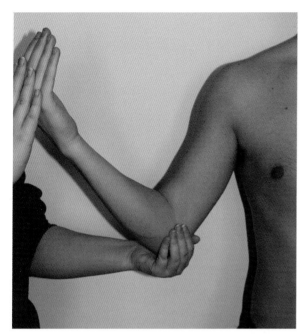

Fig. 3.45 External rotation lag sign tests the integrity of the supraspinatus and infraspinatus tendons. The examiner passively moves the patient's affected arm into external (lateral) rotation, and then releases the hold. The patient should be able to hold the arm in this position (negative test), and if unable to, the arm drifts into medial rotation denoting a positive test and suggesting pathology in the posterolateral cuff.

and do not always produce symptoms. Symptomatic patients present with a history of gradual onset pain and loss of arm function caused either by sport, occupation, or direct trauma. They complain of localised pain to the deltoid region (ache), which worsens with activity. On examination, a painful arc may or may not be present, and one or two resisted muscle tests will be painful and weak.[21,30]

Other tests that assess for cuff pathology are the external rotation lag sign test which assesses the integrity of the posterolateral cuff (SST and IST) (Fig. 3.45), and the lift-off test, the belly-press test, and the bear hug test which assess the anterior cuff (SSC)[29,31] (Fig. 3.46).

Tendinopathy

On ultrasound, tendinopathy can manifest as focal or global changes within a tendon that do not resolve when the transducer is tilted or angled. These changes appear as thickening or thinning of the tendon with loss of the normal fibrillar pattern and a general reduction in echogenicity or focal hypoechoic areas (Fig. 3.47). These changes can be subtle, and comparison to the contralateral side is again useful to support the diagnosis. Doppler imaging has proven useful in the diagnosis of tendinopathy in other anatomical areas; however, this is not the case with the rotator cuff tendons where its value is minimal.[8,17]

Calcific Tendinopathy

Calcific tendinopathy is the pathological deposition of calcium hydroxyapatite crystals within tendons. The exact pathogenesis of this condition is unclear with several theories proposed but many consider it a sequelae of tendon degeneration/necrosis and tears.[9]

On ultrasound, it appears as echogenic foci within the substance of the tendon with or without acoustic shadowing. Microcalcifications are commonly identified within tendinopathic tendons and these are often too small to cast an acoustic shadow, whereas larger foci can be "hard" (shadowing) or "soft" (minimal or no shadowing). There are four distinct phases associated with calcific tendinopathy and the contrasting appearances observed on ultrasound correspond to the changes that occur within the calcific deposits throughout this process[17,32]:

- Stage one—deposition/formative. For unknown reasons, a segment of the tendon undergoes fibrocartilaginous change causing the deposition of soft, chalk-like calcium.
- Stage two—calcific or latent "resting" phase. At this stage, the calcium becomes hard and on ultrasound it appears as a well-defined, echogenic area within the tendon that casts an acoustic shadow (Fig. 3.48). It can be asymptomatic but if it is large, mass effect may result in pain due to impingement.
- Stage three—resorptive. The calcium begins to be reabsorbed and becomes soft and paste-like. On ultrasound it still appears hyperechoic, but it becomes more amorphous and subtle with minimal or no acoustic shadowing (Fig. 3.49). This stage can be extremely painful as there may be crystal leakage into the bursa, resulting in acute bursitis which may last for several weeks.
- Stage four—reparative/post calcific. Following resorption of the calcium, the normal tendon structure is restored.

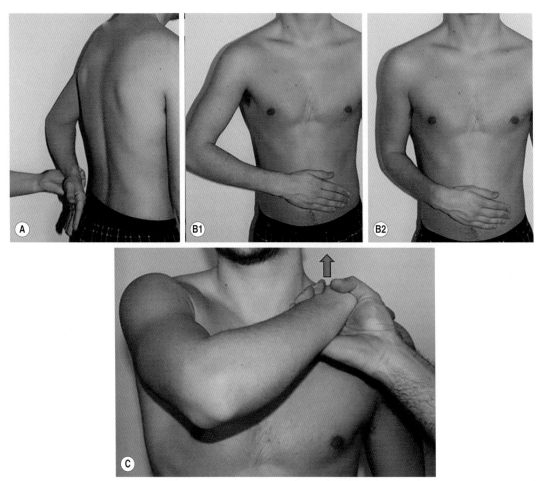

Fig. 3.46 **Subscapularis Physical Examination Maneuvers.** **(A)** Gerber's lift off test used to test for isolated subscapularis tear. The patients arm is placed behind their back with the dorsum of the hand in the lumbar region. The hand is raised off the back and the test is positive if the patient cannot maintain the position. **(B)** Belly press or "Napoleon" test. Hand on stomach maintaining an internally rotated position. **(B1)**, if the elbow moves backwards and the wrist flexes when the patient presses on to their abdomen the subscapularis is considered weak **(B2)**. **(C)** Bear hug test. The hand of the affected extremity placed on top of the contralateral shoulder and the elbow pointing anteriorly. The examiner tries to lift the hand off the patient's shoulder while the patient resists external rotation.[6] This test is considered positive when the examiner can externally rotate the arm while the patient is trying to actively maintain internal rotation.

Rotator Cuff Tendon Tears

The RC tendons are strap-like structures that have three dimensions: length, width, and thickness. When you look at the tendon end on, you are looking at it in its short axis and you can appreciate its width and thickness; looking at the tendon from the side (its long axis) allows you to assess its length and thickness (Fig. 3.50).

By applying this analogy to RC tendons, practitioners can accurately assess and report tears by evaluating them in all three dimensions—width, thickness, and length (proximal retraction). This is important as tear size has an impact on postoperative functional outcome and successful tendon healing, as does patient age and level of activity and the degree of fatty infiltration/atrophy of the RC muscles.[33]

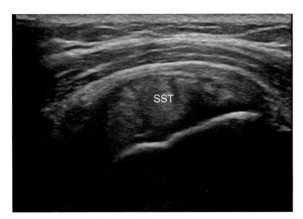

Fig. 3.47 Tendinopathic supraspinatus tendon *(SST)* which is thickened, has lost its normal fibrillar pattern, and demonstrates a global reduction in echogenicity.

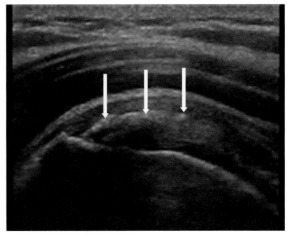

Fig. 3.49 "Soft" calcific tendinopathy *(white arrows)* appears hyperechoic but it becomes more amorphous and subtle with minimal or no acoustic shadowing.

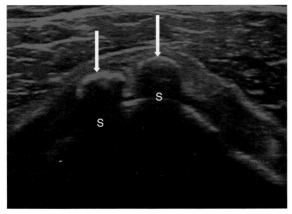

Fig. 3.48 Calcific Tendinopathy. Calcific phase: the calcium appears as well-defined, echogenic areas within the tendon substance that are convex superiorly *(arrows)* and cast clear acoustic shadows *(S)*. Note how the posterior shadowing obscures the deeper tissues.

The most common site of RC tears is the anterior aspect of the distal SST tendon, adjacent to the RI. This region of the tendon is also referred to as the anterior free edge or the anterior leading edge. Isolated tears of the SSC and IST tendons are less common and usually present as extensions of SST tears: anterior extension into the SSC and posterior extension into the IST. The exception to this is isolated SSC tears caused by recurrent or traumatic anterior dislocation of the shoulder. Tears of the TM tendon are very rare in isolation but can

occasionally be seen associated with massive RC tears and joint degeneration.[6,9,34,35]

RC tears can be divided into two categories: partial thickness tears and full thickness tears.

Partial thickness (PT) tears. On ultrasound, PT tears appear as hypoechoic or anechoic defects within the tendon which do not traverse the full thickness of the tendon so there is only partial disruption of the fibrillar pattern.[6,7,34] These tears can be subdivided into:

- Articular, undersurface, or joint surface tears—the tear is confined to the deep fibres of the tendon but the more superficial aspect of the tendon remains intact (Fig. 3.51).
- Bursal surface tears—the deeper fibres of the tendon remain intact and the tear is demonstrated in the superficial fibres of the tendon most closely related to the SASD bursa (Fig. 3.52).
- Intrasubstance tears—the deep and superficial tendon retains its normal structure and fibrillar pattern and the tear is located within the substance of the tendon[34,35] (Fig. 3.53).

The tendon defect should be clearly defined in both the long (LS) and short (TS) axis to confirm the presence of a tear as this avoids the possibility of inaccuracies due to anisotropy. Measurements of the width of the tear should be taken in TS and its length or proximal retraction in LS. The thickness or depth of the tear is evaluated in both the long and short axis and although it is not

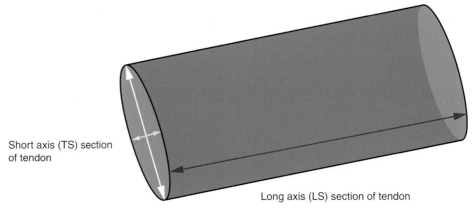

Fig. 3.50 The rotator cuff tendons are sheet-like structures and have three dimensions. They have a length *(red arrow)*, a width *(white arrow)*, and a thickness *(yellow arrow)*.

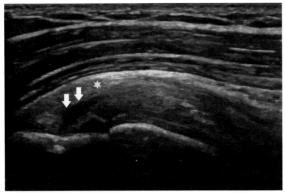

Fig. 3.51 Partial Thickness Articular Surface Tear of the SST Tendon. The anechoic tear is confined to the deep fibres of the tendon *(white arrows)* but the more superficial aspect of the tendon remains intact *(yellow star)*. (From Fawcett R, et al. Ultrasound-guided subacromial–subdeltoid bursa corticosteroid injections: a study of short- and long-term outcomes. Clin Radiol. 2018;73(8):e7-12.)

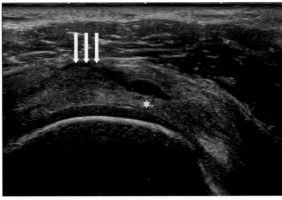

Fig. 3.52 Partial Thickness Bursal Surface Tear. The tear is demonstrated originating in the superficial fibres of the tendon most closely related to the subacromial-subdeltoid (SASD) bursa *(white arrows)*. The deeper fibres *(yellow star)* remain intact.

always common practice to measure the thickness of a PT tear, providing this information as a percentage of the complete tendon thickness is advised as this may affect surgical treatments. For example, PT tears which affect over 50% of the normal tendon thickness may be managed as if they are full thickness defects.

Other more subtle signs of a PT tear that may be evident on ultrasound are focal thinning with loss of convexity, or flattening of the superficial surface of the tendon (if the tear is large), fluid in the SASD bursa, and cortical irregularity at the greater tuberosity deep to the tear. There may be a bright cartilage sign deep to the tear caused by increased through transmission of the sound waves. This would only be evident in the presence of large PT tears.[8,9]

Full thickness (FT) tears. FT tears are described as tears that traverse the full thickness of the tendon from the bursal to the articular surface. Appearances on

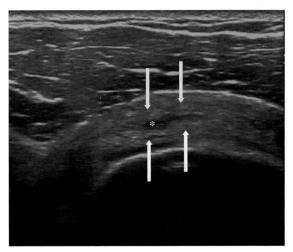

Fig. 3.53 Partial Thickness Intrasubstance Tear. The anechoic defect is evident within the substance of the tear *(*)* but the deep *(white arrows)* and superficial *(yellow arrows)* aspect of the tendon retains its normal fibrillar pattern.

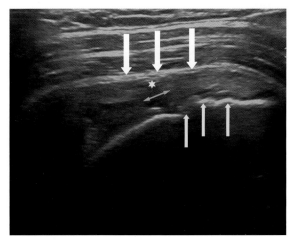

Fig. 3.54 Longitudinal (long) section of proximal full thickness tear demonstrating flattening of the tendon *(white arrows)* at the site of the tear *(yellow star)* and associated cortical irregularity of the humeral head *(yellow arrows)*. In acute tears, fluid is often demonstrated in the tendon gap and this allows measurement of the degree of separation *(blue arrow)*.

ultrasound are variable depending on the chronicity of the tear, but often an anechoic or hypoechoic defect is demonstrated within the tendon extending from the articular to the bursal surface with discontinuity of the fibrillar pattern. There is often loss of the convexity of the superior surface of the tendon with obvious flattening of the tendon at the site of the tear and associated cortical irregularity of the humeral head. In acute tears, fluid is often demonstrated in the tendon gap[8,9,34,35] (Fig. 3.54).

It is much easier to diagnose acute full thickness tears it simple fluid or fluid containing low level echoes is present as the margins of the tear are clear in both the short and long axis (Fig. 3.55A,B); however, if the defect is filled with echogenic debris or synovium, or if the overlying deltoid muscle herniates into the tendon gap as with chronic tears, diagnosis and accurate assessment becomes much more challenging. Additionally, FT tears can range from large tears that involve the full width of the tendon with obvious proximal retraction to tiny "pin point" tears with no notable retraction. Often with these challenging tears, the common secondary signs such as flattening of the tendon, fluid in the LHB tendon sheath, and/or SASD bursa, cortical changes of the humeral head and the bright cartilage sign can help to guide the practitioner and careful examination can often aid diagnosis.[2]

◎ TOP TIP

Positioning the patient's arm in extreme internal rotation, i.e., crass position (see Fig. 3.31), places the SST tendon under increased tension and this may increase the size of the defect in small, full thickness tears, allowing more accurate visualisation and assessment.

Having established that the tear is FT, confirmed in both the short (TS) and long (LS) axis views, the following information should be obtained and reported:
- Location of the tear, which tendon(s) is/are involved, and what aspect of the tendon is affected
- Size of the tear
- Evidence of fatty infiltration/atrophy of the relevant muscle(s)

Most tears commence in the SST tendon, and these can present as either:
- Leading edge tears (also referred to as anterior leading edge or free edge tears), which manifest as defects in the fibres immediately adjacent to the rotator interval whilst the posterior fibres of the tendon remain intact (Fig. 3.56)
- Central tears (mid-substance or crescent), which occur within the more posterior aspect of the tendon with the anterior fibres and the IST tendon fibres

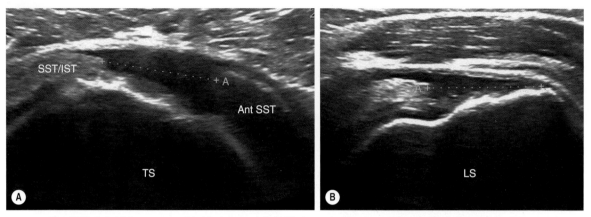

Fig. 3.55 Full thickness central (midsubstance) fluid-filled tear in **(A)** short (TS) and **(B)** long (LS) axis. Due to the presence of fluid the width of the tear can be clearly measured in the TS plane and the degree of proximal retraction in the LS plane *(blue calipers). IST,* Infraspinatus; *LS,* longitudinal; *SST,* supraspinatus; *TS,* transverse.

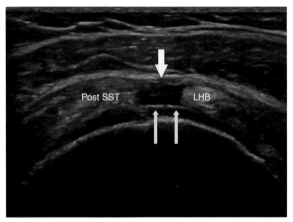

Fig. 3.56 Anterior leading-edge tear in the supraspinatus *(SST)* tendon *(white arrow),* located in the fibres immediately adjacent to the rotator interval *(LHB)* whilst the posterior fibres *(Post SST)* of the tendon remain intact. Note the flattening of the tendon and the bright cartilage sign *(yellow arrows).* (From Fawcett R, et al. Ultrasound-guided subacromial–subdeltoid bursa corticosteroid injections: a study of short- and long-term outcomes. Clin Radiol. 2018;73(8):e7-12.)

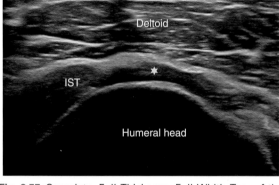

Fig. 3.57 Complete, Full Thickness, Full Width Tear of the SST Tendon. Bursal fluid *(yellow star)* is noted separating the deltoid muscle from the humeral head with no SST tendon fibres evident. The IST tendon is intact *(IST). IST,* Infraspinatus; *SST,* supraspinatus. (From McCreesh KM, Riley SJ, Crotty JM. Acromio-clavicular joint cyst associated with a complete rotator cuff tear - a case report. Man Ther. 2014;19(5):490-493.)

remaining intact. This is best appreciated in TS (see Fig. 3.55A)

- Complete tears or tendon ruptures which affect the full width and thickness of the tendon with no intact fibres visible. Fluid is often seen in the tendon gap (Fig. 3.57), and these tears may or may not extend into the IST tendon. Chronic or old complete tears result in the "bare tuberosity" or "deltoid to bone"

sign where the SST tendon is absent, there is no fluid or synovium present within the SASD and as such there is nothing to separate the deltoid from coming into direct contact with the humeral head (Fig. 3.58).

As with PT tears the width of a tear is measured in TS and the calipers are placed at the anterior aspect of the tear, across the defect to the posterior intact margin of the tendon (see Fig. 3.55A). A complete tear

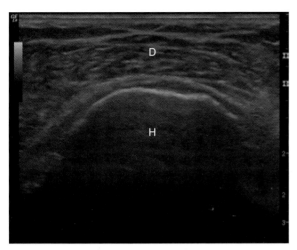

Fig. 3.58 Chronic Complete Tear SST Tendon. "Bare tuberosity" or "deltoid to bone" sign where the SST tendon is absent. There is very little or no fluid or synovium present within the SASD and as such there is nothing to separate the deltoid *(D)* from coming into direct contact with the humeral head *(H)*. *SASD,* Subacromial-subdeltoid; *SST,* supraspinatus.

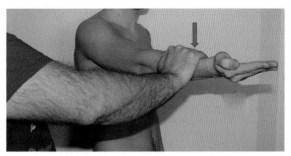

Fig. 3.59 Speed's Test. The patients shoulder is flexed to 90 degrees with the elbow extended, the hand is supinated. The patient is asked to resist downward pressure by the practitioner. The test is positive for long head biceps if pain is reproduced.

is diagnosed if the tear extends across the full width of the tendon. In regards to the SST, this would be from the RI and extending more than 2 cm posteriorly as this is the normal width of the SST tendon. SST tears over 2 cm in width indicate involvement of the IST tendon. Proximal retraction is appreciated in LS and can be measured by placing the calipers at the insertion site, across the defect, to the intact aspect of the tendon (see Fig. 3.55B). If the proximal stump is not visible because it has retracted beyond the acromion, the degree of retraction cannot be accurately assessed. In tears that occur in the proximal aspect of the tendon, the degree of tendon separation can be assessed in the long axis (see Fig. 3.54).

Assessing the RC muscles for evidence of fatty infiltration/atrophy is not routine practice in all centres as surgeons will often request magnetic resonance imaging (MRI) prior to shoulder surgery even if an ultrasound has previously been performed. This is because MRI is considered more accurate in the assessment of muscle architecture. However, comparing the echogenicity of the SST to the trapezius and the IST to the deltoid muscles allows the practitioner to provide the referrer with a subjective evaluation of the degree of fatty infiltration and any reduction in muscle bulk.[33]

Long Head of Biceps (LHB) Tendon

Clinically, patients present with local pain over the anterior aspect of the shoulder in the area just under the anterior deltoid which can be diffuse and vague. The clinical tests used to detect LHB pathology are Speed's (Fig. 3.59) and Yergason's tests (Fig. 3.60), though each test lacks specificity. An accurate history would determine whether the lesion was degenerate or traumatic in onset.

LHB pathology rarely presents in isolation and is often associated with RC pathology. SST and SSC tendon tears can disrupt the supporting sling that maintains the LHB in the bicipital groove, causing mechanical instability.[2] Pathological conditions include:

- Tendinopathy—on ultrasound, the tendon appears hypoechoic and thickened with or without neovascularisation.
- Tenosynovitis—appearances of the tendon may suggest tendinopathy but in addition there is fluid distension/thickening of the tendon sheath, usually with hyperemia and pain on palpation/during scanning (Fig. 3.61).
- Tears—partial thickness intrasubstance tears or splits can be challenging to diagnose on ultrasound but appear as hypoechoic or anechoic linear clefts within the substance of the tendon (Fig. 3.62). Full ruptures of the tendon present as an empty groove with no evidence of medial dislocation of the tendon or in acute proximal ruptures, the tendon may be visible in the bicipital groove but will not be visible at the rotator interval. Fluid can sometimes

be seen in the empty tendon sheath. The "Popeye" sign, or bulging of the biceps muscle belly, will be commonly seen in cases of LHB tendon ruptures and may be clinically diagnosed as a possible mass in the upper arm.

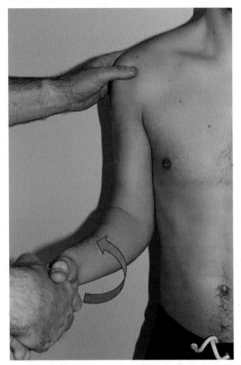

Fig. 3.60 Yergason's Test. The elbow is flexed to 90 degrees with the forearm pronated, the patient is asked to forcibly resist supination. Pain in the anterior aspect of the shoulder (bicipital groove) will indicate biceps tendinopathy or tenosynovitis.

- Dislocation—if the biceps sling fails, the LHB tendon can dislocate medially and on ultrasound the tendon can be identified in TS overlying the SSC tendon insertion. If a tear is present within the anterior SSC, the dislocated LHB can be located deep to the SSC tendon insertion (Fig. 3.63).[8,14]

Fluid within the LHB tendon sheath can be indicative of a RC tear and careful examination of the RC should ensue; however, it is important to remember that the sheath communicates with the GHJ so this could also represent joint fluid.[2]

Posterior Glenohumeral Joint (PGHJ)

The GHJ can only be clearly assessed on ultrasound at its posterior margin and as this is a deeper structure, imaging may be limited in larger patients. Common pathological conditions associated with the PGHJ are joint effusions, synovitis, and labral cysts. On ultrasound, effusions can be seen arising from the posterior joint and the main aim of the scan is to ascertain if this is a simple or a complex effusion:

- Simple effusions manifest as simple fluid collections arising from the PGHJ with no evidence of neovascularisation on Doppler assessment (Fig. 3.64).
- Complex effusions present as fluid collections that contain internal debris or synovial thickening/proliferation with possible hyperemia on Doppler. They can be inflammatory in nature or can be due to infection or haemorrhage and patient presentation will guide the diagnosis as much as the ultrasound findings.

Ganglion cysts arising from the posterior labrum can extend into the spinoglenoid notch (SGN) where they may

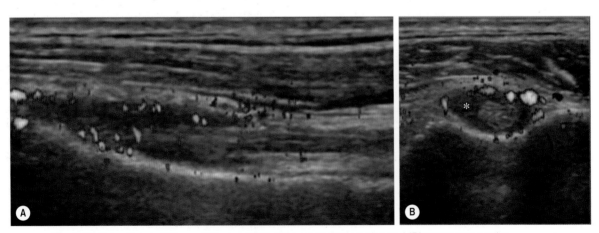

Fig. 3.61 Long Head of Biceps Tenosynovitis. (A) Longitudinal section and **(B)** transverse section.

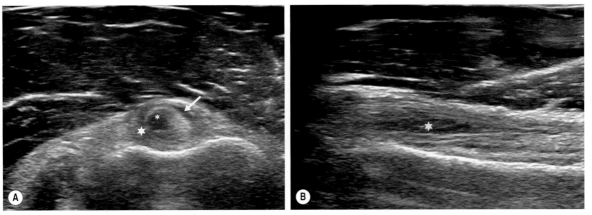

Fig. 3.62 Long Head of Biceps Partial Tear. (A) Note the hypoechoic defect in the transverse plane *(yellow star)* and **(B)** the hypoechoic linear cleft in the longitudinal plane *(yellow star)* within the substance of the tendon. On image (A), fluid distension *(white arrow)* and thickening *(white star)* of the tendon sheath is evident in keeping with tenosynovitis.

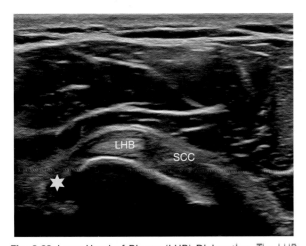

Fig. 3.63 Long Head of Biceps (LHB) Dislocation. The LHB tendon *(LHB)* has dislocated medially out of the bicipital groove *(yellow star)*. A tear is present within the anterior subscapularis (SSC) tendon *(SCC)* so the dislocated LHB is located deep to the SSC tendon insertion.

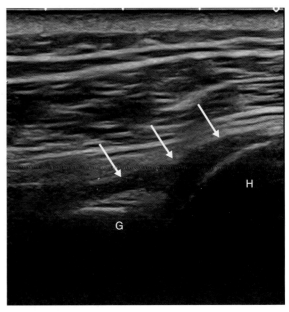

Fig. 3.64 Glenohumeral joint (GHJ) effusion, noted as a simple fluid collection arising from the PGHJ *(white arrows)*. *G*, Glenoid; *H*, humeral head.

compress the suprascapular nerve. This results in atrophy and weakness of the IST muscle and is more common in throwing athletes. On ultrasound, the anechoic cyst can be seen within the SGN, confirming the diagnosis.

Acromioclavicular Joint (ACJ)

The ACJ is not imaged routinely in all centres but excluding or confirming painful joint arthropathy can be useful.

Typically, the pain is felt on palpation of the joint and becomes worse during a range of occupational or recreational sporting activities, performing press-ups, bench pressing, or carrying weights on that shoulder. The main clinical test is the scarf test (Fig. 3.65).

Degenerative changes are relatively common at this joint and on ultrasound osteophytes appear as articular

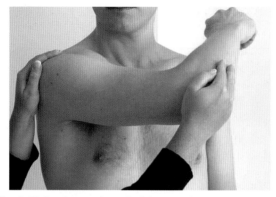

Fig. 3.65 Scarf test, also called the cross-body adduction arm test or acromioclavicular compression test. The examiner horizontally adducts the arm from a 90 degrees forward flexion position. The test is positive if pain is reproduced.

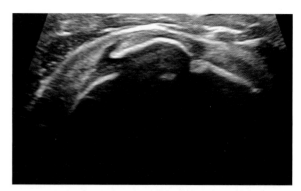

Fig. 3.67 Humeral Head Avulsion Fracture. Careful imaging in two planes plus correlation with clinical presentation and contralateral scanning can help to distinguish this from calcific tendinopathy.

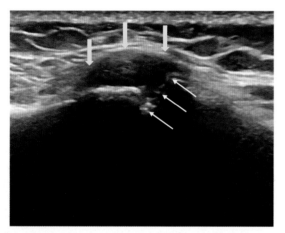

Fig. 3.66 Acromioclavicular Joint Arthropathy. Articular surface irregularities (white arrows) with capsular distension (yellow arrows).

surface irregularities with or without capsular distension or joint effusion (Fig. 3.66). In the case of effusion or capsular distension, Doppler assessment should be undertaken and may show active synovitis, which may be seen both in inflammatory arthritis and in symptomatic osteoarthritis.[7] When imaging the ACJ, firm probe pressure should be applied to the joint to observe if this elicits pain and this should be documented in the report. Pain on palpation is a more significant and useful observation than degenerative changes alone.

FRACTURES

Although ultrasound alone is not the modality of choice for the posttraumatic shoulder, patients commonly present for scan with a history of injury and suspected torn rotator cuff. It is not uncommon for experienced sonographers to pick up bony changes, especially around the greater tuberosity of the humerus, which would suggest bony avulsion (Fig. 3.67). This can occur in relatively young patients with significant trauma where the tendon is strong and remains intact, but the greater tuberosity is avulsed. It may also occur in older patients who fall directly onto their shoulder, causing avulsion of the greater tuberosity or even fracture of the humeral neck or shaft. In cases of suspected fracture, it is important to follow up with additional imaging to confirm the injury and full extent of damage.

MANAGEMENT AND OTHER IMAGING

The current options for the treatment of shoulder pain attributed to rotator cuff pathology, bursal pathology, LHB tendinopathy, or joint arthropathy are nonsteroidal antiinflammatory drugs, rehabilitation physiotherapy, pain relieving interventional techniques, and surgery.[3,21]

Rehabilitation

The aim of physiotherapy treatment is to reduce pain and restore the functional use of the arm and this may be used alone, or in refractory cases, in conjunction with other less conservative interventions to provide long-term solutions to pain and disability.

Interventional Techniques

Interventional techniques are also utilised to relieve pain if rehabilitation and other medication have been

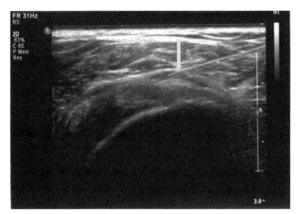

Fig. 3.68 The needle is demonstrated in the subacromial bursa *(yellow arrow)* and local anaesthetic mildly distends the bursa, proving correct needle placement prior to injection of steroid.

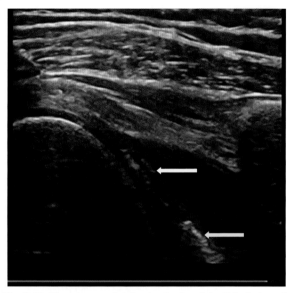

Fig. 3.69 Glenohumeral Joint Aspiration. It is clinically beneficial to aspirate the maximum amount of fluid from an affected joint or bursa. If being performed therapeutically, once all fluid has been aspirated, a corticosteroid can be injected. *White arrow,* Needle; *yellow arrow,* injectate following aspiration.

unsuccessful, as a pain-relieving measure in patients who are not surgical candidates, as temporary pain relief in patients awaiting surgery, and finally as a diagnostic tool.[36]

There are several pain-relieving interventional procedures that are commonly performed for shoulder pain:

- Injection of local anaesthetic (LA): as a diagnostic measure to determine origin of pain. In cases where the site of pain is not obvious, LA can be injected into one site and the level of pain relief measured after a few minutes.
- Injection of LA and corticosteroid: e.g., a subacromial bursal injection (Fig. 3.68) used in the management of impingement/bursitis, LHB injection for tenosynovitis, ACJ injections for OA, or GHJ injections for AC (frozen shoulder) and OA. In cases of recalcitrant AC, large volume hydrodilatation of the joint capsule is favored, where a large volume of saline is injected to distend the joint, followed by corticosteroid.
- Aspiration of large fluid collections (Fig. 3.69): rather than administering drugs when the needle is in place, fluid is instead removed. Utilising ultrasound confirms the diagnosis of an effusion within a swollen, painful joint and also identifies complications such as loculation or synovial proliferation within the effusion.
- Barbotage for calcific tendinopathy: barbotage works by repeated injection and aspiration of small volumes of local anaesthetic into the calcification to break it

up from the inside. The degree of success to this procedure depends on how hard or soft the calcification is. If it has a paste-like centre, aspiration and washout is possible. If it is truly solid, then fenestration (dry needling) of the deposit is the only option. Injection of corticosteroids into the bursa commonly follows this procedure as the free calcium may cause an acute bursitis.

Additional Imaging

Plain X-ray still plays a valuable role in shoulder imaging, and its importance should not be overlooked. It should be included as a primary imaging investigation for trauma to confirm or exclude fracture and dislocation, and in older patients (older than 50) to rule out OA as a cause of movement restriction and pain. An X-ray shows the mature calcification present in calcific tendinopathy[32] (Fig. 3.70), upward shift of the humeral head in the presence of a large rotator cuff tear, and downward shift of the humeral head in patients with bleeding inside the joint. It can also detect bone tumours which would almost certainly be missed on ultrasound.

MRI is frequently requested in patients with cuff tears prior to surgery even if a previous ultrasound scan

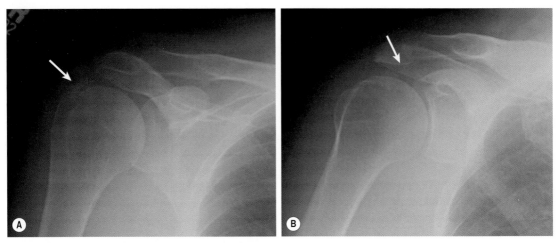

Fig. 3.70 X-ray Demonstrating the Resorptive Phase of Calcific Tendinitis. **(A)** Internal and **(B)** external rotation views of the right shoulder demonstrate globular areas of hazy, ill-defined calcifications *(arrows)* in the region of the supraspinatus tendon.[32] (Image taken from Siegal D, Wu JS, Newman JS, del Cura JL, Hochman MG. Calcific tendinitis: a pictorial review. Can Assoc Radiol J. 2009;60(5):263-272.)

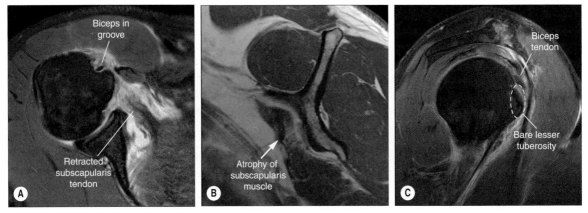

Fig. 3.71 Shoulder Magnetic Resonance Image. **(A)** Axial image showing the biceps tendon in the groove with an obvious retracted tear of the subscapularis tendon. **(B)** Sagittal image showing grade 2 fatty infiltration of the subscapularis muscle. **(C)** Sagittal image showing a bare lesser tuberosity. (Images from Lee J, Shukla DR, Sánchez-Sotelo J. Subscapularis tears: hidden and forgotten no more. J Shoulder Elbow Surg. 2018;2(1);74-83. https://www.sciencedirect.com/science/journal/24686026)

has been performed. MRI may provide additional information regarding the degree of retraction of the torn tendon and fatty infiltration or atrophy of the associated muscle (Fig. 3.71). These factors, along with the size of the tendon tear, may assist the surgeon with preoperative planning. Establishing the condition of the tendons is also crucial in cases where patients have severe OA and require a shoulder replacement as this may predict the long-term postoperative outcome.

Ultrasound scanning may not be achievable when patients have severely restricted movement and, in these cases, MRI may be preferable as it is not as dependent on patient position to achieve diagnostic information.

MR arthrography (MRA) is the imaging of choice for glenohumeral instability as it provides excellent detail of the ligamentous, cartilaginous, and labral structures.

The main use for computed tomography (CT) in the evaluation of the shoulder is to assist surgeons in planning surgeries in patients with OA or fractures.[16,33]

Surgical Management

In patients where the more conservative approach of physiotherapy and/or interventional steroid injections have failed, surgery may be considered although its success cannot be guaranteed.

Surgeries commonly performed around the shoulder include capsular release in refractory adhesive capsulitis, subacromial decompression to increase space around the rotator cuff tendons, repair or debridement of rotator cuff tears, and various types of joint replacement.[23]

▌ MULTIPLE CHOICE QUESTIONS

1. Which of the following tendons comprise the rotator cuff?
   a) Supraspinatus, infraspinatus, long head of biceps, and subscapularis
   b) Supraspinatus, infraspinatus, subscapularis, and teres minor
   c) Supraspinatus, infraspinatus, teres minor, and deltoid
2. Why does the patient externally rotate their arm when imaging the subscapularis tendon?
   a) To move the tendon from underneath the acromion
   b) To move the tendon from underneath the greater tuberosity
   c) To move the tendon from underneath the coracoid process
3. Which tendon of the rotator cuff is most often affected by pathology?
   a) Infraspinatus
   b) Subscapularis
   c) Supraspinatus

4. Which clinical test is most often utilised to assess the AC joint?
   a) Scarf test
   b) Neer's test
   c) Gerber's lift off test
5. The current options for the treatment of shoulder pain attributed to rotator cuff pathology, bursal pathology, LHB tendinopathy, or joint arthropathy are:
   a) nonsteroidal antiinflammatory drugs, rehabilitation physiotherapy, pain relieving interventional techniques, and surgery
   b) acupuncture, rehabilitation physiotherapy, pain relieving interventional techniques, and surgery
   c) rehabilitation physiotherapy, pain relieving interventional techniques, massage, and surgery

REFERENCES

1. Minns Lowe CJ, Moser J, Barker K. Living with a symptomatic rotator cuff tear 'bad days, bad nights': a qualitative study. BMC Musculoskelet Disord. 2014;15:228.
2. Hanusch BC, Makaram N, Utrillas-Compaired A, Lawson-Smith M, Rangan A. Biceps sheath fluid on shoulder ultrasound as a predictor of rotator cuff tear: analysis of a consecutive cohort. J Shoulder Elbow Surg. 2016;25:1661–1667.
3. Diercks R, Bron C, Dorrestijn O, et al. Guidelines for diagnosis and treatment of subacromial pain syndrome. Acta Orthop. 2014;85(3):314–322. Available at: https://doi.org/10.3109/17453674.2014.920991.
4. Soames R, Palastange N. Anatomy and Human Movement Structure and Function. 7th ed. London: Elsevier; 2019.

5. Smith MJ, Rogers A, Amso N, Kennedy J, Hall A, Mullaney P. A training, assessment and feedback package for the trainee shoulder sonographer. Ultrasound. 2015; 23:29–41.
6. Allen GM, Wilson DJ. Ultrasound of the shoulder. Eur J Ultrasound. 2001;14:3–9.
7. Girish G, Lobo LG, Jacobson JA, Morag Y, Miller B, Jamadar DA. Ultrasound of the shoulder: asymptomatic findings in men. Am J Roentgenol. 2011;197:713–719.
8. Read JW, Perko M. Shoulder ultrasound: diagnostic accuracy for impingement syndrome, rotator cuff tear, and biceps tendon pathology. J Shoulder Elbow Surg. 1998;7(3):264–271.
9. Allen GM. Shoulder ultrasound imaging-integrating anatomy. Biomechanics and disease processes. Eur J Radiol. 2008;68:137–146.

10. Sconfienza LM, Orlandi D, Fabbro E, et al. Ultrasound assessment of the rotator cuff cable: comparison between young and elderly asymptomatic volunteers and interobserver reproducibility. Ultrasound Med Biol. 2012;38(1):35–41.

11. Burkhart SS, Esch JC, Jolson RS. The rotator crescent and rotator cable: an anatomic description of the shoulder's "suspension bridge". Arthroscopy. 1993;9(6):611–616.

12. ESSR. Musculoskeletal Ultrasound Technical Guidelines I. Shoulder. Available at: https://essr.org/content-essr/uploads/2016/10/shoulder.pdf.

13. BMUS. Guidelines for professional ultrasound practice. 2019. Available at: https://www.bmus.org/static/uploads/resources/Guidelines_for_Professional_Ultrasound_Practice_v3_OHoz76r.pdf.

14. Skendzel JG, Jacobson JA, Carpenter JE, Miller BS. Long head of biceps brachii tendon evaluation: accuracy or preoperative ultrasound. Am J Roentgenol. 2011;197:942–948.

15. Beggs I. Shoulder ultrasound. Semin Ultrasound CT MR. 2011;32:101–113.

16. Jacobson JA. Musculoskeletal ultrasound: focused impact on MRI. Am J Roentgenol. 2009;193:619–627.

17. Ingwersen KG, Hjarbaek J, Eshoej H, Larsen CM, Vobbe J, Juul-Kristensen B. Ultrasound assessment for grading structural tendon changes in supraspinatus tendinopathy: an inter-rater reliability study. BMJ. 2016;6:1–8.

18. Rees JD, Stride M, Scott A. Tendons-time to revisit inflammation. Br J Sports Med. 2014;48(21):1553–1557.

19. McFarland EG, Maffulli N, Del Buono A, Murrell GA, Garzon-Muvdi J, Petersen SA. Impingement is not impingement: the case for calling it 'rotator cuff disease'. Muscles Ligaments Tendons J. 2013;3(3):196–200.

20. Funk L. Shoulder examination tests. 2020. Available at: https://www.shoulderdoc.co.uk/section/497. Accessed February 6, 2020.

21. Atkins E, Keer J, Goodlad E. A Practical Approach to Musculoskeletal Medicine. Assessment, Diagnosis and Treatment. 4th ed. London: Elsevier; 2015:8

22. Perry J. Anatomy and biomechanics of the shoulder in throwing, swimming, gymnastics and tennis. Clin Sports Med. 1983;2:255.

23. Hohmann E, Shea K, Scheiderer B, Millett P, Imhoff A. Indications for arthroscopic subacromial decompression. A level V evidence clinical guideline. Arthroscopy. 2020;36(3):913–922.

24. Lewis JS. Frozen shoulder contracture syndrome - aetiology, diagnosis and management. Man Ther. 2015;20(1):2–9.

25. Tandon A, Dewan S, Bhatt S, Jain AK, Kumari R. Sonography in diagnosis of adhesive capsulitis of the shoulder: a case–control study. J Ultrasound. 2017;20(3):227–236. doi:10.1007/s40477-017-0262-5.

26. Teng A, Liu F, Zhou D, He T, Chevalier Y, Klar RM. Effectiveness of 3-dimensional shoulder ultrasound in the diagnosis of rotator cuff tears: a meta-analysis. Medicine. 2018;97(37):1–7.

27. Lewis JS. Subacromial impingement syndrome: a musculoskeletal condition or a clinical illusion? Phys Ther Rev. 2013;16(5):388–398.

28. Daghir AA, Sookur PA, Shah S, Watson M. Dynamic ultrasound of the subacromial–subdeltoid bursa in patients with shoulder impingement: a comparison with normal volunteers. Skeletal Radiol. 2012;41:1047–1053.

29. Hurschler C, Wülker N, Windhagen H, Hellmersa N, Plumhoffa P. Evaluation of the lag sign tests for external rotator function of the shoulder. J Shoulder Elbow Surg. 2004;13(3):298–304.

30. Magee DJ. Orthopedic Physical Assessment. 6th ed. London: Elsevier; 2014:273.

31. Lee J, Shukla DR, Sánchez-Sotelo J. Subscapularis tears: hidden and forgotten no more. J Shoulder Elbow Surg. 2018;2(1);74–83.

32. Siegal D, Wu JS, Newman JS, del Cura JL, Hochman MG. Calcific tendinitis: a pictorial review. Can Assoc Radiol J. 2009;60(5):263–272.

33. Hebert-Davies J, Teefey SA, Steger-May K, et al. Progression of fatty muscle degeneration in atraumatic rotator cuff tears. J Bone Joint Surg Am. 2017;99:832–839.

34. McAuliffe S, McCreesh K, Purtill H, O'Sullivan K. A systematic review of the reliability of diagnostic ultrasound imaging in measuring tendon size: is the error clinically acceptable? Phys Ther Sport. 2017;26:52–63.

35. Namdari S, Donegan RP, Dahiya N, Galatz LM, Yamaguchi K, Keener JD. Characteristics of small to medium-sized rotator cuff tears with and without disruption of the anterior supraspinatus tendon. J Shoulder Elbow Surg. 2014;23:20–27.

36. Fawcett R, Grainger, Robinson P, Jafari M, Rowbotham. Ultrasound-guided subacromial–subdeltoid bursa corticosteroid injections: a study of short- and long-term outcomes. Clin Radiol. 2018;73(8):e7–12. Available at: https://www.clinicalradiologyonline.net/article/S0009-9260(18)30137-5/fulltext. doi:10.1016/j.crad.2018.03.016.

4

Ultrasound of the Elbow and Forearm

Nicki Delves and Sara Riley

CHAPTER OUTLINE

LEARNING OBJECTIVES

After reading this chapter you should understand:
- The gross anatomy of the elbow and the relevant ultrasound appearances.
- How to direct the ultrasound findings to the clinical indications.
- Normal variants that may mimic pathology.
- When ultrasound as a stand-alone modality is inappropriate
- Common pathology and the basics of rehabilitation in injury/chronic conditions.

INTRODUCTION

Scanning of the elbow and forearm should be directed by the clinical indications rather than an evaluation of the entire region. Consequently, this chapter will discuss the anatomy, ultrasound technique, and normal appearances in four anatomical regions, although in practice more than one compartment may require attention depending on the clinical scenario.

Examples of common pathology will also be discussed.

The nerves are easily identified around the elbow and forearm and can be assessed for pathology/compression, which may be a cause of upper limb neurological symptoms. These will therefore be included in detail in this chapter.

The elbow can be difficult to scan from an ergonomic perspective, and consideration will be given to variations in patient positioning.

ELBOW JOINT

Anatomy

There are three articular surfaces between the humerus, the ulna, and the radius.

The hinge joint of the humeral trochlea with the trochlear notch of the ulna on the medial aspect allows flexion and extension.

The pivotal joint of the humeral capitulum, with the head of the radius on the lateral aspect and, centrally, the pivotal joint of the radioulnar articulation in the sigmoid notch of the ulna, allow flexion and extension of the elbow, and pronation and supination of the forearm (Fig. 4.1).

Movement is limited by bony, ligamentous structures and muscle action, making the elbow one of the most stable joints. The articular surfaces, with exception of

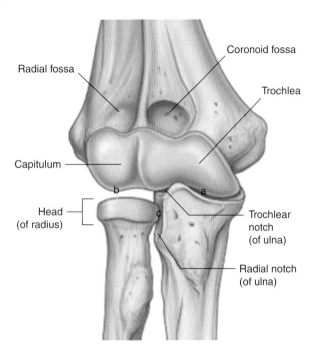

Fig. 4.1 Anterior view of the elbow joint. *a,* Ulnar-trochlear joint; *b,* radio-capitellar joint; *c,* radioulnar articulation. (From Drake RL. Gray's Anatomy for Students. 3rd Ed. London: Churchill Livingstone, Elsevier; 2015.)

the anterolateral aspect of the radial head, are covered with hyaline cartilage which is approximately 2 mm thick.[1] The elbow joint is innervated by the median, musculocutaneous, radial, and ulnar nerves.

The entire joint is invested by a capsule which extends anteriorly from the humeral shaft, superior to the radial and coronoid fossae, and posteriorly, superior to the olecranon fossa. It envelops the joint and radial head distally, inserting into the coronoid process of the ulna at the annular ligament and olecranon (Fig. 4.2).

This capsule is reinforced by the lateral (radial) and medial (ulnar) collateral ligaments which lie deep to the respective common extensor and flexor tendon origins, anteriorly by the bulk of the brachialis muscle and posteriorly by the triceps muscle. The inner surface of the capsule is enveloped by synovial membrane and synovial "out-pouch" recesses, increasing the synovial lining of the joint. These are important structures to examine for several pathological conditions where quantitative and qualitative evaluations are required,[2] including effusions, synovitis, and loose bodies. There are fat pads

(hyperechoic on ultrasound) within these recesses which, although intra-articular and subcapsular, are extrasynovial and will be displaced away from the joint by an effusion.[2,3] The largest is the anterior recess which extends over the radial and coronoid fossae. The posterior olecranon recess is within the olecranon fossa and the annular recess envelops the radial neck (Fig. 4.3).

Ultrasound Technique and Normal Ultrasound Appearances

There are several alternative positions for scanning the elbow joint. If scanning with a fixed position machine and a couch, lying the patient supine with the arm at their side is comfortable for both the patient and the operator. Initially the elbow is fully extended and hand supinated. This works well for the right elbow. For the left elbow, the patient could either lie with their feet at the head end of the couch or alternatively sit side onto the couch (Fig. 4.4), with the arm propped on a bolster/support on the couch.

> ◎ **TIP**
>
> Using a bolster allows unhindered access to many parts of the elbow, without the hand-held probe catching on the couch.

As a routine, examinations should include transverse, longitudinal, and oblique planes extending at least 5 cm proximal and distal of the ulnar-trochlear joint.[4] Initially place the transducer in a transverse section (TS) at the level of distal humerus. The hypoechoic hyaline cartilage is visualised showing an undulating "clam shell" appearance of the articular surface of the distal humerus (Fig. 4.5). This view is particularly helpful when assessing for osteophytosis and cartilage reduction in osteoarthritis.

> ◎ **TIP**
>
> Toggle the probe superior/inferior, left/right, keeping perpendicular to the wavy joint line to fully assess the hyaline cartilage.

Longitudinal sections (LS) of the radio-capitellar and ulnar-trochlear joints are more useful when looking for effusions and synovitis (Figs. 4.6 and 4.7). Slight flexion of the elbow may be required as full extension

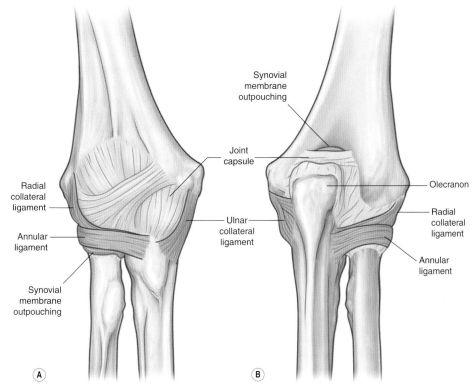

Fig. 4.2 Elbow joint capsule. Anterior **(A)** and posterior **(B)** aspects of right elbow joint capsule and radial and ulnar collateral ligaments. (From Soames R, Palastanga N. Anatomy of Human Movement, Structure and Function. 7th ed. London: Elsevier; 2019:106.)

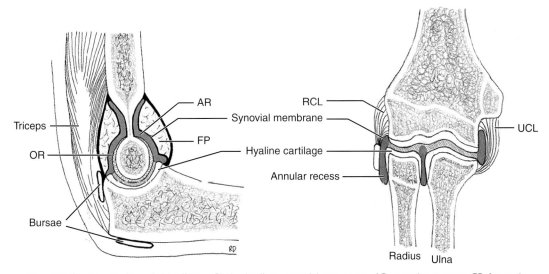

Fig. 4.3 Sectional view right elbow. *Dark shading*, synovial recesses. *AR,* anterior recess; *FP,* fat pad; *OR,* olecranon recess; *RCL,* radial collateral ligament; *UCL,* ulnar collateral ligament. (Drawing courtesy Rhiannon Delves.)

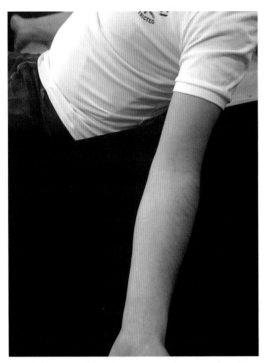

Fig. 4.4 Patient position for scanning left anterior elbow.

can cause compression of the joint structures against brachialis preventing visualisation of a joint effusion and compression of neovascularity if present. Dynamic assessment during passive supination and pronation of the forearm allows a thorough assessment of the radial head/recess.[1,3,4]

> **TIP**
>
> Scan beyond the capsular insertions, particularly at the radial head, as the synovial recesses fold well beyond the joint line and an effusion may only be evident within the distal fold.

The posterior joint recess within the olecranon fossa is the most sensitive site for small effusions. This should be examined with the patient's elbow slightly flexed, preferably with the tip of the elbow pointing to the floor, thus demonstrating fluid accumulation within the dependent joint recess. A comfortable position involves the patient sitting on the couch facing away from the operator. The transducer is placed on the dorsal aspect of the arm, in LS, just superior to the olecranon process (Fig. 4.8).

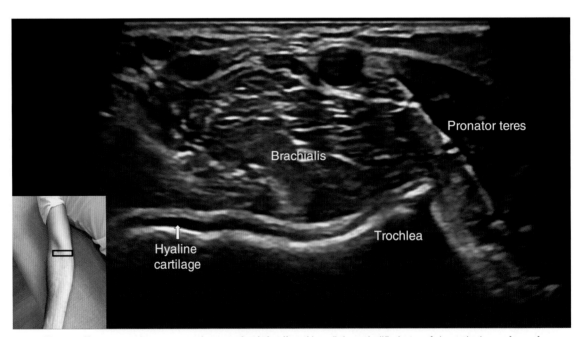

Fig. 4.5 Transverse image over the anterior joint line. Note "clam shell" shape of the articular surface of the distal humerus. Insert: supine patient/probe position.

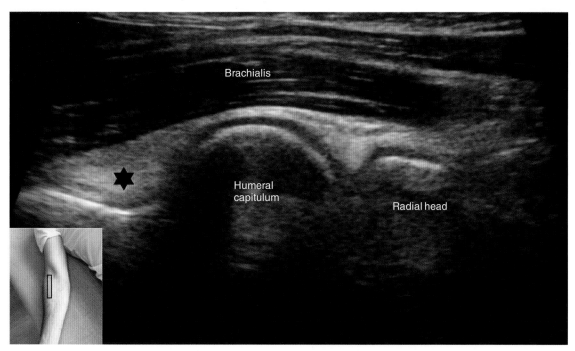

Fig. 4.6 Longitudinal section over the radio-capitellar joint. Anterior fat pad *(star)*. Insert: patient/probe position.

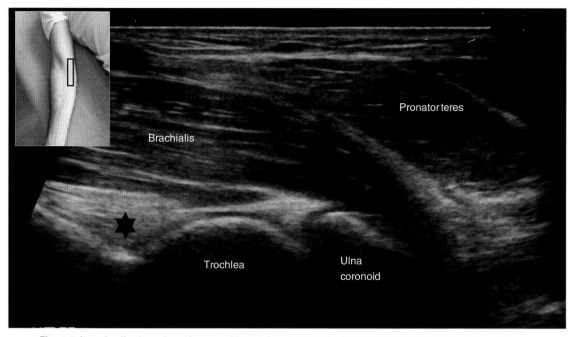

Fig. 4.7 Longitudinal section ulnar-trochlear joint. Anterior fat fad *(star)*. Insert: patient/probe position.

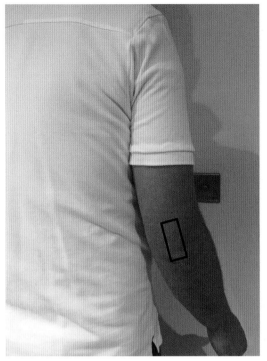

Fig. 4.8 Patient position for the posterior joint recess. Alternative scanning position with the tip of the elbow dependent.

The distinctive concavity superior to the bony outline of the trochlea is the olecranon fossa (Fig. 4.9). Care should be taken not to compress away fluid from the joint.

ANTERIOR STRUCTURES

The anterior muscles, biceps brachii and brachialis, lie in the antecubital fossa between the brachioradialis muscle laterally and the pronator teres medially (Fig. 4.10). The more commonly injured is biceps brachii; however, tears within brachialis can mimic biceps injury clinically and brachialis should be included in the examination, especially if the biceps is normal.

Biceps Brachii and Bicipitoradial Bursa

Anatomy

The biceps brachii muscle has two muscle bodies, the short and long heads, which flex the elbow and supinate the forearm, respectively.[5] It originates within the shoulder from the corocoid process of the scapula and the supraglenoid tubercle and inserts onto the posteromedial aspect of the radial tuberosity in the forearm via a

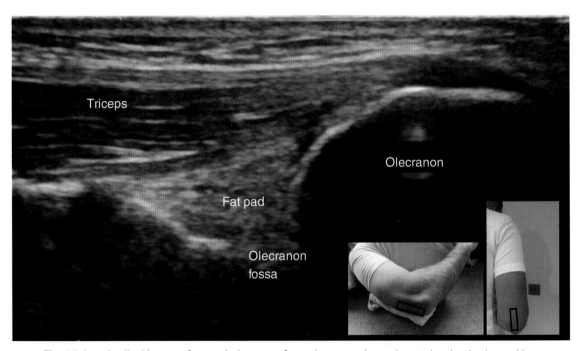

Fig. 4.9 Longitudinal image of normal olecranon fossa. Insert: supine and seated patient/probe position.

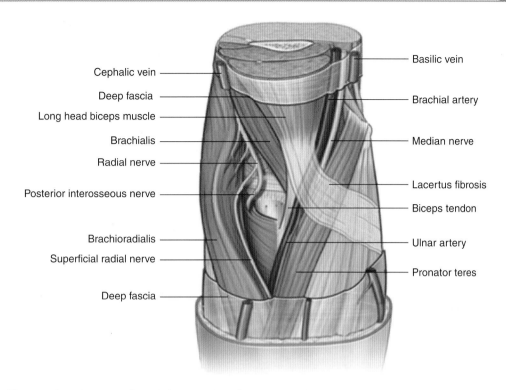

Fig. 4.10 Anterior view of the right arm. (From Soames R, Palastanga N. Anatomy of Human Movement, Structure and Function. 7th ed. London: Elsevier; 2019:108.)

distal tendon, with components from both the long and short heads. The distal short (SH) and long head (LH) tendon components are fused in close rotated apposition, forming a tendon (biceps tendon [BT]) of 6 to 7 cm in length, lying lateral to the brachial artery before diving deeper and obliquely to its insertion onto the radius[6] (Fig. 4.11).

The SH tendon is more superficial and inserts distal to the LH tendon insertion onto the radial tuberosity (Fig. 4.12), producing a more favorable lever than the LH, particularly when starting flexion from a fully extended position.[7] The LH tendon is more commonly involved in injury, with partial tears frequently involving just this portion, leaving the SH fibres intact.

A 2-cm long mid-tendon "critical zone" (Fig. 4.13) is subject to radial/ulnar impingement in pronation, and is exacerbated by osteophytosis if present. Its relative hypovascularity makes it prone to rupture. Rarer selective disruption of the short head component can occur with a forced flexion against an eccentric load injury.[8,9]

Biceps brachii has a separate attachment, the lacertus fibrosus, or biceps aponeurosis, which is a flattened fibrous fascia originating from the superficial aspect of the bicipital musculotendinous junction, expanding over pronator teres, the median nerve, and brachial artery before inserting into the deep fascia of the medial forearm (see Fig. 4.11). This acts as a stabiliser of the distal tendon and is less commonly involved in injury.[1]

The bicipitoradial bursa (BRB) lies on the radial aspect of the BT and is not normally visible. When inflamed, for example from attritional osteophytosis of the radius, the BRB may distend as an effusion along and around the distal BT. This is noted particularly on pronation when the BT squeezes the bursa against the radius (Fig. 4.14). This could imitate "tenosynovitis" of the distal BT; however, as the BT is covered with an extra synovial paratenon, not a synovial sheath, this should not be considered as a sheath effusion (see later Pathology section).[1]

Labels on figure:
Cephalic vein
Deep fascia
Long head biceps muscle
Brachialis
Radial nerve
Posterior interosseous nerve
Brachioradialis
Superficial radial nerve
Deep fascia
Basilic vein
Brachial artery
Median nerve
Lacertus fibrosis
Biceps tendon
Ulnar artery
Pronator teres

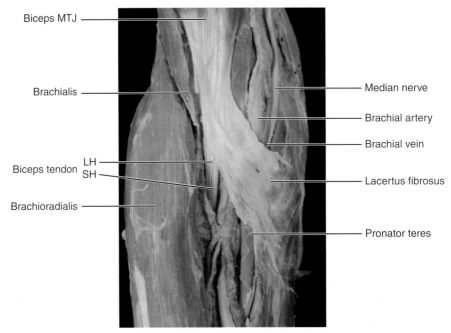

Biceps MTJ

Brachialis

Biceps tendon LH SH

Brachioradialis

Median nerve

Brachial artery

Brachial vein

Lacertus fibrosus

Pronator teres

Fig. 4.11 Cadaveric specimen right anterior elbow, demonstrating two parts of the biceps tendon. *LH,* Long head portion; *MJT,* musculotendinous junction; *SH,* biceps short head. (Courtesy Dept of Anatomy, Brighton and Sussex Medical School, credit A.)

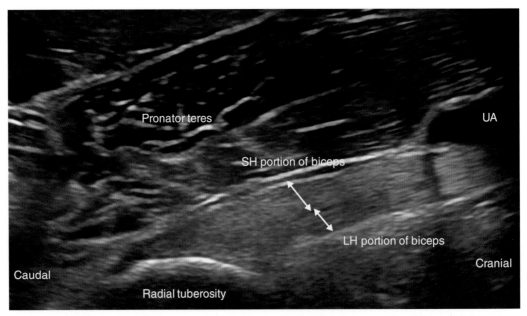

Fig. 4.12 Distal biceps insertion. Longitudinal scan distal biceps insertion, showing two components: short head *(SH)* and more proximally inserting long head *(LH)*. *UA,* Ulnar artery.

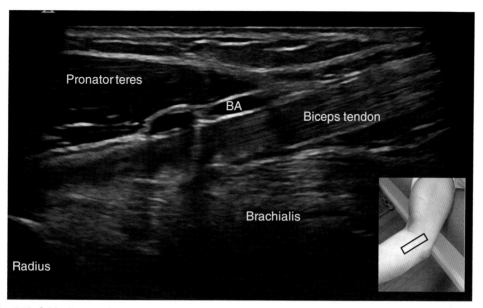

Fig. 4.13 Critical zone of biceps. Medial to lateral longitudinal section probe tilt. *BA,* Brachial artery. Insert: patient/probe position.

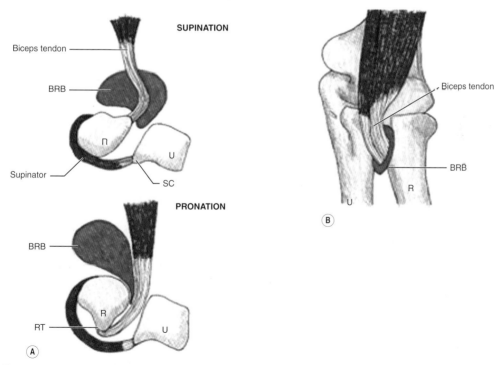

Fig. 4.14 Bicipitoradial bursa. (A) Schematic transverse section at the level of the radial tuberosity *(RT)* in supination and pronation. This shows the relationship of the bicipitoradial bursa *(BRB)* wrapping the distal biceps and the associated distention from the radial origin on pronation. **(B)** Longitudinal section anterior view. *R,* Radius; *SC,* supinator crest; *U,* ulna. (Drawings courtesy Rhiannon Delves.)

Ultrasound Technique and Normal Appearances

The patient is supine or seated, with the arm outstretched and supinated and elbow slightly flexed.

The distal BT is difficult to scan due to its superficial to deep travel, but an intact distal BT can be palpated by using a Hook test – hooking your index finger around the side of the tendon in the elbow crease, which may also help with orientation.

Fixed flexion deformities due to osteo- or inflammatory arthritis, posterior impingement, or those with high muscle bulk, can make visualisation of the distal biceps especially tricky. Consequently, a few different techniques can be utilised to enable assessment of the whole of the tendon.

Start with the transducer in TS over the mid upper arm. Assess the short and long head biceps brachii muscle bellies which should be of similar size. If one is more echogenic and significantly smaller than the other, indicating muscle atrophy, this may be the first clue of a tear of the corresponding tendon. Moving the transducer caudally, note the musculotendinous junction and the emerging form of the ovoid or dumbbell-shaped echogenic BT anterolateral to the brachial artery with the thin fascia of lacertus fibrosus overlying the artery (Fig. 4.15).

TIP

In the absence of trauma, muscle atrophy may be an indication of denervation injury or insult.

Due to anisotropy, the BT quickly becomes difficult to follow in TS, as it dives deeper. At this point it should be interrogated in LS to its insertion onto the radial tuberosity. This can also be challenging, and there are several approaches discussed here which, in combination, can help demonstrate the tendon in its entirety:

- **Anterior.** Maintaining the arm in an extended, supinated position facilitates imaging of the proximal BT in LS lateral to the brachial artery. By using a large amount of gel under the proximal end of the probe and heeling-in the distal end, the BT becomes more perpendicular to the probe. Dynamic assessment is performed in resisted flexion which can help visualise muscle and tendon retraction, particularly in difficult cases.
- **Medial.** Place the transducer in LS just distal of the slightly flexed elbow. Angle across the pronator teres muscle and brachial/ulnar artery from a medial to lateral approach, using these structures as an acoustic window (Figs. 4.13 and 4.16). Use resisted flexion to assess whether the tendon is intact. This view can also be achieved by scanning from a lateral to medial approach, using the brachioradialis muscle as a window.[7,10,11]
- **Posterior** (cobra view). The transducer is placed in TS on the proximal posterior forearm over the radial head. Move distally over the supinator muscle to bring both the radius and ulna into view. This will be 4 to 5 cm distal to the lateral epicondyle. Undertake passive supination/pronation. In full pronation the insertion of the distal BT will be visualised (Fig. 4.17).

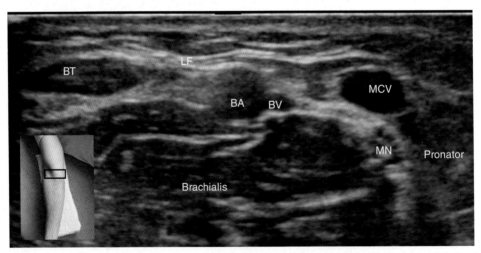

Fig. 4.15 Transverse scan anterior elbow, just distal of the musculotendinous junction. *BA*, Brachial artery; *BT*, biceps tendon; *BV*, brachial vein; *LF*, lacertus fibrosus; *MCV*, medial cubital vein; *MN*, medial nerve. Insert: patient/probe position.

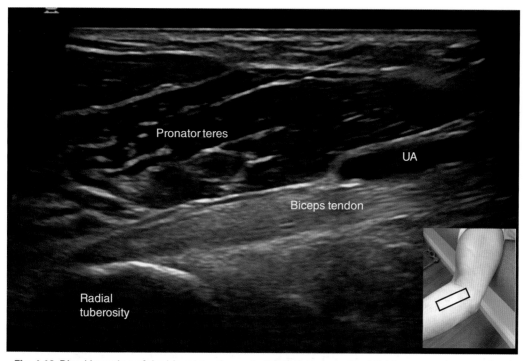

Fig. 4.16 Distal insertion of the biceps tendon onto the radial tuberosity. *UA*, Ulnar artery. Insert: patient/probe position.

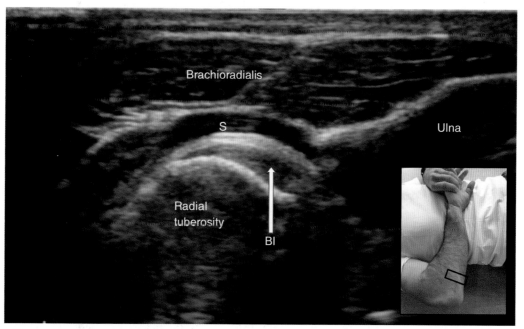

Fig. 4.17 Pronated "Cobra position". Arrow pointing to the insertion of the biceps tendon. *BI*, Biceps insertion; *S*, supinator. Insert: patient/probe position.

This view is used to confirm or refute full avulsion from the tuberosity and for assessment of osteophytosis around the biceps insertion which may be a cause of proximal radial-ulnar impingement.[1,11] In this position, a distended BRB may also be evident.

Brachialis
Anatomy
Brachialis is the deepest muscle of the anterior elbow; it flexes the elbow and is innervated by the musculocutaneous nerves. It originates from the anterior mid-distal shaft of the humerus (Fig. 4.18). It consists of two components: the superficial component inserting onto the ulnar tuberosity which is a roughening immediately distal to the coronoid process, and the deep portion, which inserts slightly more proximally with a short flat tendon and muscular insertion onto the anterior joint capsule, making it more likely to be involved in joint injury, e.g., posterior dislocation of the elbow.[12]

Ultrasound Technique and Normal Appearances
The patient is positioned with the elbow extended and hand supinated as for the anterior joint structures. When scanned in LS, the brachialis muscle is visible

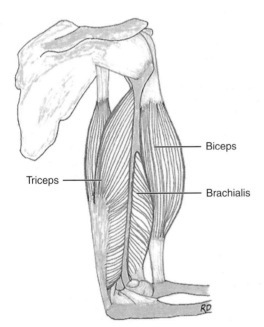

Fig. 4.18 Schematic drawing to demonstrate the relationship of the major arm muscles. (Drawing courtesy Rhiannon Delves.)

anterior to the joint structures (Fig. 4.19). Care should be taken to avoid anisotropy of the distal insertion. Dynamic assessment to help with visualisation of muscle injury is performed with resisted flexion and pronosupination.[7,12]

 TIP

General Scanning Tips for Nerves

- The rule of very light probe contact applicable to all superficial structures is less relevant when scanning nerves. Although nerves do distort with anisotropy, they do not distort to probe pressure. Relative firm pressure can be helpful in identifying them.
- It can be easy to get lost when scanning nerves. If so, go back to an anatomical point where you can identify the nerve. For example, go back to the medial epicondyle for the ulnar nerve or the spiral groove of the humerus for the radial nerve and trace up and down.
- Many nerves are accompanied by blood vessels; use Doppler as a guide.
- Most nerves are easier to follow in TS, but calibre change due to pathology should be evaluated in LS as well as TS.
- Use a sweep scan of the region initially before focusing on a specific region to get your eye in.

Median and Anterior Interosseous Nerves
Anatomy
The median nerve (MN) is a branch of the medial and lateral cords of the brachial plexus. It innervates pronator teres, palmaris longus, flexor carpi radialis, flexor digitorum superficialis, and distally, structures in the hand.

The MN passes down the anteromedial upper arm in the neurovascular bundle with the brachial artery. The median nerve continues medial to the brachial artery and passes under the lacertus fibrosus, remaining between pronator teres and brachialis (Fig. 4.20). At the distal cubital fossa, it normally traverses between the larger superficial humeral head and smaller deep ulnar head of pronator teres, progressing deep to the sublimis fascia which is the proximal fascial bridge of flexor digitorum superficialis (FDS). It then travels distally between the superficial and deep flexor muscles towards the carpal tunnel at the wrist.

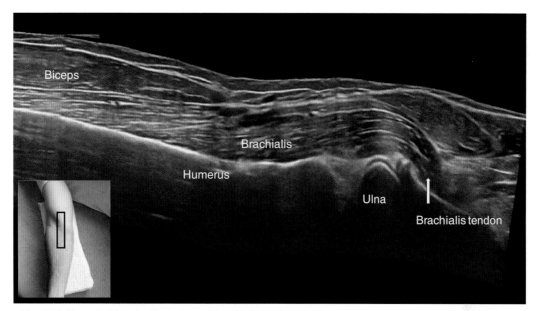

Fig. 4.19 Extended longitudinal view of brachialis at the anterior elbow. Insert: patient/probe position.

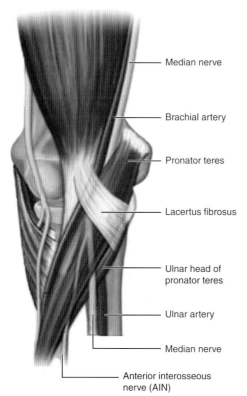

Fig. 4.20 Anterior right arm anatomy. Median nerve with anterior interosseous nerve branch. (From https://radiologykey.com)

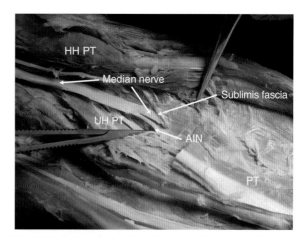

Fig. 4.21 Cadaveric section right anterior elbow. Pronator teres cut and reflected. *AIN*, Anterior interosseous nerve; *HH PT*, humeral head of pronator teres; *PT*, pronator teres; *UH PT*, ulnar head of pronator teres. (Courtesy Dept. of Anatomy, Brighton and Sussex Medical School, credit A.)

The anterior interosseous nerve (AIN) is a purely motor nerve supplying the flexor pollicis longus, pronator teres, and lateral flexor digitorum profundus muscles. It branches off the median nerve approximately 5 cm below the elbow crease at the level of the sublimis fascia (distal edge of the pronator teres) (Fig. 4.21).

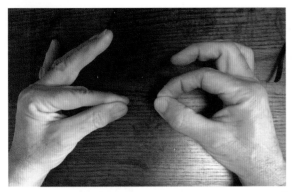

Fig. 4.22 Anterior interosseous nerve impingement. *Left,* abnormal; *right,* normal.

Compression neuropathy of the AIN, may be suggested by loss of bulk of the innervated muscles[7] and inhibition of the thumb and index finger coordination to form an "O" (Fig. 4.22).

Ultrasound Technique and Normal Appearances

The patient's arm is supinated, elbow extended.

In TS over the medial upper third of the upper arm, medial of the biceps bulk, identify the MN and adjacent brachial artery (Fig. 4.23).

Graded compression helps to differentiate arteries from the associated veins and the superficial basilic vein, which lies medially and superficially. Trace the MN in TS to the cubital fossa. At the elbow crease note the lateral to medial, "BAM" relationship, of the Biceps, brachial Artery and Median nerve[13] (Fig. 4.24).

Follow the MN distally in LS and TS as it passes anteromedial to brachialis, extending between the two heads of pronator teres (Figs. 4.25 and 4.26).

Look carefully at the distal edge of the pronator where the FDS (sublimis) commences. This is the location of the sublimis fascia (Fig. 4.27).

It will not be visible as a structure, but its location should be appreciated as it can be a source of compression of the MN or AIN. Distally, the MN can be identified between the superficial and deep flexor muscles of the forearm to the carpal tunnel at the wrist.

Anterior Forearm Musculature

The superficial and deep flexor muscles of the wrist, FDS (mentioned earlier) and flexor digitorum profundus (FDP), lie in the anterior compartment of the forearm. Their distal tendons are important structures for ultrasound assessment and are discussed in Chapter 5. The tendinous origins are discussed further in the next section.

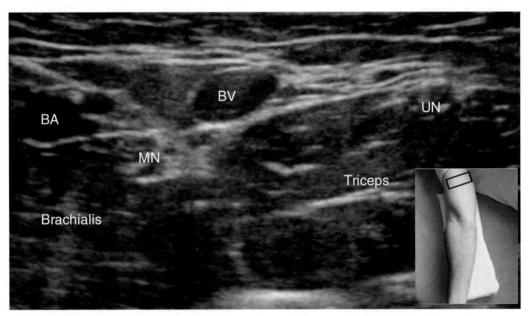

Fig. 4.23 Transverse image medial upper arm. *BA,* Brachial artery; *BV,* basilic vein; *MN,* median nerve; *UN,* ulnar nerve. Insert: patient/probe position.

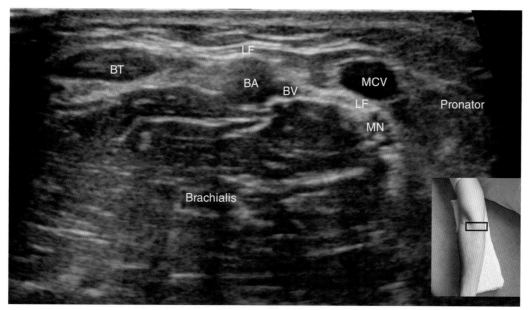

Fig. 4.24 Transverse scan at the elbow crease. "BAM" relationship, lateral to medial. *BA,* Brachial artery; *BAM,* biceps, brachial artery, and median nerve. *BT,* biceps tendon; *BV,* brachial vein; *LF,* lacertus fibrosus; *MN,* median nerve; *MCV,* medial cubital vein. Insert: patient/probe position.

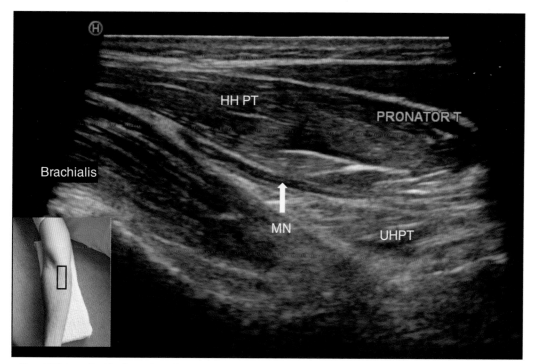

Fig. 4.25 Longitudinal section distal elbow. *HH PT,* Humeral head of pronator teres; *MN,* median nerve; *UHPT,* ulnar head of pronator teres. Insert: patient/probe position.

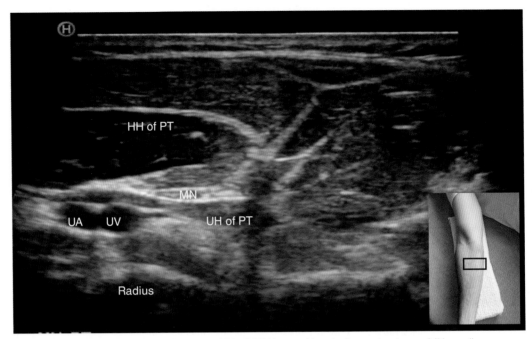

Fig. 4.26 Transverse proximal forearm. *HH of PT,* Humeral head of pronator teres; *MN,* median nerve; *UA,* ulnar artery; *UV,* ulnar vein; *UH of PT,* ulnar head of pronator teres. Insert: patient/probe position.

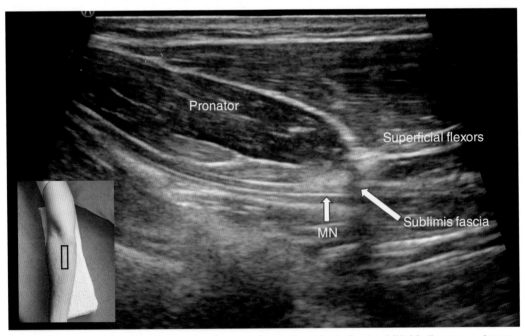

Fig. 4.27 Longitudinal section anterior forearm, level of sublimis fascia. *MN,* Median nerve. Insert: patient/probe position.

The FDP muscles can be differentiated from FDS on ultrasound in the anterior forearm in TS by asking the patient to flex just the tips of the fingers.[1]

MEDIAL STRUCTURES

Anatomy

Ulnar Collateral Ligament

The medial (ulnar) collateral ligament (UCL), is a three-part triangle of ligamentous bands (see Fig 4.28). The most prominent, and important in constraining valgus stress, is the anterior band which originates from the medial epicondyle and inserts into the medial coronoid process of the ulna.

Common Flexor Origin

There are four superficial flexor muscles of the hand and wrist that arise from the medial epicondyle as the common flexor origin (CFO).

This common tendon overlies the UCL. They appear as a merged origin, but the individual tendon order from anteromedial to posterolateral is flexor carpi radialis, palmaris longus, FDS, flexor carpi ulnaris (FCU) (Fig. 4.29).

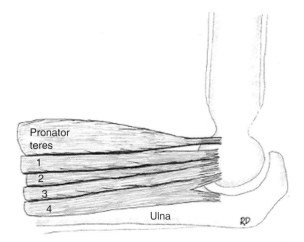

Fig. 4.29 Schematic Drawing Medial Elbow, Common Flexor Origin. *1,* flexor carpus radialis; *2,* palmaris longus; *3,* flexor digitorum superficialis; *4,* flexor carpus ulnaris. (Drawings courtesy Rhiannon Delves.)

The deeper flexors, digitorum profundus, have a common origin attaching to the coronoid and the anterior interosseous membrane.

Ulnar Nerve

The ulnar nerve (UN) is a branch of the medial cord of the brachial plexus. It innervates the FCU and FDP muscles in the forearm, wrist, and hand. It descends the anteromedial upper arm in a neurovascular bundle with the MN, brachial artery, and basilic vein, lying posterior to the brachial artery. In the distal third of the upper arm, the UN deviates medially and enters the posterior compartment, adjacent to the medial head of the triceps to pass into the cubital tunnel deep to the stabilizing cubital tunnel fascial sheet, the Osbourne retinaculum. Approximately 1 cm distal, the UN enters the proper cubital tunnel, under the arcuate ligament between the humeral and ulnar heads of FCU and continues in close proximity to the FCU to the wrist (Figs. 4.30 and 4.31).

During elbow flexion there is traction and compression of the UN against the medial epicondyle. If there is laxity or a tear of the Osbourne retinaculum, subluxation, or sometimes dislocation of the nerve, can occur and may be symptomatic. Asymptomatic subluxation or dislocation, considered a normal variant, can also occur with the nerve occasionally dislocating superficial to the CFO.[14] In some patient's subluxation represents a

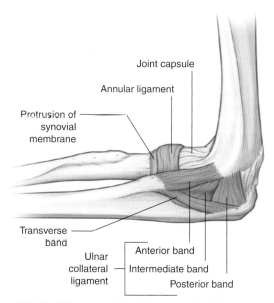

Fig. 4.28 Medial aspect right elbow showing joint capsule and ulnar collateral ligament. (From Soames R, Palastanga N. Anatomy of Human Movement, Structure and Function. 7th ed. London: Elsevier; 2019:107.)

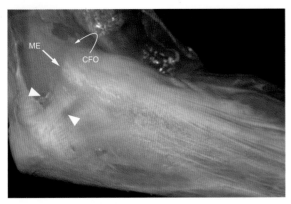

Fig. 4.30 Dissection of the medial elbow, *Arrowheads*, Osbourne retinaculum; *CFO*, common flexor origin; *ME*, medial epicondyle. (From De Maeseneer M, et al. Ultrasound of the elbow with emphasis on detailed assessment of ligaments, tendons and nerves. Eur J Radiol. 2015;84(4):671-681.)

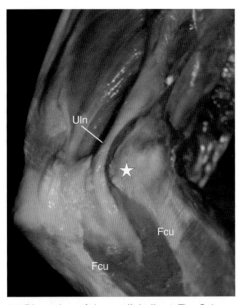

Fig. 4.31 Dissection of the medial elbow. The Osbourne retinaculum has been removed. *Fcu*, Heads of the flexor carpus ulnaris; *star*, medial epicondyle; *Uln*, Ulnar nerve. (From De Maeseneer M, et al. Ultrasound of the elbow with emphasis on detailed assessment of ligaments, tendons and nerves. Eur J Radiol. 2015;84(4):671-681.)

significant finding, particularly if nerve thickening is present. "Snapping" triceps syndrome, with subluxation of the medial head of triceps or an anatomical variant of the anconeus epitrochlearis replacing the Osbourne retinaculum, can be symptomatic causes.[7,15,16] The UN should be of moderately uniform, round calibre

throughout the tunnel, although some normal ovoid distortion can be seen on full flexion. Overall diameter should be less than 8 mm; rarely the nerve may be bifid or trifid.[17]

Ultrasound Technique and Normal Appearances

The scan technique for the medial joint, UCL, and CFO are similar. There are variable tried and tested patient positions for accessing the medial elbow (Fig. 4.32). A comfortable position for the patient and operator is with the patient supine and the arm externally rotated, elbow flexed, with a small pad under the arm to raise it from the couch to allow probe access (Fig. 4.32C). In this position, the region can be scanned and the flexion for dynamic assessment controlled passively. Flexion enables further external rotation and better access than a straight elbow.

This is good for the right arm. For the left arm, the patient can lie with the head to the foot of the bed or the other side of the couch from the operator, facing away (Fig. 4.32A), although control of the probe, without arm support, makes this position more awkward for the operator.

UCL and CFO

Initially palpate the medial epicondyle. Place the probe in long axis to the forearm over the epicondyle. Identify the characteristic bony epicondyle and the joint space. The anterior bundle of the UCL is near perpendicular to the beam and immediately deep to the adjacent CFO. Both are fibrillar in appearance, but the UCL is slightly more hyperechoic. The slightly different attachment of both should be appreciated. A minimum 70-degree flexion of the elbow improves the visualisation of the taut UCL[7] (Fig. 4.33).

The CFO is best scanned in LS. It will appear shorter than the common extensor origin of the lateral elbow.

Ulnar Nerve (UN)

The UN should be traced in TS, starting proximal to the cubital tunnel until distal to the heads of FCU, in full extension and in varying degrees of flexion for assessment of stability (Figs. 4.34 and 4.35). Dislocation may only be demonstrated on full flexion, so it is important to observe the UN in TS, whilst passively bending the elbow to full flexion.

Palpate the olecranon and medial epicondyle and scan between them in LS for alignment of the UN. Follow the nerve proximally and distally (Fig. 4.36).

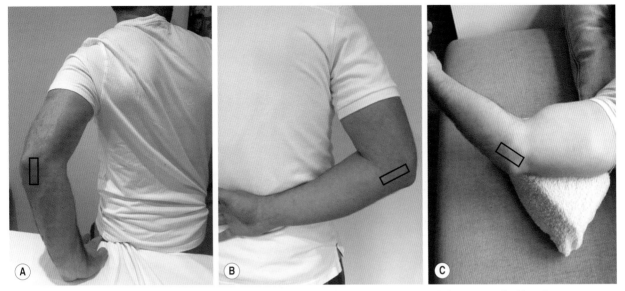

Fig. 4.32 (A–C) Alternative patient positions for scanning the medial elbow and ulnar nerve. Position C enables controlled flexion by the operator.

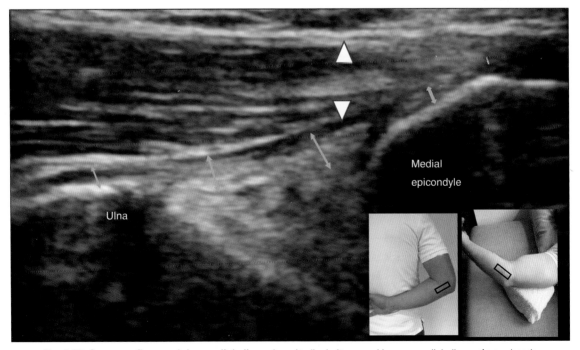

Fig. 4.33 Common flexor origin, medial elbow. Longitudinal ultrasound image medial elbow. *Arrow heads,* Common flexor tendons; *blue arrows,* ulnar collateral ligament. Insert: alternative patient/probe position, erect or supine.

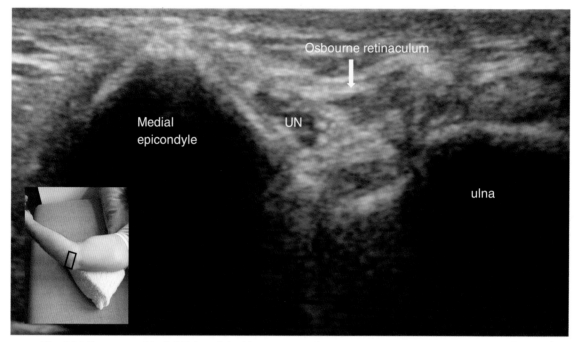

Fig. 4.34 Transverse Medial Epicondyle. Note overlying Osbourne retinaculum. *UN*, Ulnar nerve. Insert: patient/probe position.

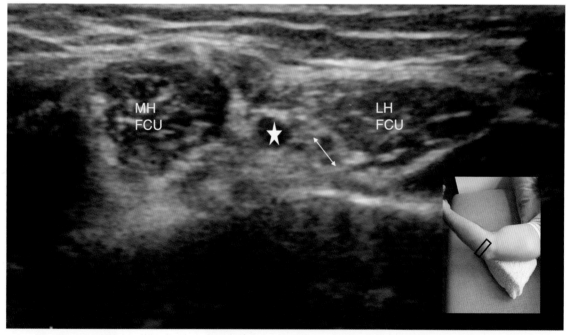

Fig. 4.35 Transverse Scan Through the Bellies of the Flexor Carpus Ulnaris *(FCU)*. *Double arrow*, Ulnar nerve; *LHFCU*, lateral head of FCU; *MHFCU*, medial head of the FCU; *star*, superior ulnar collateral artery. Insert: patient/probe position.

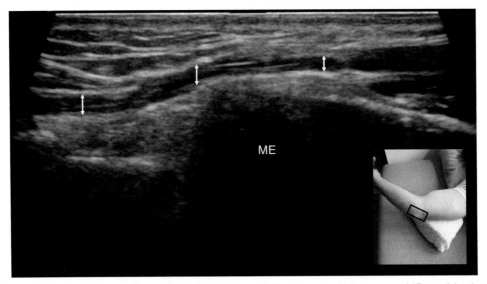

Fig. 4.36 Longitudinal scan through the cubital tunnel. *Double arrows,* Ulnar nerve. *ME,* medial epicondyle. Insert: patient/probe position.

POSTERIOR STRUCTURES

Anatomy

Bursae

There are three main bursae in the posterior aspect of the elbow, but they may not be visualised on ultrasound when normal:

Superficial olecranon bursa—lies between olecranon and subcutaneous tissue.

Sub-tendinous olecranon bursa—lies between olecranon and the triceps brachii (Fig. 4.37).

Intratendinous olecranon bursa—variably lies in the triceps brachii tendon.

Triceps Brachii

The triceps muscle consists of the lateral, long, and medial heads. The lateral and long heads converge into an aponeurosis that is lateral and more superficial than the medial head. This converging tendon inserts onto the olecranon, approximately 1.5 cm distal to the tip, increasing the point of contact and strength of this major elbow extensor. The medial head has a deeper more medial insertion onto the olecranon, remains muscular to the insertion, and is consequently less commonly injured. However, hypertrophy of the medial head of triceps or an accessory medial head can cause extrinsic impingement of the ulnar nerve.[16,17]

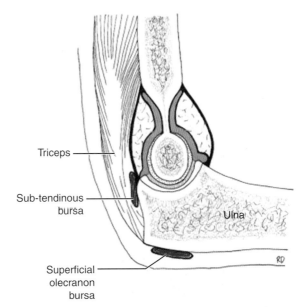

Fig. 4.37 Sectional sketch right elbow with olecranon bursae. (Drawing courtesy Rhiannon Dolves.)

Triceps tears may occur at the musculotendinous junction or avulsions from the olecranon. Tendinopathy of the triceps tendon can occur in overuse injuries and in patients with seronegative arthropathy (see Rheumatology chapter).

Ultrasound Technique and Normal Appearances

Elbow flexed, patient's hand across waist.

Scan the posterior distal humerus, in LS, just superior to the elbow joint. Identify the distinctive concavity of the olecranon fossa (see Fig. 4.9). At this level (Fig. 4.38), the central tendon of the triceps aponeurosis has an echogenic fibrillar appearance compared with the less echogenic muscle. The medial head of the triceps is noted more medially, with the muscle extending to the insertion. The different insertions can be particularly appreciated in TS (Fig. 4.39).

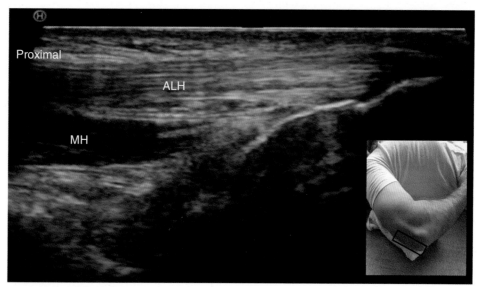

Fig. 4.38 Longitudinal section, triceps tendon. *ALH,* Aponeurosis long head; *MH,* muscular medial head. Insert: patient position.

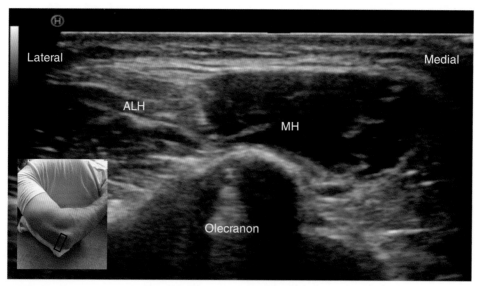

Fig. 4.39 Transverse section, distal triceps. *ALH,* Aponeurosis long head; *MH,* medial head. Insert: patient/probe position.

LATERAL STRUCTURES

Anatomy

Radial (Lateral) Collateral Ligaments

The radial (lateral) collateral ligament complex (RCL) is a Y-shaped, three-part complex. The annular ligament both originates and inserts into the radial notch of the ulnar and encircles the radial head. The RCL originates from the lateral epicondyle and inserts into the annular ligament. The lateral ulnar collateral ligament (LUCL) originates from the lateral epicondyle and inserts into the superior crest of the ulna, blending with the annular ligament (Fig. 4.40).

Common Extensor Origin (CEO)

Four of the extensors of the hand and wrist have a common origin on the anterolateral surface of the lateral epicondyle. This overlies the RCL. The extensor carpi radialis brevis and the extensor digitorum communicans make up most of the CEO, with the extensor digitorum minimi and extensor carpi ulnaris contributing only minor components. The extensor carpi radialis longus originates separately from the posterior superior supracondylar ridge (Fig. 4.41A,B).

Ultrasound Technique and Normal Appearances

The patient's elbow is flexed, hand in neutral or internally rotated.

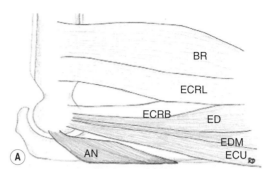

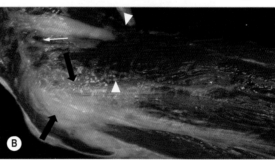

Fig. 4.41 Lateral elbow. (A) Schematic drawing of the common extensor origin. *AN*, Anconeus; *BR*, brachioradialis; *ECRB*, extensor carpus radialis brevis; *ECRL*, extensor carpi radialis longus; *ECU*, extensor carpus ulnaris; *ED*, extensor digitorum; *EDM*, extensor digiti minimi. (B) Dissection exposing the right extensor origin. *Black arrows*, Common extensor origin; *small arrow*, supracondylar ridge; *white arrow heads*, ECRL and brachioradialis. (A, Drawings courtesy Rhiannon Delves. B, From De Maeseneer M, et al. Ultrasound of the elbow with emphasis on detailed assessment of ligaments, tendons and nerves. Eur J Radiol 2015;84(4):671-681.)

Palpate the lateral epicondyle. Place the transducer over and just distal of the lateral epicondyle in line with the forearm to image the CEO in LS. Appreciate the subtle difference in appearance of the CEO overlying the radial collateral ligament (Figs. 4.42 and 4.43). Use light pressure otherwise the Doppler signal from any pathological neovascularity may be suppressed.

RADIAL NERVE AND ADJACENT MUSCULATURE

Anatomy

The radial nerve (RN) is a branch of the posterior cord of the brachial plexus. It provides motor innervation to the triceps brachii and extensors muscles of the fore-

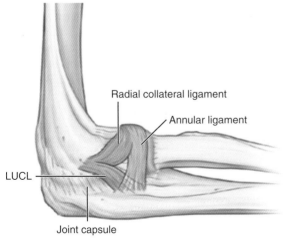

Fig. 4.40 Lateral aspect of the elbow. *LUCL*, Lateral ulnar collateral ligament. (From Soames R, Palastanga N. Anatomy of Human Movement, Structure and Function. 7th ed. London: Elsevier; 2019:106.)

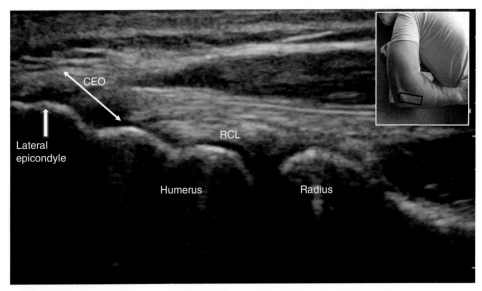

Fig. 4.42 Longitudinal section lateral elbow. Radial collateral ligament *(RCL)* and the common extensor tendon between the double arrows *(CEO)*. Insert: patient/probe position.

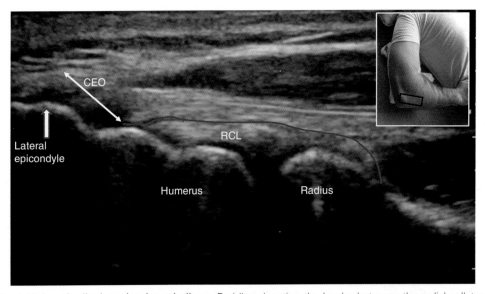

Fig. 4.43 Longitudinal section lateral elbow. Red line denoting the border between the radial collateral ligament *(RCL)* and the common extensor tendon *(CEO)*. Insert: patient/probe position.

arm and sensory innervation to the skin of the posterior forearm and part of the hand. The RN has a spiral route compared to the median and ulnar nerves, passing from medial to lateral posterior to the humeral shaft, within the spiral groove, making it susceptible to injury from adjacent fractures of the shaft of the humerus. It then passes on the lateral aspect of the arm, between the brachialis and brachioradialis muscles, to the anterolateral aspect of the cubital tunnel. At the superior edge of the supinator muscle, it divides into

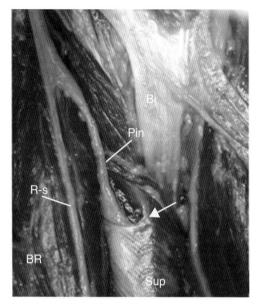

Fig. 4.44 Branches of the right radial nerve (brachioradialis and superficial radial nerve reflected). *Arrow*, Arcade of Frohse; *Bi*, biceps; *BR*, brachioradialis; *Pin*, posterior interosseous nerve; *R-s*, superficial radial nerve; *Sup*, supinator. (From De Maeseneer M, et al. Ultrasound of the elbow with emphasis on detailed assessment of ligaments, tendons and nerves. Eur J Radiol 2015;84(4):671-681.)

the motor portion, the posterior interosseous (PIN), and the sensory superficial radial nerve. The supinator muscle, the deepest muscle of the lateral elbow, encircles the radial head. It has two heads: the superficial head originates from the lateral epicondyle and the deep head from the supinator crest of the ulna. Between these two heads the PIN branch of the RN traverses from a superior anterolateral position to a posterior location in the forearm.[1] In 35% of people, the superior edge of the superficial supinator head unites with a fibrous layer, the Arcade of Frohse, which can be a site of attritional compression of the RN.[18]

The superficial branch of the RN remains in close alignment with the under surface of the brachioradialis muscle to the wrist (Figs. 4.10 and 4.44).

Ultrasound Technique and Normal Appearances

Patient's arm in supination, hand in pronation.

To find the RN, start in TS along the anterolateral aspect of the arm, lateral to brachialis and medial to brachioradialis (Fig. 4.45). Trace back up to the spiral

groove, then down again to the superior edge of the supinator, where the nerve bifurcates (Fig. 4.46). The RN nerve appears as several smaller nerve fascicles, compared with the more rounded median and ulnar nerves.

The PIN then runs obliquely through the supinator to the posterior forearm (Fig. 4.47). The superficial RN remains alongside the underside of the brachioradialis to the wrist (Fig. 4.48).

REPORTING TERMINOLOGY FOR NORMAL FINDINGS

- No evidence of a joint effusion or synovial proliferation. Normal smooth appearance of the hyaline cartilage, no evidence of osteophytosis seen, although intraarticular pathology cannot be excluded.
- The common flexor and extensor origins and corresponding ulnar and radial collateral ligaments are of normal appearance.
- Normal appearance of the antecubital fossa, anterior flexors, specifically the biceps brachii and brachialis.
- Normal distal insertion of the biceps. No evidence of bicipitoradial bursitis.
- No olecranon bursitis, normal triceps insertion.
- The ulnar nerve is of uniform diameter throughout the cubital tunnel and stable within the groove on full flexion.

PATHOLOGY

Pathological conditions relating to the elbow can be traumatic, degenerative, autoimmune, overuse injuries, or related to anomalous variants. We will discuss the more commonly presenting conditions.

Ligamentous tears and laxity can be assessed with dynamic ultrasound, but unless scanned by experienced hands, will require magnetic resonance imaging for diagnostic evaluation and assessment of intra-articular pathology.

Bony fractures can be detected with ultrasound. An acute fracture site may show sharp cortical disruption, in contrast to a more irregular nodular appearance of degenerative changes at the joint line. With an undisplaced fracture, there may be little separation of the bone, but there will be periosteal thickening and possibly associated hyperemia. Fibrocartilaginous callus formation may be evident from 7 to 14 days.[19] A simple effusion/lifting of the fat pad

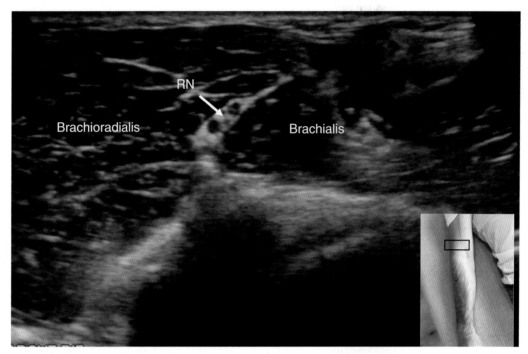

Fig. 4.45 Transverse scan showing the radial nerve between the brachioradialis and brachialis muscle bellies. Upper arm supinated, hand pronated. *RN*, Radial nerve. Insert: patient/probe position.

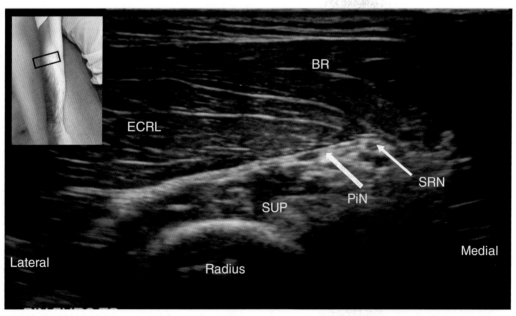

Fig. 4.46 Transverse scan. Division of the radial nerve into the posterior interosseous nerve *(PIN)* and superficial radial nerve *(SRN)*. *BR*, Brachioradialis; *ECRL*, extensor carpus radialis longus; *SUP*, supinator. Insert: patient/probe position.

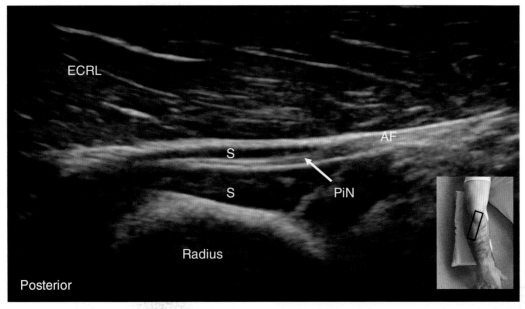

Fig. 4.47 Longitudinal oblique scan. *AF,* Arcade of Frohse; *ECRL,* extensor carpus radialis longus; *PIN,* posterior interosseous nerve; *S,* supinator. Insert, patient/probe position.

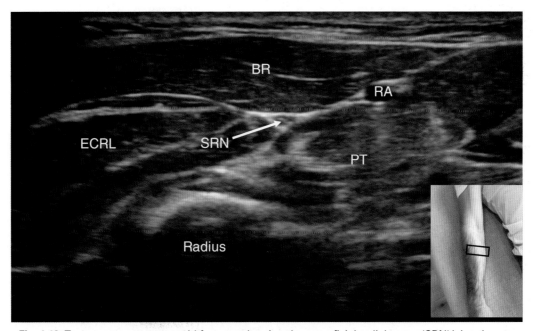

Fig. 4.48 Transverse scan upper mid forearm showing the superficial radial nerve *(SRN)* lying deep to brachioradialis *(BR)*. *ECRL,* Ext carpus radialis longus; *PT,* pronator teres; *RA,* radial artery. Insert: patient/probe position.

in the olecranon fossa may indicate fracture of the radial head following trauma. All suspected fractures should be confirmed with further imaging, usually with X-Ray.

Joint Effusion

An elbow effusion (Fig. 4.49) may be cystic and simple in nature, being completely anechoic. A more complex and particulate effusion (e.g., proteinaceous, haemorrhagic, inflammatory, or infectious content) will be more reflective and heterogenous but still maintain echolucency with degrees of posterior enhancement. An effusion should be compressible, adjacent to the articular surface and seen separately from the peripheral

capsule and fat pads during dynamic compression. Synovial hypertrophy is noncompressible, extending close to the articular surface but originates close to the capsular walls, has irregular margins and sometimes associate hyperemia (Fig. 4.50). These appearances are nonspecific and as always, history is key in considering differentiation and clinical significance. Clinical management depends on the underlying cause.

Lateral/Medial Epicondylitis/Tendinopathy

Tendinopathy of the common extensor tendons at the lateral epicondyle or common flexor tendons at the medial epicondyle are known as tennis elbow or golfer's elbow, respectively.

Symptoms have often been referred to as lateral or medial epicondylitis, although strictly this is a condition of the tendon rather than the epicondyle. The symptoms are acute focal pain over the respective epicondyle, particularly with gripping, sometimes extending down the forearm. It is a degenerative condition of the common tendon caused by repetitive overuse activity with typical ultrasound features including thickening of the tendon, neovascularity, and sometimes small partial tears (Figs. 4.51 and 4.52). It is a painful, often poorly managed condition that may take months or years to resolve. Chronic symptoms associated with tendinopathy may respond well to graded isometric, concentric/eccentric loading exercises of wrist flexion/extension which can be combined with extracorporeal shock wave therapy[20] and corticosteroid injection in some cases. However, there is concern that whilst corticosteroid

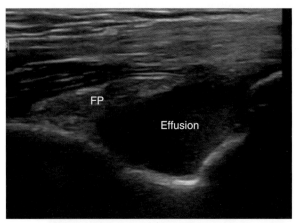

Fig. 4.49 Joint effusion in the olecranon fossa. *FP,* Fat pad.

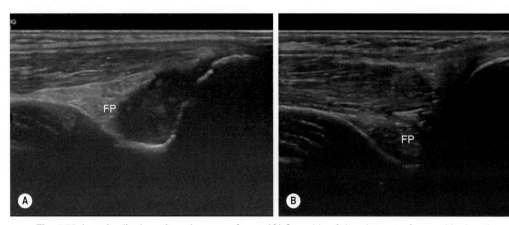

Fig. 4.50 Longitudinal section olecranon fossa. **(A)** Synovitis of the olecranon fossa with elevation of the fat pad. **(B)** Normal contralateral olecranon fossa. *FP,* Fat pad.

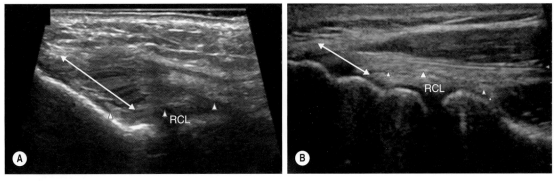

Fig. 4.51 Lateral epicondylitis. *Double arrow,* Common extensor origin. **(A)** Tendinopathic thickened echolucent tendon with disruption to fibrillar pattern. **(B)** Normal study. *Triangles,* Underlying radial collateral ligament *(RCL).*

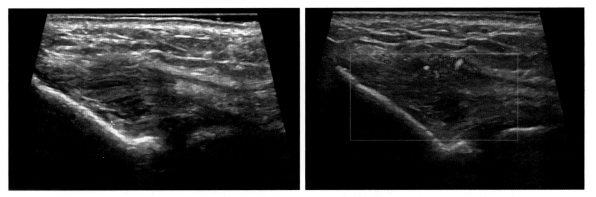

Fig. 4.52 Same patient as Fig. 4.51A, with clear intrasubstance tears and hyperemia of the extensor carpi radialis brevis and extensor digitorum communis portion of the common extensor origin.

injections may improve pain and functional outcomes in the short term, the long-term consequence may exacerbate further tendon degeneration. Injection of autologous blood or plasma rich protein are proving the most effective treatments in the longer term.[21,22]

Acute tendon rupture of the CFO or CEO is more likely to occur due to sports injury in a background of tendinopathy. In cases of acute traumatic tears within the tendon itself rather than at the musculotendinous junction, early increases in loading may cause the formation of mediocre scar tissue. After 6 to 8 weeks, or earlier in musculotendinous injury, progressive loading can be cautiously started.

Occasionally, these symptoms can be due to a more widespread inflammatory arthropathy such as psoriatic arthritis and, although ultrasound appearances may be similar, the clinical history may be atypical.

REPORT—RIGHT LATERAL EPICONDYLITIS

Clinical History: Works as chef, pain right lateral elbow, query soft tissue injury

US Forearm Rt:

Right-handed chef. Focal pain over right lateral epicondyle. The right common extensor origin (CEO) is swollen, of overall decreased reflectivity with focal anechoic areas in keeping with tendinopathy and small intratendinous tears.

There is marked neovascularity of the more anterior-superficial portion of the CEO, those more associated the extensor carpi radialis brevis.

The underlying radial collateral ligament and lateral ulnar collateral ligament are of normal appearance.

There is no joint effusion.

Summary: Appearances in keeping with right CEO tendinopathy.

Distal Biceps Tendon Tear

Distal biceps injury is usually as a result of a fall or from lifting a heavy weight. It is important to establish if there has been a partial or full thickness tear (i.e., both tendon portions), whether this involves an avulsion from the radial tuberosity, or whether a full or partial tear has occurred proximally, leaving an intact attachment to the radial tuberosity, as this could influence surgical intervention. Proximal retraction of both biceps muscle bulks is associated with full thickness tears. If there is involvement of the lacertus fibrosus (LF), with a tear close to the musculotendinous junction, there is likely to be marked proximal retraction of the biceps muscle as well as abnormal thickening of the LF (comparison should be made with the contralateral side).[1]

Surgical intervention is a clinical decision on an individual case basis. Conservative treatment may be considered in patients with low demand, but supination (long head portion), and to a lesser extent elbow flexion (short head portion), strength will be reduced. As with all partial tears, a period of relative rest should be followed by progressive strengthening.

The images shown in Figs. 4.53–4.55A show an example of a proximal full thickness tear of both the short and long biceps tendon heads, with the LF remaining intact. The torn retracted conjoint tendon/muscle causes a clinical "reverse Popeye" sign when the elbow is flexed against resistance. In this particular case, a stump of intact tendon remains attached at the radial insertion (Figs. 4.55 and 4.56).

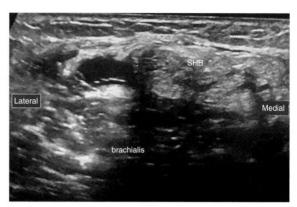

Fig. 4.54 Same case as Fig. 4.53. Transverse section over right biceps proximal of the myotendinous junction, showing retraction and atrophy of the short head muscle bulk. The long head portion had retracted proximal of this image. *SHB,* Short head biceps

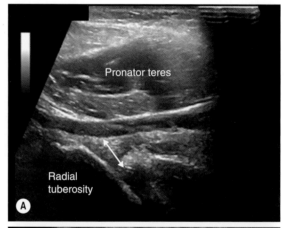

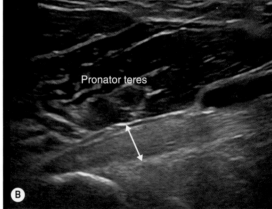

Fig. 4.55 (A) Same case as Figs. 4.53 and 4.54. Distal insertion of the biceps with disruption to the normal fibrillar pattern due to a proximal tear and retraction of this portion of distal tendon. **(B)** Comparative example of normal distal biceps.

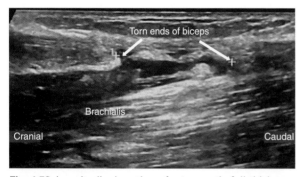

Fig. 4.53 Longitudinal section of a traumatic full thickness tear of the distal biceps.

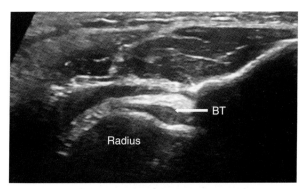

Fig. 4.56 Same case as Figs. 4.53 and 4.54, in the "cobra" scan position, confirming an intact distal biceps *(BT)* attachment.

REPORT—TEAR OF THE DISTAL BICEPS TENDON

Clinical History: Lifting weights. Pain and "Popeye sign"? ruptured distal biceps.

US Upper arm Rt:

Injury 6 days ago

There is marked disruption and a complex echolucent collection, which is likely to represent blood, at the musculotendinous junction of the distal biceps. Dynamic scanning during passive resisted flexion confirms a complete tear involving both the long head and short head portions.

There is retraction of the distal portion of the tendon. The insertion onto the radial tuberosity remains intact.

The lacertus fibrosus remains intact.

Summary: Proximal full thickness tear of the distal biceps.

Bicipitoradial Bursitis

As discussed previously, the BRB is located on the radial aspect of the biceps insertion[23] and is not visible when normal. Osteophytosis at the radial tuberosity can cause attritional bursitis as in the following case (Figs. 4.57 and 4.58). Clinical management of bursitis will vary but may include rest, isometric loading, an injection of steroid for short-term relief, preferably under ultrasound guidance, or possibly surgical intervention to remove the source of impingement.

Olecranon Bursitis

The olecranon bursal sac within the subcutaneous tissue overlying the olecranon process of the elbow

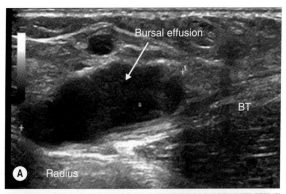

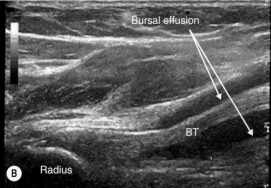

Fig. 4.57 (A) Longitudinal section biceps *(BT)* insertion with distended bicipitoradial bursa. **(B)** Same case, showing extension of the effusion surrounding the tendon, mimicking a sheath effusion.

REPORT—BICIPITORADIAL BURSITIS

Clinical History: Right antecubital fossa painless lump.

US Rt elbow:

The palpable lump in the antecubital fossa is a thin-walled anechoic, avascular lesion extending along the length of the distal biceps tendon to the musculotendinous junction. This has the typical appearance of a moderate bicipitoradial bursa. The biceps tendon is intact, but there is evidence of distal insertional tendinopathy and osteophytosis of the radial tuberosity.

Summary: Appearances in keeping with attritional bicipitoradial bursitis.

---

contains a small amount of fluid that is not visible when normal. Bursitis refers to an inflammatory process where there is proliferation of bursal tissue and fluid, which may be painful. Causes include excessive leaning on the elbow, the so called "student elbow,"

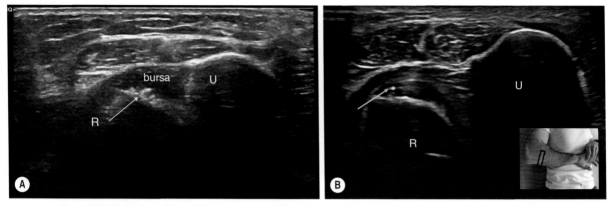

Fig. 4.58 "Cobra" position. **(A)** Same case as Fig. 4.57, showing marked radial osteophytosis with tendino-pathic distal tendon and bicipitoradial bursitis. **(B)** Different case, showing minor asymptomatic osteophytosis, normal tendon, no bursitis. *R*, Radius; *U*, Ulna. Insert, patient/probe position.

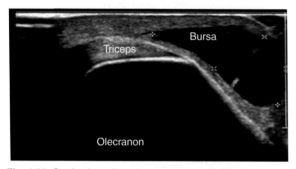

Fig. 4.59 Sagittal section olecranon bursal effusion.

REPORT—OLECRANON BURSITIS

Clinical History: Swelling over elbow, ? Bursitis.

US Rt elbow:

Mr. B reports that the swelling has been present for several months following trauma to the elbow. The swelling has reduced a little in size and is no longer painful.

There is a 3.5 cm × 2.0 cm × 1.5 cm unilocular, anechoic, thin-walled collection overlying the olecranon process of the elbow. There is no associated vascularity to suggest an acute inflammatory process or any echogenic foci to suggest loose bodies.

Summary: The appearance is in keeping with a recalcitrant olecranon bursal effusion.

---

acute or repetitive trauma, infection, or systemic autoimmune conditions such as rheumatoid arthritis or gout. On ultrasound there will be a unilocular or multiloculated collection, superficial to the olecranon process, which may be thin-walled and anechoic (Fig. 4.59), or thick-walled with obvious synovial proliferation, with or without associated hyperemia, occasionally containing loose bodies. For clinical management, as always, history is important. Mild compression of the tissues with or without aspiration and avoiding the cause of pressure on the area is often effective management.

Triceps Tear

This is a less common tendon injury due to the large insertional area of the tendon onto the olecranon, which can also make it difficult to differentiate clinically from other conditions (e.g., tennis elbow). Triceps tendon tears are usually caused by excessive force trying to bend the elbow whilst the triceps is performing extension (e.g., during a pushing activity), more commonly in the male 30 to 50 age group. Tears usually occur at the tendon-osseous junction and less so at the myotendinous junction. With ultrasound imaging there will be disruption and loss of the normal fibrillar pattern of the tendon/muscle fibres with an effusion or complex blood-filled collection within the torn component (Figs. 4.60–4.62). A full thickness tear involves all three heads, including the less commonly torn medial head, and requires surgical intervention.[24] Partial tears are often managed conservatively considering function, patient expectation, and coexisting conditions.

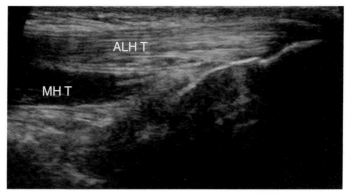

Fig. 4.60 Longitudinal section normal triceps tendon for comparison. *ALH T,* Aponeurosis lateral/long head of triceps; *MH T,* muscular medial head.

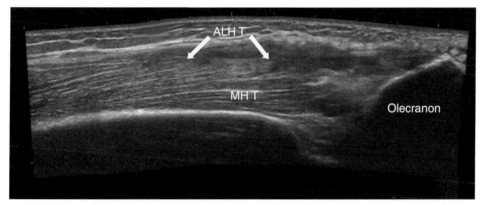

Fig. 4.61 Triceps tear. Longitudinal section view of triceps brachii, with a retracted tear of the aponeurosis of the lateral/long head. The medial fibres remain intact. *ALH T,* Aponeurosis of lateral/long head of triceps; *MH T,* medial head of triceps.

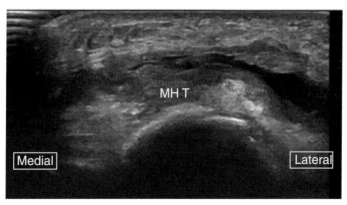

Fig. 4.62 Transverse view over left distal triceps, showing fluid within the tear of the lateral head, with the medial head remaining attached.

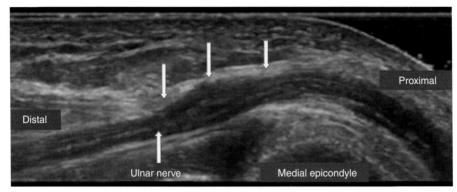

Fig. 4.63 Longitudinal ulnar nerve through the cubital tunnel. Note swelling and loss of parallel fascicular reflectivity. *Arrows* marking the extent of the Osbourne retinaculum (see normal ulnar nerve Fig. 4.36).

REPORT—TRICEPS TEAR

Clinical History: Pain elbow region following workout at the gym.

US Rt arm:

Injury 14 days ago. The specific point of pain is over the distal triceps where there is disruption and proximal retraction of the lateral/long head of the triceps tendon. There is an anechoic collection within the torn components, in keeping with an effusion or blood collection. The gap between the torn components extends to approx. 3 cm. In comparison with the contralateral side, the lateral head of triceps muscle bulk is smaller and of abnormally increased reflectivity in keeping with atrophy. The medial head maintains the normal fibrillar pattern remains intact.

Summary: Large retracted tear of the lateral/long head of triceps tendon but the medial head remains intact.

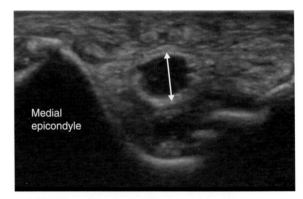

Fig. 4.64 Transverse scan of the abnormal ulnar nerve. *Double arrow,* Swollen ulnar nerve, with loss of normal "sponge-like" reflectivity (see normal ulnar nerve, Fig. 4.34).

Cubital Tunnel Syndrome

The ulnar nerve is subject to pressure and stretching injury against the medial tunnel boundaries, particularly if the elbow remains in the flexed position for extended times, e.g., whilst asleep. The nerve becomes swollen and hypoechoic with loss of the normal fascicular linear pattern. There may be a significant change in calibre of the nerve, proximal, through, and distal of the cubital tunnel (Figs. 4.63 and 4.64).

Dislocation of the nerve from the tunnel may be evident on full elbow flexion. Identifying this is important, not only if surgical intervention is being considered, but also if therapeutic injections of the CFO are being undertaken, as the nerve may lie superficial to the CFO on flexion.

Always consider the possibility of extrinsic space–occupying lesions, such as osteophytosis, effusions, or anomalous muscles, that may be causing extrinsic compression.[16,17]

Consider medial epicondylitis as a differential cause for the medial elbow pain and assess the common flexor origin whilst examining the region.

Conservative management is often effective, particularly in mild cases, with rest and education of behavior modification being the most important factors. Splinting may also have a role along with specific exercises to mobilise the ulnar nerve. Symptomatic cases of dislocation will require surgical opinion and may involving ulnar nerve transposition surgery.[25]

REPORT—ULNAR NERVE NEURITIS

Clinical History: Pain right elbow with tingling to ring and little finger, which wakes her at night.

US Rt elbow:

Mrs. B~reports her pain is worse at night. She sleeps with her arm bent under her pillow.

There is fusiform swelling of the ulnar nerve throughout the cubital tunnel. The nerve is of decreased reflectivity with loss of fascicular pattern in keeping with oedema. The nerve is of normal calibre proximal to the Osbourne retinaculum and returns to normal calibre distal to the heads of the flexor carpi ulnaris muscle. There is no evidence of an extrinsic lesion compressing the nerve. There is no evidence of anomalous musculature. On full flexion, the nerve remains stable within the cubital tunnel.

Summary: Appearances in keeping with ulnar nerve neuritis.

⊚ SUMMARY OF TIPS FOR THE CHAPTER

1. Use a bolster under the elbow to allow unhindered probe access.
2. Toggle over the joint to view perpendicular to the hyaline cartilage.
3. Scan distal of the capsular insertions, especially at the radial head, as the synovial recesses extend beyond the joint line.
4. In the absence of trauma, muscular atrophy may indicate denervation injury.
5. Proximal retraction of the distal biceps bulk is associated with full thickness tears.

MULTIPLE CHOICE QUESTIONS

1. Which part of the distal biceps tendon is more commonly involved in traumatic injury?
   a) Short head portion
   b) Lacertus fibrosis
   c) Long head portion

2. What is the most sensitive site for detecting an elbow joint effusion?
   a) Cubital fossa
   b) Radial fossa
   c) Olecranon fossa

3. How would one dynamically assess the integrity of the distal biceps whilst scanning?
   a) Hook test
   b) Resisted flexion
   c) Resisted extension

4. What does the anatomical acronym BAM stand for?
   a) Brachioradialis, artery, median nerve
   b) Brachialis, artery, median nerve,
   c) Biceps, artery, median nerve

5. If a traumatic biceps tendon injury is suspected, but excluded, what other structure should be assessed?
   a) Brachioradialis
   b) Brachialis
   c) Bicipitoradial bursa

REFERENCES

1. Bianchi S, Martinoli C. Ultrasound of the musculoskeletal system. Berlin Heidelberg: Springer-Verlag; 2007:350–407.
2. Martinoli C, Della Casa Alberighi O, Di Minno G, et al. Development and definition of a simplified scanning procedure and scoring method for Haemophilia Early Arthropathy Detection with Ultrasound (HEAD-US). Thromb Haemost. 2013;109(6):1170–1179.
3. Jacobson JA. Fundamentals of radiology: fundamentals of musculoskeletal ultrasound. Philadelphia: Elsevier; 2018.
4. Beggs I, Bianchi S, Bueno A, et al. Musculoskeletal ultrasound technical guidelines. European Society of Musculoskeletal Radiology; 2006. Available at; https://essr.org/content-essr/uploads/2016/10/elbow.pdf
5. Jarrett CD, Weir DM, Stuffmann ES, Jain S, Miller MC, Schmidt CC. Anatomic and biomechanical analysis of the short and long head components of the distal biceps tendon. J Shoulder Elbow Surg. 2012;21:942–948.
6. Tagliafico A, Michaud J, Capaccio E, Derchi LE, Martinoli C. Ultrasound demonstration of distal biceps tendon bifurcation: normal and abnormal findings. Eur Radiol. 2010;20(1):202–208.

7. Tagliafico AS, Bignotti B, Martinoli C. Elbow US: anatomy, variants, and scanning technique. Radiology. 2015;275(3):636–650.

8. Seiler JG III, Parker LM, Chamberland PD, Sherbourne GM, Carpenter WA. The distal biceps tendon. Two potential mechanisms involved in its rupture: arterial supply and mechanical impingement. J Shoulder Elbow Surg. 1995;4:149–156.

9. Voleti PB, Berkowitz JL, Konin GP, Cordasco FA. Rupture of the short head component of a bifurcated distal biceps tendon. J Shoulder Elbow Surg. 2017;26:403–408.

10. Kalume Brigido M, De Maeseneer M, Jacobson JA, Jamadar DA, Morag Y, Marcelis S. Improved visualisation of the radial insertion of the biceps tendon at ultrasound with a lateral approach. Eur Radiol. 2009;19(7):1871–1821.

11. Giuffre BM, Lisle DA. Tear of the distal biceps brachii tendon: a new method of ultrasound evaluation. Australas Radiol. 2005;49(5):404–406.

12. Tagliafico A, Michaud J, Perez MM, Martinoli C. Ultrasound of distal brachialis tendon attachment: normal and abnormal findings. Br J Radiol. 2013;86(1025): 20130004.

13. De Maeseneer M, Brigido MK, Antic M, et al. Ultrasound of the elbow with emphasis on detailed assessment of ligaments, tendons, and nerves. Eur J Radiol. 2015;84(4): 671–681. Available at: http://dx.doi.org/10.1016/j.ejrad. 2014.12.007.

14. Michelin P, Leleup G, Ould-Slimane M, Merlet MC, Dubourg B, Duparc F. Ultrasound biomechanical anatomy of the soft structures in relation to the ulnar nerve in the cubital tunnel of the elbow. Surg Radiol Anat. 2017;39: 1215–1221.

15. Martinoli C, Perez MM, Padua L, et al. Muscle variants of the upper and lower limb (with anatomical correlation). Semin Musculoskelet Radiol. 2010;14(2):106–121.

16. O'Hara JJ. *Ulnar nerve compression* at the elbow caused by a prominent *medial head* of the *triceps* and an anconeus epitrochlearis. J Hand Surg Br. 1996;21(1): 133–135.

17. Miller TT, Reinus WR. Nerve entrapment syndromes of the elbow, forearm and wrist. AJR Am J Roentgenol. 2010;195:585–594.

18. Xiao TG, Cartwright MS. Ultrasound in the evaluation of radial neuropathies at the elbow. Front Neurol. 2019; 10:216.

19. Marsell R, Einhorn TA. The biology of fracture healing. Injury. 2011;42(6):551–555. doi:10.1016/j.injury.2011.03.031.

20. Buchbinder R, Green S, Youd JM, Assendelft WJJ, Barnsley L, Smidt N. Shock wave therapy for lateral elbow pain. Cochrane Database Syst Rev 2005;(4): CD003524. doi:10.1002/14651858.CD003524.pub2.

21. Hastie G, Soufi M, Wilson J, Roy B. Platelet rich plasma injections for lateral epicondylitis of the elbow reduce the need for surgical intervention. J Orthop 2018;15(1): 239–241.

22. Houck DA, Kraeutler MJ, Thornton LB, McCarty EC, Bravman JT. Treatment of lateral epicondylitis with autologous blood, platelet-rich plasma, or corticosteroid injections: a systematic review of overlapping meta-analyses. Orthop J Sports Med. 2019;7(3): 2325967119831052.

23. Draghi F, Gregoli B, Sileo C. Sonography of the bicipito-radial bursa: a short pictorial essay. J Ultrasound. 2012;15(1):39–41. doi:10.1016/j.jus.2012.02.003.

24. Tagliafico A, Gandolfo N, Michaud J, Perez MM, Palmieri F, Martinoli C. Ultrasound demonstration of distal triceps tendon tears. Eur Radiol. 2012;81(6):1207–1210.

25. Catalano LW III, Barron OA. Anterior subcutaneous transposition of the ulnar nerve. Hand Clin. 2007;23(3): 339–344.

5

Ultrasound of the Hand and Wrist

Sophie Cochran, Sara Riley, and Mark Maybury

LEARNING OBJECTIVES

After reading this chapter you should have gained an understanding of:
- Relevant anatomical structures of the hand and wrist
- Ultrasound technique and normal appearances of the hand and wrist including tips and pitfalls
- Clinical tests and dynamic assessment which may help interpret findings
- Common pathologies and their ultrasound appearances
- The place of other imaging modalities

INTRODUCTION

Like most musculoskeletal ultrasound, assessment of the hand and wrist is often focused to answer a specific question relevant to the history and clinical examination.

PATIENT POSITIONING, EQUIPMENT, AND PHYSICAL EXAMINATION

Patient comfort and operator ergonomics are both important when considering scanning positions. These are discussed in more detail in Chapter 10. A pad/cushion to raise the hand/wrist away from the examination surface may increase manoeuverability and help with dynamic assessment.

Advances in technology have led to the development of small footprint, high frequency transducers[1] which are ideally suited to imaging the small, superficial structures of the hand and wrist in detail.

Physical examination can be challenging in patients presenting with wrist and hand pain because there may be considerable overlap in symptoms from structures that are closely related. The origins of many of the muscles responsible for actions of the hands are within the forearm/elbow; extending the scan to include these areas may be necessary for a comprehensive examination. Taking a brief clinical history and asking about injury, triggers, and the site and spread of pain may supplement clinical information provided on the request card, helping to direct the ultrasound examination.

The wrist can be separated into zones for examination purposes.[2] Fig. 5.1 presents a comprehensive list of pathologies that can occur within the five zones. It is worth noting that some symptoms are not exclusive to each condition/compartment and that not all pathologies listed can be diagnosed with ultrasound.

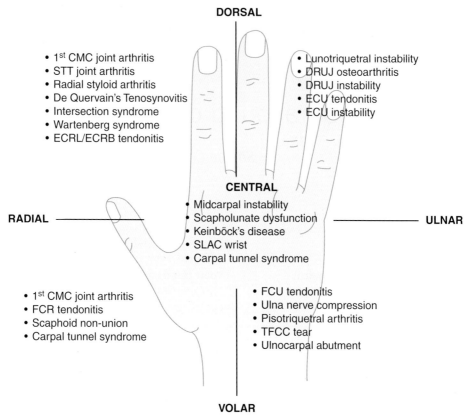

DORSAL

- 1st CMC joint arthritis
- STT joint arthritis
- Radial styloid arthritis
- De Quervain's Tenosynovitis
- Intersection syndrome
- Wartenberg syndrome
- ECRL/ECRB tendonitis

- Lunotriquetral instability
- DRUJ osteoarthritis
- DRUJ instability
- ECU tendonitis
- ECU instability

CENTRAL
- Midcarpal instability
- Scapholunate dysfunction
- Keinböck's disease
- SLAC wrist
- Carpal tunnel syndrome

RADIAL   **ULNAR**

- 1st CMC joint arthritis
- FCR tendonitis
- Scaphoid non-union
- Carpal tunnel syndrome

- FCU tendonitis
- Ulna nerve compression
- Pisotriquetral arthritis
- TFCC tear
- Ulnocarpal abutment

VOLAR

Fig. 5.1 Pathologies occurring in the five zones of the wrist. *CMC,* carpometacarpal; *DRUJ,* distal radio-ulnar joint; *ECRB/ECRU,* extensor carpi radialis brevis/ extensor carpi radialis longus; *ECU,* extensor carpi ulnaris; *FCR,* flexor carpi radialis; *FCU,* flexor carpi ulnaris; *SLAC,* scaphoid lunate advanced collapse; *STT,* scaphotrapeziotrapezoid; *TFCC,* triangular fibrocartilage complex.

JOINTS OF THE WRIST AND HAND

Anatomy

The wrist (carpus) is composed of the radioulnar, radio-carpal, ulnocarpal, midcarpal, and carpometacarpal synovial articulations (Fig. 5.2).[3]

Fibrocartilage separates many of the bones of the wrist. The fibrocartilage which extends between the base of the ulnar head, the lunate and triquetrum bones, deep to the extensor carpi ulnaris (ECU) tendon, is part of the stabilising triangular fibrocartilage complex (TFCC) which includes the radioulnar and ulnocarpal ligaments.[4]

Intrinsic and extrinsic ligaments run between the bony articulations of the wrist, most of which are difficult to

visualise with ultrasound due to their size and anatomical position. Confirmation of the presence of a ligament on ultrasound (comparable with the asymptomatic side) is often useful to a referrer, although it is not a guarantee of injury/pathology and magnetic resonance imaging (MRI) may be the preferred imaging modality.[5,6]

In the fingers, the metacarpophalangeal (MCP), proximal interphalangeal (PIP), and distal interphalangeal (DIP) joints are synovial articulations with prominent dorsal joint recesses. In contrast, there are only two joints in the thumb; MCP and interphalangeal (IP) joints. Each joint is stabilised by ulnar and radial collateral ligaments. The volar plates are ligamentous intra-articular structures which reinforce the joints, limiting hyperextension.

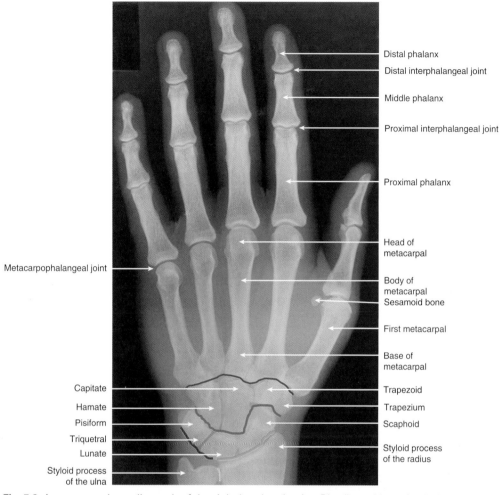

Fig. 5.2 Anteroposterior radiograph of the right hand and wrist. *Blue line;* midcarpal articulations; *green line;* radiocarpal articulations; *purple line:* ulnocarpal articulations; *red line;* carpometacarpal articulations; *yellow line;* radioulnar articulations.

Technique and Ultrasound Appearances

Figure 5.3 demonstrates the bony surface anatomy of the dorsal and volar wrist. These landmarks can help locate structures during an ultrasound examination.

Joints

Ultrasound referrals to assess all the joints of the hand and wrist are usually for diagnostic evaluation of clinically occult inflammation. Joint assessment for inflammatory arthropathy is explained in more detail in Chapter 10. Ultrasound examination of an individual joint is more likely following injury or to assess the origin/nature of a soft tissue swelling.

The joints of the wrist are assessed in longitudinal section from the dorsal surface where they are most superficial. It is worth noting that thin synovial folds may be seen arising from the joints which are normal and should not be mistaken for synovial hypertrophy[7,8] (Fig. 5.4). If the wrist is flexed during a dynamic scan, these normal folds should disappear.

Joints of the digits can be examined from the dorsal or palmar/volar aspects; however, the dorsal approach is considered the most effective, as the tight capsule/volar plate on the volar surface can compress fluid, synovial

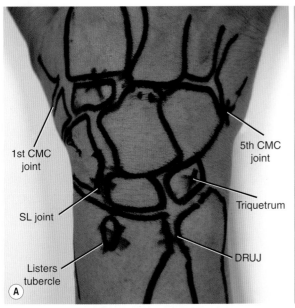
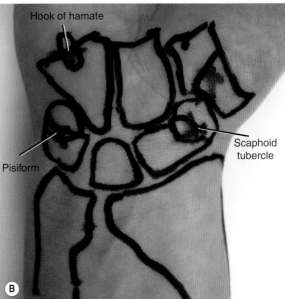

Fig. 5.3 Bony surface anatomy of the wrist. **(A)** Dorsal. **(B)** Volar. *CMC,* carpometacarpal; *DRUJ,* distal radioulnar joint; *SL,* scapholunate.

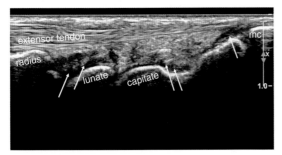

Fig. 5.4 Wrist articulations. Longitudinal section dorsal wrist, from the radiocarpal articulation between the radius and lunate, midcarpal, to the base of the metacarpal *(mc).* Folds of synovium *(arrows).*

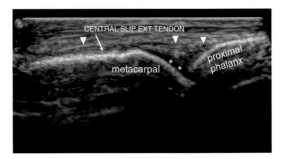

Fig. 5.5 Longitudinal section normal metacarpophalangeal joint. *Arrows,* proximal synovial recess; *arrowheads,* joint capsule; **,* cartilage.

hypertrophy, and neovascularity, all signs of joint inflammation (Figs. 5.5 and 5.6). Using a systematic approach in both longitudinal and transverse sections, care should be taken to ensure that as much of the joint as possible is assessed by including the ulnar and radial aspects. Grey scale and Doppler imaging should be used to assess for inflammatory changes (see Chapter 10). It is particularly important to avoid excessive transducer pressure, as this inhibits the identification of effusion and neovascularity.

The volar plates are identified by placing the transducer longitudinally over the volar/palmar aspect of the

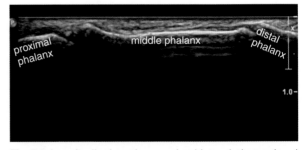

Fig. 5.6 Longitudinal section proximal interphalangeal and distal interphalangeal joints.

joints. They appear as a triangular hyperechoic structure superficial to the articular cartilage[7,8] (Fig. 5.7).

Ligaments

Two of the ligaments which can be readily evaluated with ultrasound are the ulnar collateral ligament of the thumb (UCL) and the scapholunate ligament in the wrist.

The UCL of the thumb is examined by placing the patient's hand palm down and rotating the thumb so that the radial aspect is in contact with the examination surface (Fig. 5.8A). The transducer is then placed longitudinally across the ulnar aspect of the MCP joint, near the soft tissue/webbing between the thumb and index

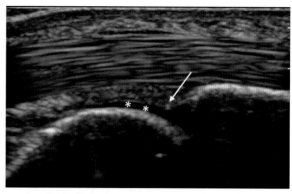

Fig. 5.7 Volar aspect of the metacarpophalangeal joint. *Arrow*, Volar plate; *, cartilage.

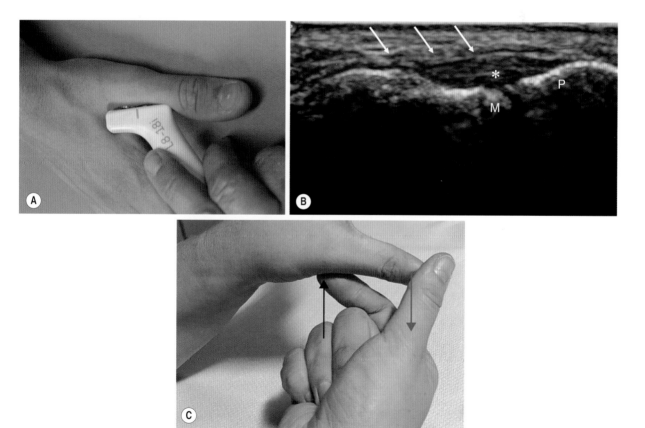

Fig. 5.8 Ulnar collateral ligament. (A) Probe position for ulnar collateral ligament (UCL) of the thumb. **(B)** UCL *(*)* extending between the metacarpal *(M)* and proximal phalanx *(P)* with the overlying adductor aponeurosis *(arrows)*. **(C)** Photo demonstrating the method for stressing the thumb UCL with the operators index finger exerting gentle pressure upwards and their thumb exerting gentle pressure downwards.

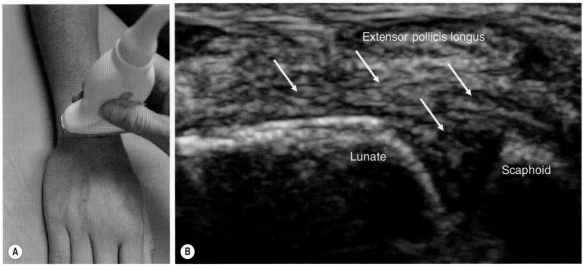

Fig. 5.9 Scapholunate ligament. **(A)** Transverse section wrist **(B)** shows the components of the SLL *(arrows).*

finger. The normal UCL is a hyperechoic band spanning the ulnar side of the MCP joint (Fig. 5.8B). The smooth concavities on the bone surface of the distal metacarpal and proximal phalanx are the footprints of the ligament attachments.[6,9]

Dynamic assessment during the ultrasound examination, using the clinical thumb abduction stress test can help identification of pathology. This test is performed by raising the patient's hand on a pad/cushion and leaving the thumb in free air; while scanning, stabilise the metacarpal of the affected hand and apply varus strain force (radial deviation) to the phalanx, causing tensioning in the UCL (Fig. 5.8C).

The scapholunate (SLL) ligament is scanned with the palm of the hand down over a cushion or raised so there is slight flexion of the wrist. By locating Lister's tubercle (see Fig 5.13) with the transducer in transverse (Fig 5.9A) the surfaces of the radius and ulna can be seen. Scan slowly distally until the surfaces of three bones can be seen: from the radial side these are the scaphoid, lunate, and triquetrum. The normal SLL appears as a hyperechoic, fibrillar structure extending between the scaphoid and lunate (Fig. 5.9B).[9–11]

Dynamic assessment: stressing SLL can be achieved by asking the patient to form a fist during the scan, though it is worth noting that there is considerable variation in the normal width of these joints and their

reaction to stress; comparison with the unaffected wrist is suggested.

DORSAL HAND AND WRIST TENDONS (AND ADJACENT STRUCTURES)

Anatomy

The extensor retinaculum is a strong fibrous/ligamentous band which maintains the position of the dorsal wrist tendons (Fig. 5.10)[3]. It attaches laterally to the radius and medially to the triquetral and pisiform. Fibrous septae from the retinaculum run deep towards the radius to form six fibro-osseous compartments, which contain the extensor tendons.

From the radial to ulnar aspect, the six tendon compartments (I–VI) have separate synovial sheaths, shown in green in Fig. 5.10, which can be up to 7 cm in length and terminate at the level of the proximal metacarpals.[9] Distally over the digits, the tendons have a thin superficial covering of synovium, a paratenon rather than a full sheath.

Compartment I contains the extensor pollicis brevis (EPB) and abductor pollicis longus tendons (APL).[12] It is aligned with the base of the first metacarpal and forms the lateral/radial border of the anatomical snuff box (Fig. 5.11).

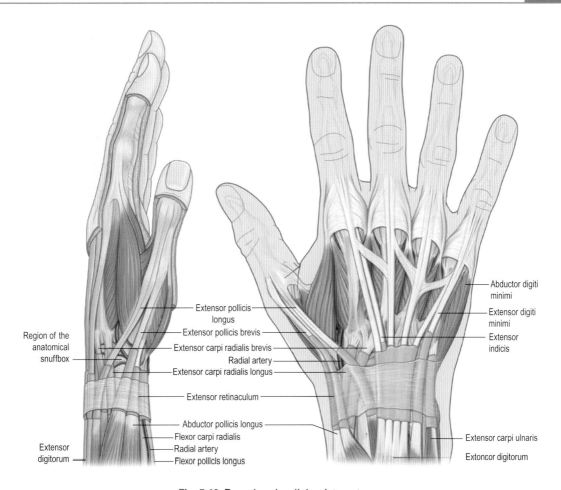

Extensor pollicis longus

Extensor pollicis brevis

Extensor carpi radialis brevis

Radial artery

Extensor carpi radialis longus

Region of the anatomical snuffbox

Extensor retinaculum

Abductor pollicis longus

Flexor carpi radialis

Radial artery

Flexor polllcls longus

Extensor digitorum

Abductor digiti minimi

Extensor digiti minimi

Extensor indicis

Extensor carpi ulnaris

Extoncor digitorum

Fig. 5.10 Dorsal and radial wrist anatomy.

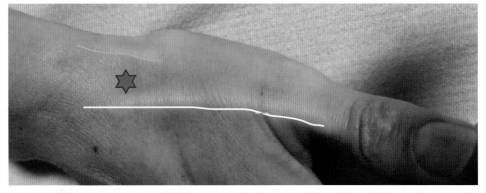

Fig. 5.11 Photo of the right hand depicting the anatomical snuff box. *Green line;* lateral/radial border of the anatomical snuff box—extensor compartment I; *blue star;* centre of the anatomical snuff box—extensor compartment II, also the location of the radial neurovascular bundle; *white line;* dorsal/ulna border of the anatomical sniff box—extensor compartment III.

Anatomical variations include multiple slips of APL which should not be confused with synovial hypertrophy or longitudinal tendon splitting.[10] The EPB and APL tendons may be separated by a vertical septum and these patients may be more susceptible to stenosing De Quervain's tenosynovitis (see Pathology).

Compartment II contains the extensor carpi radialis brevis (ECRB) and extensor carpi radialis longus (ECRL) tendons. This compartment lies within the centre of the anatomical snuff box. Anatomic variations include an accessory ECR tendon, seen in 10% to 24% of individuals, running within extensor compartment II or more rarely through a separate fascial tunnel.[13]

Compartment III contains the extensor pollicis longus (EPL) tendon on the radial aspect of Lister's tubercle. This helpful landmark is located on the dorsal aspect of the distal radius. Another tip which can aid the identification of this compartment is that it forms the dorsal/ulnar border of the anatomical snuff box.

Compartment IV contains the extensor tendons of digits 2 to 4. These are extensor digitorum communis (EDC), a conjoined tendon proximally, which divides into four extensor digitorum longus (EDL) slips distally, and extensor indicis proprius (EIP) which aids extension of the index finger.

Compartment V contains extensor digiti minimi (EDM), the little finger tendon.[11]

Compartment VI contains the extensor carpi ulnaris (ECU) tendon which lies within the ulnar groove, lateral to the ulnar styloid process – a palpable projection of bone extending distally from the dorsal surface of the ulna.[11]

The radial artery, nerve, and veins lie on the radial aspect of the wrist within the anatomical snuff box.[11]

At the dorsal aspect of each of the four fingers, the central slip of the EDL tendon attaches to the base of the middle phalanx, whereas slips of the extensor tendon that contribute to the lateral bands attach to the distal phalanx. The MCP joints have an overlying aponeurotic sheet or extensor hood, which consists of transverse-oriented sagittal bands that stabilise the extensor tendons (Fig. 5.12).[3,12]

The EIP tendon joins the ulnar side of the index EDL tendon at the level of the metacarpal head of the index finger. The EDM tendon divides into two as it crosses the hand and finally joins the EDL tendon of the fifth finger where the conjoined tendons insert at the dorsal extensor expansion.[6,7]

Technique and Normal Ultrasound Appearances

With the palm of the hand down and the transducer in the transverse position, the starting point is Lister's tubercle (Fig. 5.13) on the distal radius.

From this point it is then easy to move between the different extensor tendon compartments shown in panoramic view in Fig. 5.14.[11] If Lister's tubercle is not present on the initial ultrasound image, moving the transducer slowly proximally or distally will bring it in to view.

It may be necessary to vary the wrist position to enable access and better dynamic assessment of some of the wrist compartments. For instance, the tendons in compartment I are best examined with the patient's wrist in a lateral position (thumb up) (Fig. 5.15). Compartment II can be assessed either with the wrist in a lateral (thumb up) position or with the hand palm down (Fig. 5.16).[11] It is important to note that the tendons of compartment II are crossed in the forearm at an angle of 60 degrees, by the musculotendinous junctions of the first extensor compartment (approximately 4cm proximal to Lister's tubercle). This can be the site of pain due to excessive friction between the two compartments and is known as proximal intersection syndrome. In this condition there may be tenosynovitis of the tendons in compartment II (see pathology section) and therefore it may be necessary to extend the examination into the forearm.

In compartment III, EPL is easily located on the ulnar side of Lister's tubercle and as the dorsal/ulnar border of the anatomical snuff box.

As this tendon is followed distally to its insertion, it can be seen to cross superficial to the tendons within compartment II (Fig. 5.17). Pain at the intersection of compartments II and III is known as distal intersection syndrome (see pathology section).

The tendons within compartment IV and V (Fig. 5.18) can be followed distally to the fingers. Moving each finger whilst scanning the tendons in transverse at the wrist may help define each individual tendon.

It is worth noting that the extensor retinaculum is at its thickest over compartment IV at the wrist, creating a hypoechoic band which may be mistaken for tenosynovitis by less experienced operators (see Fig. 5.18A).

Another pitfall that may simulate tenosynovitis at the wrist is misinterpreting the normal hypoechoic muscle at the musculotendinous junction as effusion. This can be avoided by confirming the normal tapering of muscle tissue in two imaging planes.[9–11,13] Ascertaining if direct palpation

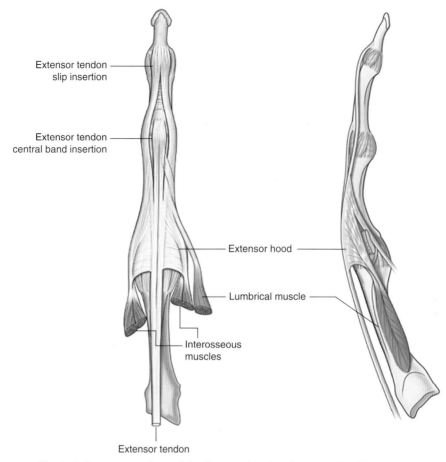

Extensor tendon
slip insertion

Extensor tendon
central band insertion

Extensor hood

Lumbrical muscle

Interosseous
muscles

Extensor tendon

Fig. 5.12 Extensor tendons of the fingers showing the central and lateral slips.

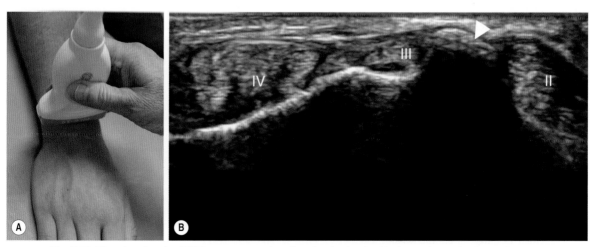

Fig. 5.13 Lister's tubercle. **(A)** Transverse section dorsal wrist level with the probe at the level of Lister's tubercle. **(B)** Lister's tubercle *(arrowhead)* with the adjacent II, III, and IV extensor compartments.

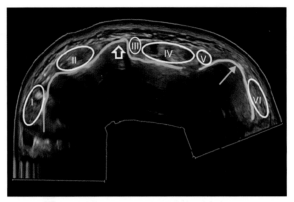

Fig. 5.14 Transverse section dorsal wrist. The six extensor compartments are numbered and outlined with white circles. *Blue arrow;* ulna styloid process; *blue line;* surface of the ulna; *green line;* surface of the radius; *white arrow;* Lister's tubercle.

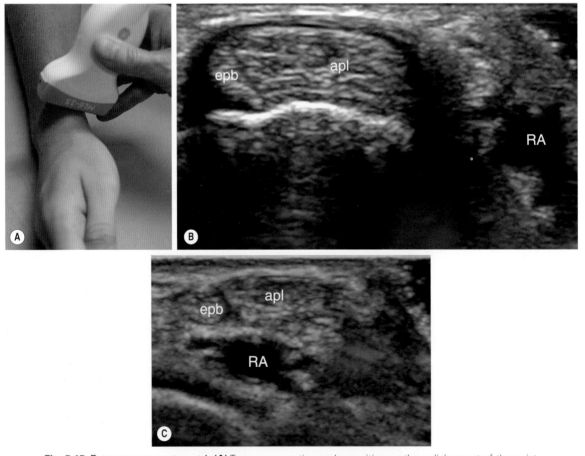

Fig. 5.15 Extensor compartment I. (A) Transverse section probe position on the radial aspect of the wrist, thumb up. Relationship of the radial artery *(RA)*, abductor pollicis longus *(apl)*, and extensor pollicis brevis tendons *(epb)* in **(B)** the proximal and **(C)** distal wrist.

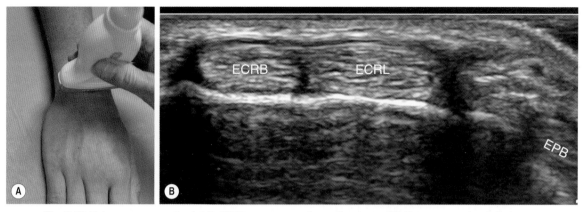

Fig. 5.16 Extensor compartment II. **(A)** Transverse section palm down. **(B)** Extensor carpi radialis longus *(ERCL)*, on the radial side, and extensor carpi radialis brevis *(ECRB)* on the ulnar side. *EPB*, extensor pollicis brevis.

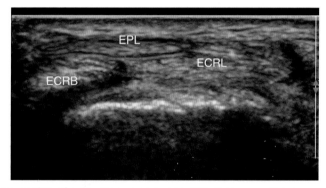

Fig. 5.17 Transverse section of extensor compartments II/III. Extensor pollicis longus *(EPL)* crosses over the extensor carpi radialis longus *(ECRL)* and extensor carpi radialis brevis *(ECRB)* tendons.

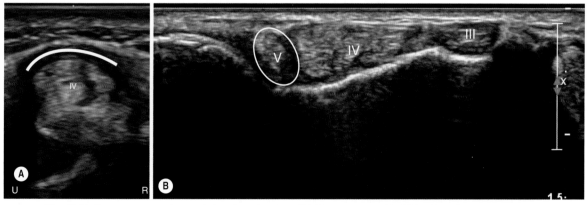

Fig. 5.18 Transverse sections of the dorsal wrist. **(A)** Compartment IV. *White line* shows retinaculum. *U,* Ulna aspect; *R,* radial aspect. **(B)** Compartments III, IV, V. (Extensor digit minimi outlined by a *white circle*.)

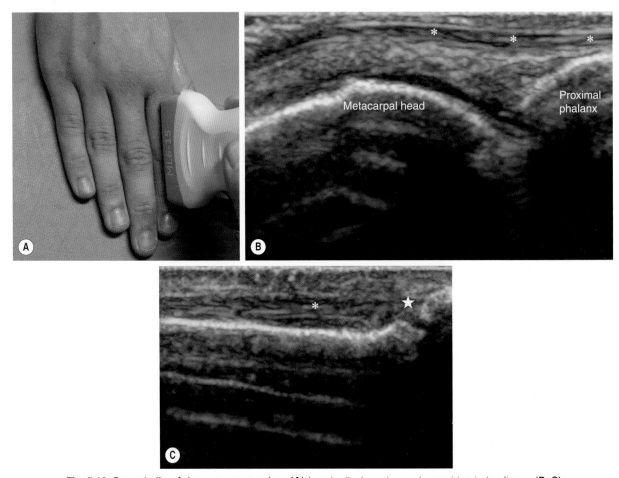

Fig. 5.19 Central slip of the extensor tendon. **(A)** Longitudinal section probe position index finger. **(B, C)** Extensor tendon central slip *(*)*, showing the insertion at the base of the middle phalanx *(star)*.

causes pain and comparisons with the nonsymptomatic side can be useful to avoid a false-positive diagnosis.

When following the extensor tendons distally into the fingers in longitudinal section, they are seen to taper into fine central and lateral band-like structures making them much more difficult to assess (Figs. 5.19 and 5.20).

In transverse section the extensor hoods of the digits are located at the level of the MCP joint/base of the proximal phalanx. They appear as thin echogenic fibrillar structures on ultrasound. In transverse section, the central slip of the extensor tendon should sit in a central position over the metacarpal head (Fig. 5.21).

On the dorsal aspect of each fingertip, distal to the DIP joint is the nail bed, which is seen on ultrasound in longitudinal section, deep to the fingernail (see Fig. 5.20).

It is important to recognise the normal appearances/vascularity of this structure as it can vary but should be comparable between digits.

At the wrist, the ECU tendon in compartment VI is best examined with the patient's wrist in a lateral position (little finger up) to allow good transducer access/contact (Fig. 5.22).[11]

In pronation, ECU is located within the ulnar groove; however, in supination or ulnar deviation of the wrist, up to 50% of the tendon can lie out of the groove. Subluxation greater than 50% of the tendon width is abnormal but often asymptomatic.[10]

On the ulnar aspect of the wrist the TFCC can be identified by placing the transducer longitudinally over and in line with the dorsal aspect of the ulna, with

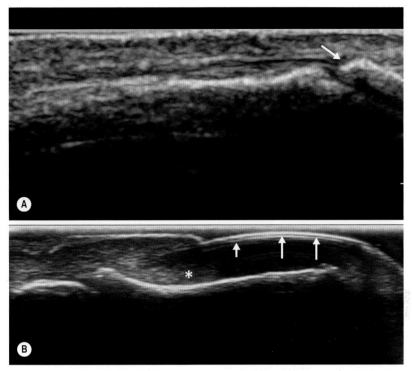

Fig. 5.20 Lateral slip of the extensor tendon and nailbed. (A) Lateral slip insertion into the distal phalanx *(arrow).* **(B)** Nailbed *(*),* nail *(arrows).*

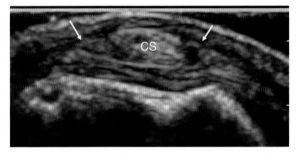

Fig. 5.21 Sagittal bands. Transverse section central slip of extensor tendon *(CS)* at the level of the metacarpal head with the overlying radial and ulnar sagittal bands *(arrows).*

the patient's hand palm down. TFCC is located just distal to the ulnar styloid process and deep to ECU and appears as a homogeneous echogenic, triangular structure (Fig. 5.23).

Individual portions of the TFCC cannot be distinguished on ultrasound and pathology cannot be excluded. The alternative investigations for tears here are arthroscopy and/or MRI.[4,6,9]

VOLAR HAND AND WRIST TENDONS (AND ADJACENT STRUCTURES)

Anatomy

Many structures enter the volar wrist through several fibro-osseous tunnels. The carpal tunnel contains the median nerve and the flexor tendons (Fig. 5.24).[3,14]

The carpal tunnel is formed by the broad ligamentous flexor retinaculum extending from the pisiform and hamate to the scaphoid and trapezium bones. Nine flexor tendons run within the carpal tunnel: four from the flexor digitorum superficialis (FDS), four from the flexor digitorum profundus (FDP) supplying the fingers, and the flexor pollicis longus (FPL) supplying the thumb. The FPL tendon lies within its own synovial sheath, whereas the eight tendons from the FDS and FDP all lie within a common synovial sheath.[14]

Superficial to the carpal tunnel in separate fibro-osseous canals and synovial sheaths lie the flexor carpi radialis (FCR), flexor carpi ulnaris (FCU), and palmaris longus (PL) tendons. PL is considered an accessory

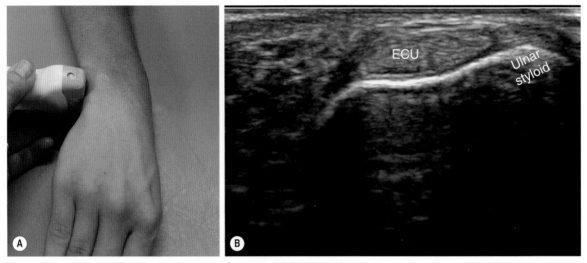

Fig. 5.22 Extensor compartment IV. **(A)** Patient and probe position. **(B)** Transverse section extensor carpi ulnaris *(ECU)*.

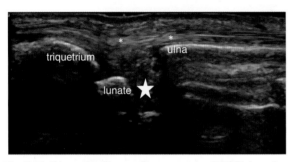

Fig. 5.23 Triangular fibrocartilage complex (TFCC). Longitudinal section TFCC *(star)*. Extensor carpi ulnaris tendon *(*)*.

tendon/muscle as it can be absent in 4% to 25% of individuals. It is important to be aware of its existence and location as it is often used in reconstructive plastic surgery.[13] The tendon may be palpated but when clinical tests are ambiguous ultrasound may be requested.[15] Anatomic variations include duplication of the tendon, and tendon/muscle reversal, where the muscle is seen at the level of the wrist and the tendon is seen proximally.[13]

The ulnar or Guyon's canal is also found on the volar aspect of the wrist. It has complex boundaries including the superficial palmar carpal ligament, the deeper flexor retinaculum, and hypothenar muscles, pisiform and pisohamate ligament, and the hook of the hamate. It contains the ulnar neurovascular bundle and in approximately 10% of individuals, the ulnar nerve bifurcates within the canal.[16]

The FDP and FDS tendons extend within the tendon sheaths (Fig. 5.25A), from the volar wrist across the palm

to the fingers. The FDS tendon splits at the PIP joint, with a slip coursing around both sides of the FDP tendon to insert on the middle phalanx; the FDP tendon inserts into the base of the distal phalanx (Fig. 5.25B,C).[3,9]

The FPL tendon lies between the lateral head of the flexor pollicis brevis (FPB) and adductor pollicis (AP) muscles before entering a fibro-osseous canal and eventually inserting into the distal phalanx of the thumb.

The flexor tendons are secured to the adjacent phalanges by a series of fibrous annular pulleys which prevent bowstringing of the tendons with flexion. The pulleys are numbered A1 to A5 and are located between the MCP and DIP joints. Smaller cruciform pulleys are located between the A pulleys along the course of the flexor tendons (Fig. 5.25D).[3,17]

The soft tissue of the fingertips on the volar aspect of distal phalanx is often highly vascular and is called the pulp.

Not to be forgotten are the intrinsic muscles of the hand, which may be the site of masses or injury (Fig. 5.26).[3]

Another structure which may be the source of pathology in the hand is the palmar fascia/aponeurosis. It is a continuation of the fascia in the forearm and has deep and superficial components which connect to the skin.[1,5,6]

Technique and Normal Ultrasound Appearances

Ultrasound of the volar aspect of the hand and wrist is performed with the patient's hand palm up.

The volar wrist structures are not as conveniently arranged for ultrasound as the dorsal anatomy and the

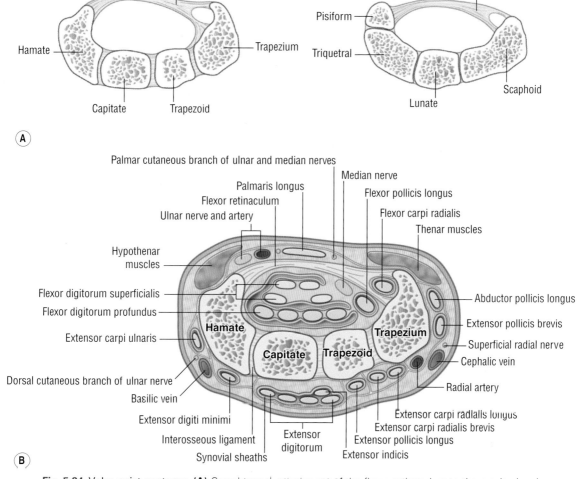

Fig. 5.24 Volar wrist anatomy. (A) Carpal tunnel, attachment of the flexor retinaculum to the proximal and distal rows of carpal bones. (B) Transverse section right wrist showing the relationships of the structures passing into the hand.

tendons can be difficult to visualise clearly at the level of the carpal tunnel due to anisotropy.[11,13] Scanning here requires careful manipulation of equipment parameters, the transducer, and/or the position of the wrist to ensure that the resultant image is optimised.

Forming the roof of the carpal tunnel, the flexor retinaculum is identified, in transverse section, as a convex, thin hypoechoic band spanning between the bony attachments (Figs. 5.27 and 5.28).[11]

The median nerve is easily identifiable in transverse section as an ovoid structure with hypoechoic fascicles deep to the retinaculum and superficial to the FDS/FDP tendons. A bifid median nerve is seen in approximately 20% of individuals.[9,13] The adjacent FCR and PL tendons are superficial to the retinaculum and should not be mistaken for the median nerve given their proximity (Fig. 5.29).[10] The median nerve courses deep in the carpal tunnel between the FDS and FDP tendons, unlike the FCR and PL, which remain superficial. The median nerve can also be followed into the forearm where it sits deep within the muscles (see Fig. 5.29B).

The tendons are examined within the carpal tunnel with the transducer in transverse section.[9,11,13] Moving the thumb will elicit movement of the FPL tendon, making it easy to identify. The finger flexor tendons lie in a bundle within the carpal tunnel, the FDS tendons

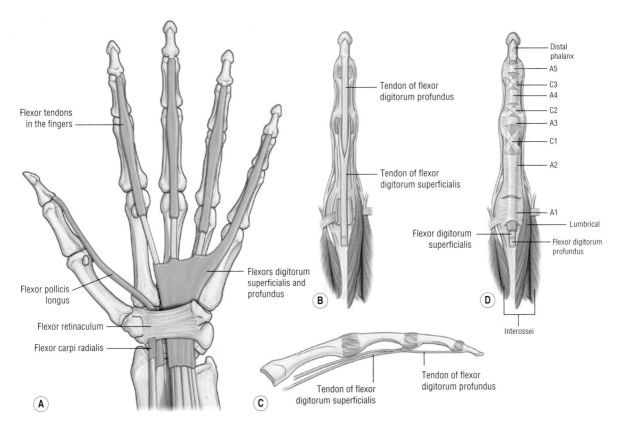

Fig. 5.25 Flexor tendon anatomy. **(A)** Tendon sheaths in green. **(B and C)** Demonstrate the insertions and relationship between the flexor digitorum superficialis and profundus tendons at the level of the fingers. **(D)** Flexor pulley system. *A*, Annular pulleys; *C*, cruciform pulleys.

sitting superficial to the FDP tendons. In the carpal tunnel, the FDS tendons for the third and fourth fingers lie superficial to the tendons for the second and fifth fingers. The FDP tendons lay side by side.[9]

It is worth noting that general movement of the individual fingers will not enable differentiation between the FDS and FDP tendons. This can be achieved by either following the tendons into the palm of the hand where the FDS lies superficial to the FDP tendon (Fig. 5.30A),[9] or by performing the specific dynamic assessment described:
- FDS—ensure that only the PIP joint of the digit is flexed and that the DIP joint remains extended[17] (Fig. 5.30B)
- FDP—ensure that only the DIP joint of the digit is flexed and that the PIP joint remains extended (Fig. 5.30C)

FDS and FDP tendons can be followed distally in transverse and longitudinal sections (Figs. 5.31 and 5.32), towards the individual digits and insertions. Due to the directional difference in the FDS and FDP

tendons, anisotropy can be a useful tool for differentiation (see Fig. 5.31).

The annular pulleys appear as a series of thin focal hypoechoic "thickenings" overlying the flexor tendons in longitudinal. In transverse, the focal hypoechoic "thickenings" surround the flexor tendons (Fig. 5.33).

On normal dynamic assessment, the flexor tendons should be seen to glide smoothly beneath the pulleys.

The cruciform pulley system is particularly difficult to visualise on ultrasound due their oblique direction and small size.[17]

The FCR and FCU tendons lie outside the carpal tunnel and are generally easier to identify and follow as they are superficial in position.[12] Incomplete assessment distally could overlook a tear of the FCR tendon which may occur at its insertion on the bases of the second and third metacarpals in the presence of osteoarthritis of the adjacent scaphoid-trapezium-trapezoid joints.[10]

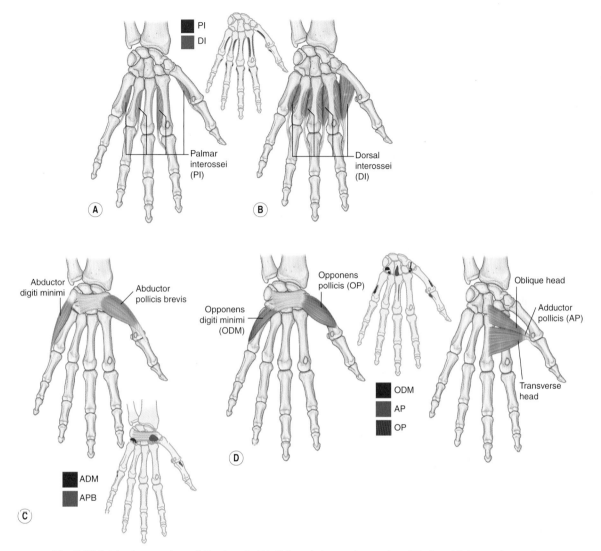

Fig. 5.26 Intrinsic muscles of the hand. **(A)** Palmar interossei muscles; **(B)** dorsal interossei muscles; **(C)** abductor pollicis brevis and abductor digit minimi muscles; **(D)** opponens digiti minimi, opponens pollicis, and adductor pollicis.

The PL tendon, if present, is usually seen at the level of the carpal tunnel and is seen in transverse section as a small ovoid tendon located superficially to the flexor retinaculum (see Fig. 5.29A).[11]

Ultrasound may be requested for examination of the ulnar nerve in Guyon's canal, usually to determine compression of the nerve at this level. The canal can be identified in transverse section towards the ulnar aspect of the wrist at the level of the proximal carpal tunnel, superficial to the flexor retinaculum (Fig. 5.34).[11,13]

Within Guyon's canal/tunnel, the ulnar nerve fascicles are easily recognised on the ulnar side of the artery and paired veins. The ulnar nerve can be followed in transverse sections distally, towards the hand, where it is seen to divide into its sensory and deep motor branches. The deep motor branch runs alongside the hook of the hamate bone. In approximately 24% of individuals, an accessory abductor digit minimi muscle is present, which arises from PL and lies in Guyon's canal and may cause compression of the ulnar nerve.[11,13]

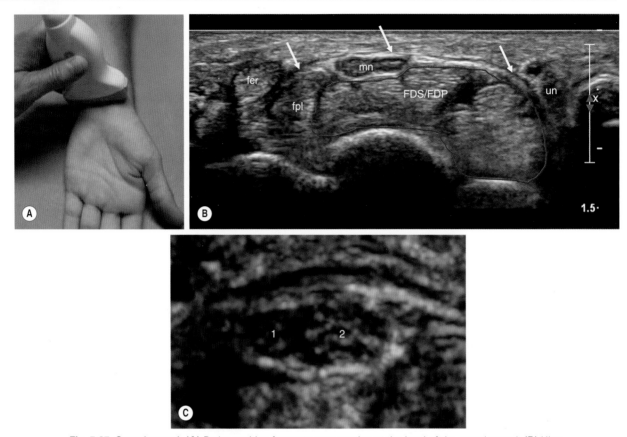

Fig. 5.27 Carpal tunnel. (A) Probe position for transverse section at the level of the carpal tunnel. **(B)** Ultrasound proximal carpal tunnel, with the flexor retinaculum *(arrows)*, median nerve *(mn)*, tendons of flexor digitorum superficialis and flexor digitorum profundus *(FDS/FDP; red outline)*, and flexor pollicis longus *(fpl)*. The flexor carpi radialis *(fcr)* tendon is outside the carpal tunnel. *un*, Ulnar nerve. **(C)** Example of a bifid median nerve *(1)* and *(2)*.

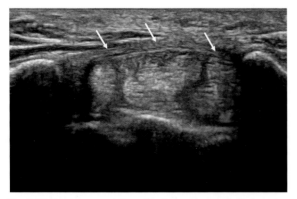

Fig. 5.28 Transverse section distal carpal tunnel. Retinaculum *(arrows)*.

> ### ◎ TIPS
>
> - Tendons of the wrist and hand are more easily identified and followed in transverse section. If they cannot be easily identified at the level of the wrist, following them from their insertions should help.
> - Dynamic assessment and comparison with the asymptomatic side is paramount in making a correct diagnosis.

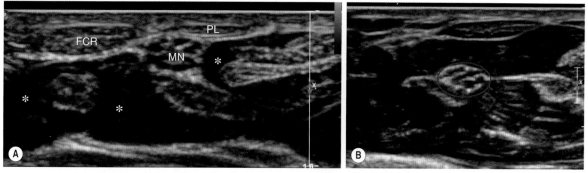

Fig. 5.29 Median nerve. (A) Transverse section proximal wrist/distal forearm showing the relationship of the median nerve *(MN)*, flexor carpi radialis *(FCR)*, and palmaris longus *(PL)* tendons. The myotendinous junction of the flexor digitorum superficialis and flexor digitorum profundus (FDS/FDP) should not be mistaken for fluid *(*)*. **(B)** Median nerve *(red outline)* deep to the forearm musculature.

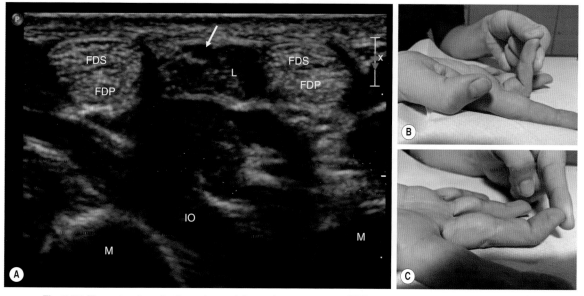

Fig. 5.30 Flexor tendons in the palm and dynamic assessment. (A) Transverse section in the palm showing the middle and index flexor tendons (FDS/FDP) and relationship to the neurovascular bundle *(arrow)*. Intrinsic muscles of the hand (*L*, lumbrical, *IO*, interosseus, and *M*, metacarpal). **(B and C)** Dynamic assessment to isolate the FDS and FDP tendons respectively. *FDS/FDP,* Flexor digitorum superficialis/flexor digitorum profundus.

PATHOLOGY

Tenosynovitis

Tenosynovitis is inflammation of the synovial lining of the tendon sheath. It is caused by mechanical overuse, infection, irritation from underlying structures such as an osteophyte or protruding portion of orthopeadic hardware, and/or inflammatory arthropathies. The inflammation can be isolated to the tendon sheath alone or it can be accompanied by tendinopathic changes and even tears within the tendons.[1,5–8,13,18]

Specific to the hand and wrist, it is worth noting that the FCU and PL tendons, as well as the distal extensor tendons of the digits and palmar portions of some

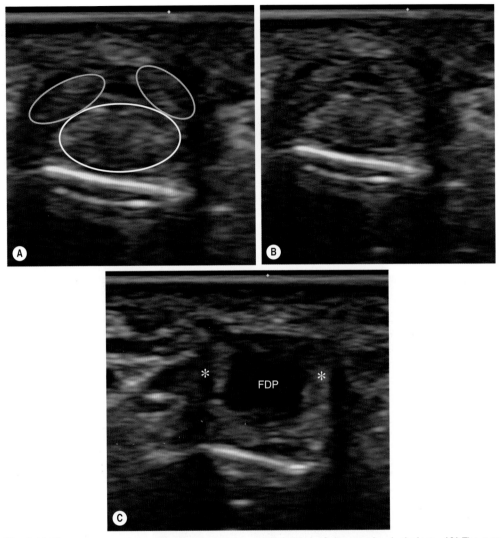

Fig. 5.31 Transverse section at the level of the proximal third of the proximal phalanx. (A) The two lateral slips of the flexor digitorum superficialis indicated in *orange,* flexor digitorum profundus indicated in *white.* **(B)** Without annotation. **(C)** Anisotropy of the flexor digitorum profundus (FDP) with the lateral slips of the flexor digitorum superficialis remaining in plane (asterisks) with normal tendon architecture.

flexor tendons, cannot be affected by tenosynovitis as they do not have full synovial sheaths.

ECU tenosynovitis raises the suspicion of inflammatory arthropathy as this tendon is not exposed to the normal mechanical strains which usually cause tenosynovitis (see Chapter 10).[6,9]

Tenosynovitis caused by infection is known as pyogenic tenosynovitis. This can be a common referral from plastic surgeons and is treated as a surgical emergency requiring washout to avoid the patient developing sepsis and/or substantial morbidity such as tendon damage, permanent loss of function, or the requirement for amputation. In some cases the infection can spread into a "horseshoe abscess" resulting from a communication between the flexor sheaths of the thumb and little fingers, which is present in many individuals. Although infective and noninfective tenosynovitis have similar ultrasound appearances, as shown in Fig. 5.35, other clinical signs and

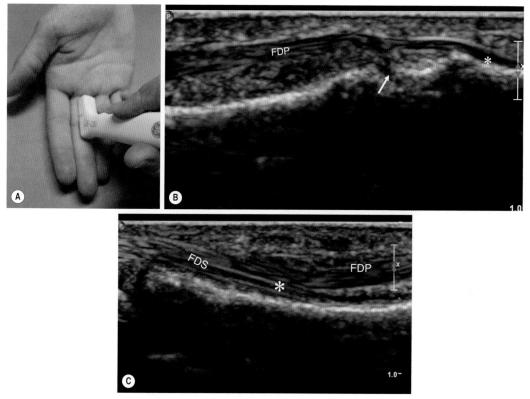

Fig. 5.32 Flexor tendon insertions. (A) Longitudinal section probe over the volar aspect of the finger. **(B)** Insertion of the FDP tendon *(*)*. The *arrow* points to the distal interphalangeal joint. **(C)** Insertion of one of the FDS slips *(*)*. *FDP,* flexor digitorum profundus; *FDS,* flexor digitorum superficialis.

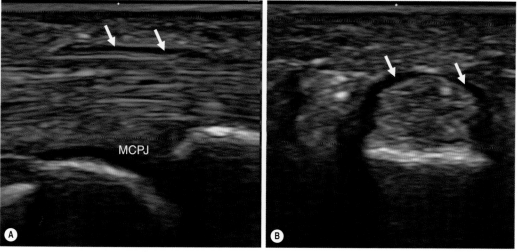

Fig. 5.33 A1 pulley. *Arrows* point to the A1 pulley of the middle finger which appears as a thin dark band. **(A)** Longitudinal section. **(B)** Transverse section. *MCPJ,* Metacarpophalangeal joint.

symptoms, such as a temperature and raised inflammatory markers, will assist its diagnosis.[2]

De Quervain's Stenosing Tenosynovitis

De Quervain's tenosynovitis or tenovaginitis is the name given to an entrapment of EPB and APL tendons within

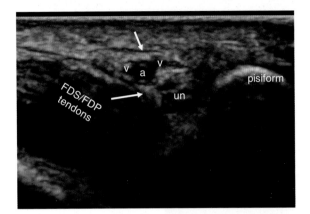

Fig. 5.34 Guyon's canal. Transverse section showing the retinaculum *(arrows)* and contents of Guyon's canal—ulnar nerve *(un)*, ulnar artery *(a)*, and ulnar veins *(v)*. *FDP,* Flexor digitorum profundus; *FDS,* flexor digitorum superficialis.

extensor compartment I. More commonly seen in women, although its cause is commonly attributed to mechanical overuse, it has an association with women who are pregnant and/or women with young children—the cause for this remains unknown *(idiopathic)*. Patients usually present with pain and swelling at the base of the thumb over extensor compartment I, which can radiate into the thumb and forearm, with symptoms exacerbated by thumb movement and gripping. Usually this is a clinical diagnosis, using clinical tests including the Finkelstein's test, Eichoff's manoeuver, and the WHAT (wrist hyperflexion and abduction of the thumb) test.[19] These tests attempt to produce a mechanical stress/shear on the tendons of EPB and APL against the overlying retinaculum or the bony floor of the radius. A positive result is indicated by reproduction of symptoms. These tests can be seen in Fig. 5.36.

Treatments include splinting, activity and workplace activity modification physiotherapy, and steroid injection, and ultrasound scanning may be requested in cases that are refractory. During the acute phase of the condition, ultrasound findings may include thickening of the tendon sheath with neovascularity (Fig 5.37) and effusion. However, thickening of the tendon and sheath

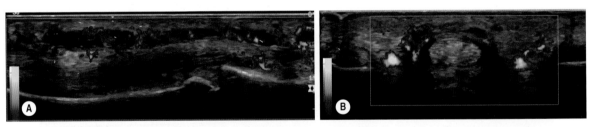

Fig. 5.35 Tenosynovitis of the ring finger flexor tendons. **A** longitudinal section, **B** transverse section. There is excessive fluid in the tendon sheath; neovascularity of the tendon/tendon sheath on Power Doppler.

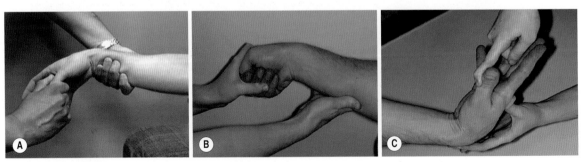

Fig. 5.36 Clinical tests for De Quervain's stenosing tenosynovitis. **(A)** Finkelstein's. **(B)** Eichoff's. **(C)** Wrist hyperflexion and abduction of the thumb (WHAT).

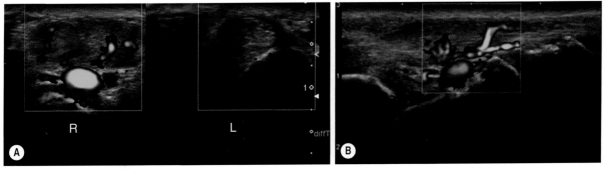

Fig. 5.37 De Quervain's tenosynovitis. **(A)** Transverse section abnormal right wrist compared with the normal left side. **(B)** Longitudinal section. The tendons in the first extensor compartment are thickened and vascularised.

is often subtle with little neovascularity, and comparison with the contralateral side may be required to confirm findings. During the chronic phase, tendinopathic changes within the tendon may become evident. As mentioned previously, EPB and APL may be separated by a vertical septum which not only makes patients more susceptible to this condition but may also account for the cause of failed steroid injections. It is therefore important to report this finding when it is identified.

Proximal/Distal Intersection Syndrome

As mentioned earlier in the technique section, where the extensor compartments cross-over in the wrist and forearm repetitive injury may cause overuse tenosynovitis. The patient presents with localised swelling and pain in the forearm or wrist, known respectively as proximal intersection syndrome (where compartments I and II cross) or the less common distal intersection syndrome (where II and III cross). On examination, crepitus can be felt when the patient moves the wrist (twisting and flexion/extension). Clinical presentation may be nonspecific therefore ultrasound may be requested to determine the precise cause of symptoms. On ultrasound there can be a loss of definition between the two compartments, hyperaemia, and associated hypoechoic soft tissue swelling due to localised oedema, as well as associated tendon changes. It is also important to assess the underlying bony surfaces for osteophytes in the case of distal intersection syndrome.[16,20]

Tendon Tear/Rupture

Tendon tears in the hand and wrist may result from chronic tendinopathy, inflammatory arthropathy, and

acute or repetitive trauma. Repetitive trauma can result from the movement of the tendon over degenerative bony surfaces or orthopeadic hardware. EPL tears in particular are a recognised complication of distal radial fractures.[18]

It is important to remember that tendon sheaths will remain in place, even when a torn tendon is completely retracted. In the acute phase of the injury, the sheath can fill with blood and debris, creating the appearance of a pseudo tendon on ultrasound. During the chronic phase of injury, once the initial inflammatory reaction has resolved, the empty tendon sheath can be mistaken for remnant of the tendon leading to misdiagnosis of a partial tear and/or atrophy. Dynamic assessment (active, passive, and against resistance), specific to the tendon under investigation, and comparison with the non-symptomatic side is of paramount importance.[10,18]

When assessing and reporting tendon tears in the hand and wrist to assist correct patient management, the most important information is whether the tear is partial or full thickness.

In a partial thickness tear, important information would include the:
- specific location of the tear in relation to palpable landmarks
- percentage of depth of the tendon involved. Comparing with the asymptomatic side can aid this

In a full thickness tear (Figs. 5.38 and 5.39) information would include the:
- location of the tear and position of the tendon ends in relation to palpable landmarks
- size of the gap/defect—it is worth noting that in the hand and wrist, tendon stump(s) can retract a long way

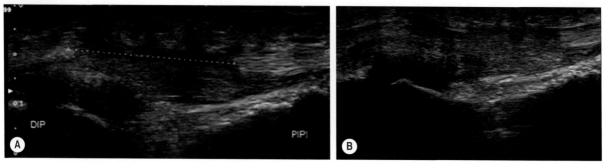

Fig. 5.38 Full thickness tear of the flexor pollicis longus tendon. (A) Showing the measurement of the gap between the tendon ends *(calipers).* **(B)** The intact proximal tendon.

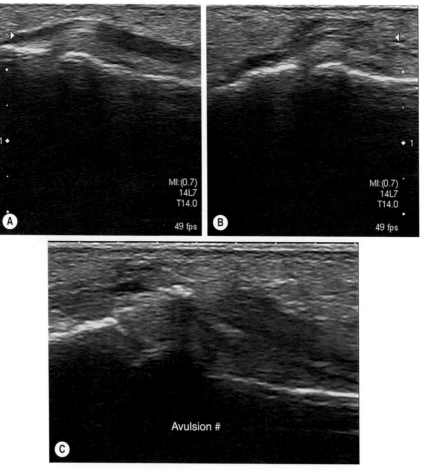

Fig. 5.39 Avulsion injury right ring finger FDP tendon. (A) Normal left ring finger FDP tendon for comparison. **(B)** Volar aspect of the left finger with no tendon at the level of the distal phalanx/DIP joint. **(C)** Bony avulsion fragment is seen in the retracted tendon end overlying the PIP joint. *DIP,* distal interphalangeal; *FDP,* flexor digitorum profundus; *PIP,* proximal interphalangeal.

- degree of tendinopathic change in the tendon ends as this can assist in management decisions around surgery
- cause of a tear, such as an underlying osteophyte or protruding portion of orthopedic hardware[18]

REPORT—FULL THICKNESS FLEXOR POLLICIS LONGUS TEAR (FIG. 5.38)

Clinical History: 2/52 cut injury to the right thumb with a Stanley knife. ? FPL tear

Ultrasound Report: There is a full thickness rupture of the FPL tendon, 6 mm proximal to the DIP joint. A gap of 16.5 mm is seen between the retracted tendon ends.

Conclusion: Full thickness tear of the FPL tendon.

REPORT—AVULSION OF THE RIGHT RING FINGER FLEXOR DIGITORUM PROFUNDUS (FIG. 5.39)

Clinical History: Patient received hyperextension injury of the DIP joint of the right fourth finger. X-rays NAD. Patient attended fracture clinic for review and unable to flex the DIP joint. ? Tendon tear

Ultrasound Report: The flexor digitorum profundus tendon of the ring finger is detached from its distal insertion and is retracted proximally to the level of the PIP joint. A small bone avulsion fragment seen.

Conclusion: Avulsion of the FDP tendon of the ring finger.

Mallet Finger

Mallet finger is a clinical deformity of the finger where there is flexion of the DIP joint (Fig. 5.40) caused by avulsion of the extensor tendon, the typical mechanism of injury being forced flexion of the DIP joint.

Patients present with pain, swelling, and an inability to extend the DIP joint. On ultrasound the extensor tendon is not identified at the distal insertion, and instead is seen slightly proximal to the joint, with or without a tiny bony fragment (avulsion fracture) and with or without inflammatory changes dependent on the time since injury. This clinical deformity can also be mimicked by degenerative changes at the DIP joint from osteoarthritis or inflammatory arthropathy (e.g., osteophytes, synovial hypertrophy, or synovitis), restricting joint extension.[7]

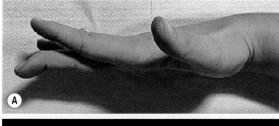
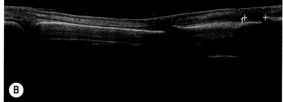
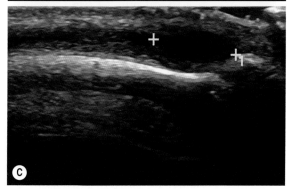

Fig. 5.40 Mallet finger. (A) Photo demonstrating the clinical appearance of Mallet finger, in this case, of the middle finger. **(B)** Panoramic view with measurement calipers showing the distance of the avulsed extensor tendon slip from the distal interphalangeal joint. **(C)** "Zoom in" to the rupture.

Sagittal Band Injuries

As mentioned, the sagittal bands form part of the stabilising aponeurotic sheet or extensor hood which overlies the MCP joints of the fingers. Sagittal bands can be injured through trauma or inflammatory diseases such as rheumatoid arthritis. In boxers, the index and middle fingers are usually affected but in patients with inflammatory arthropathies, damage to the ring and little finger sagittal bands are more common. Clinically the patient presents with a subluxation or painful clicking sensation which occurs at either the MCP or PIP joint. The tendon can be visibly seen or palpably felt to flick out of position when the patient flexes the affected finger.[9,12] On ultrasound, injury to the sagittal band itself can be difficult to visualise as the structures are tiny.

During the acute phase of the injury, it may be possible to demonstrate discontinuity of the sagittal band with focal swelling and some hyperemia evident on Doppler. A complete tear allows subluxation of the extensor tendon, usually towards the ulnar aspect of the MCP joint (Fig. 5.41) which can be appreciated clinically as well as on ultrasound. It is, however, worth noting that the index and little fingers have two extensor tendons which can sublux in different directions. Ultrasound reports should indicate if the ulnar or radial sagittal bands are involved and note any associated tendon changes present.[7,12]

Volar Plate Injuries

Hyperextension of the MCP, PIP, and DIP joints of the digits can injure the volar plate, sometimes causing avulsion or a tear, although these injuries are rare. Acutely tears appear as a hypoechoic defect within the swollen volar plate.[7,9]

Thumb Ulnar Collateral Ligament Injury

Thumb ulnar collateral ligament (UCL) injuries, also known as gamekeeper or skier's thumb, are usually caused by hyperabduction and hyperextension of the MCP joint of the thumb. Alternative mechanisms for injury include chronic overstrain/repetitive low-grade stress leading to an insufficiency in the ligament. Clinical tests can be limited due to pain and swelling; therefore, ultrasound is commonly used for the assessment of acute injury to determine if there is a tear present and the extent of retraction. This is important information for the clinician to ensure correct long-term management to avoid joint instability and osteoarthritis.[21]

When an acute/sub-acute sprain of the UCL is present, the ligament appears thickened due to oedema and haemorrhage. This can be extremely difficult to appreciate in such a small structure, but comparison with the normal contralateral side (see Fig. 5.8B) can assist.

Tears appear as a discontinuity of the ligament, usually occur at the distal insertion and can be challenging to demonstrate. Superficial to the UCL is the adductor aponeurosis: the location of the ligament in relation to the adductor aponeurosis is important. A Stener lesion (Fig. 5.42) is characterised by slippage of the torn end of the UCL superficial to the adductor aponeurosis such that now there is interposition of the adductor pollicis muscle between the UCL and the MCP joint. This prevents healing and is an indication for surgical repair, which should occur within a few days of

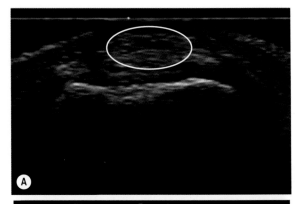

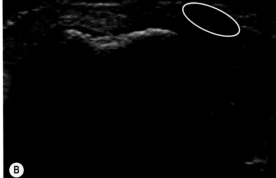

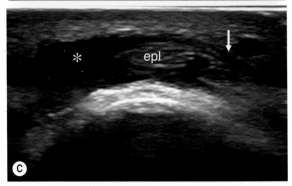

Fig. 5.41 Sagittal band injury. Transverse section images. **(A)** In this case, the extensor tendon can be seen centrally overlying the metacarpal head with the joint extended; **(B)** on flexion the extensor tendon has subluxed towards ulna side. **(C)** In another case, the radial sagittal band of the thumb is ruptured with haematoma present *(*)*. The ulnar sagittal band is intact *(arrow)*. *epl*, Extensor pollicis longus tendon.

injury to be successful. The aponeurosis can also be injured. The presence of the adductor aponeurosis can easily be confirmed with passive flexion of the interphalangeal joint where it can be identified gliding over the MCP joint with movement of the extensor tendon.

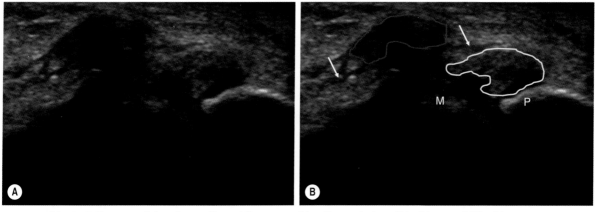

Fig. 5.42 Rupture of the ulnar collateral ligament with a Stener lesion. **(A)** without and **(B)** with annotation. *Red and yellow,* tendon stumps, *arrows* interposed adductor aponeurosis. *M,* Metacarpal; *P,* proximal phalanx.

When a tear is present there can be increased mobility in the MCP joint of the thumb, which can assist in the identification of unretracted or chronic tears on ultrasound. Caution should be taken with dynamic assessment to avoid causing a Stener lesion if a complete tear is present.[22]

REPORT—THUMB UCL RUPTURE WITH STENER LESION (FIG. 5.42)

Clinical History: ? gamekeeper's thumb Rt

Ultrasound Report: The patient found this examination very painful. There is a complete rupture of the UCL and the proximal ligament stump appears to lie superficial to the adductor aponeurosis indicating a Stener lesion.

Scapholunate Ligament (SLL) Injury

From a clinical perspective, there is a severity spectrum associated with injury to this ligament ranging from occult, to dissociation, carpal collapse, and ending in arthritis (SLAC scapholunate collapse). The degree of injury can be graded 1 to 4 by the Geissler classification. Injury to this ligament results from a fall onto an extended wrist associated with forceful ulna deviation. Pain is felt in the anatomical snuff box of the wrist or palmar scaphoid tubercle with concomitant loss of wrist range of movement and strength. Clinically, SLL disruptions are examined using the Kirk-Watson test or scaphoid shift test. This is a dynamic test which attempts to assess the integrity of the SLL by palpating the scaphoid whilst the carpal bones are moved from an

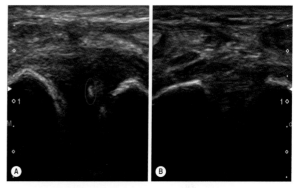

Fig. 5.43 Scapholunate ligament injury. **(A)** Transverse section thickened left SLL with tiny calcific fragment *(red outline)* following partial avulsion of the ligament; **(B)** normal right SLL. *SLL,* Scapholunate ligament.

extended and deviated position to a flexed and radially deviated position. This test can be positive in approximately 20% of the normal population, and in individuals with wrist ganglia.[23] Although MRI is normally required rather than ultrasound for full assessment of injury to the wrist ligaments, Fig. 5.43 shows an example of injury to the SLL discovered on ultrasound as the source of pain, following a fall onto a flexed wrist, not resolving with physiotherapy. This was later confirmed with MRI.

Annular Pulley Tears

Ultrasound has a major benefit over other imaging modalities in the assessment of the pulley system of the digits as it is the only modality which allows dynamic assessment. Pulley injuries/tears are common in climbers where the maximum force/load is exerted on the DIP joints, but damage can also be secondary to chronic tenosynovitis in inflammatory arthritides. Traumatic tears usually affect the ring or middle finger and most commonly are solitary affecting the A2 pulley only, although the A3 pulley can also occasionally be involved.

The torn annular pulley is not normally visualised on ultrasound, but the diagnosis is made by detection of bowstringing (a gap between the flexor tendon and bone) (Fig. 5.44). Bowstringing can be enhanced by using resisted flexion as well as comparison with an unaffected digit. During the acute phase, there may be evidence of focal tenosynovitis though this is not always the case.[7,12,18]

> **REPORT—ANNULAR PULLEY INJURY (FIG. 5.44)**
> **Clinical History:** 31-year-old builder ? right ring finger A2 pulley rupture.
> **Ultrasound Report:** There is a fluid between the flexor tendons and the underlying proximal phalanx of the right ring finger measuring 4.5 mm in flexion, in keeping with an underlying A2 pulley injury at this region. The flexor tendons are intact; however, there is also a small amount of fluid within the tendon sheath in keeping with tenosynovitis.

Trigger Finger

Trigger finger is a transient locking of the finger in flexion followed by a painful "snap" when the flexor tendon is

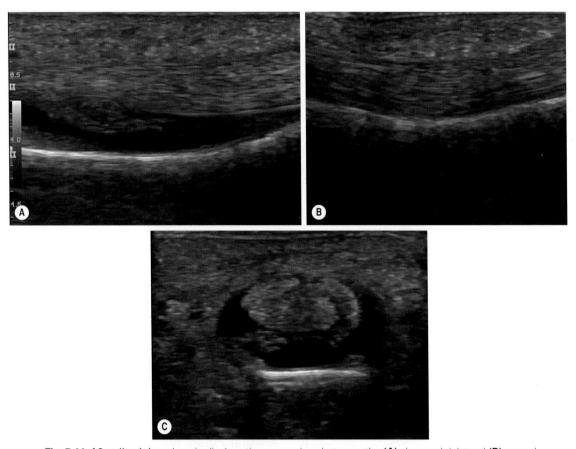

Fig. 5.44 A2 pulley injury. Longitudinal section comparison between the **(A)** abnormal right and **(B)** normal left ring finger flexor tendons at the level of the proximal phalanx. Fluid is seen lifting tendons away from the proximal phalanx. **(C)** Transverse section; fluid is also present in the right ring finger tendon sheath.

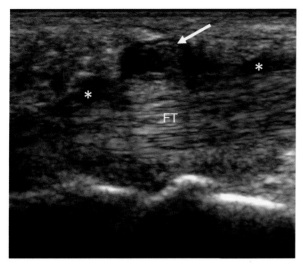

Fig. 5.45 Trigger finger right middle finger. Longitudinal section shows thickening of the A1 pulley (arrow), flexor tendons (*FT*) and tendon sheath (*).

Dupuytren's Contracture (Palmar Fibromatosis)

Dupuytren's contracture is characterised by subcutaneous nodules within the palmar aponeurosis which may eventually cause retraction and restriction of the underlying flexor tendons of one or more digits. It is seen in 1% to 2% of the population and in those affected, 42% to 60% have nodules bilaterally. Ultrasound is not required to diagnose Dupuytren's; however, it may be requested during the early stages of the disease to determine the nature of a palpable lesion in the palm. These lesions appear on ultrasound as hypoechoic nodular thickening of the palmar aponeurosis (Fig. 5.46). During early stages of the disease, the flexor tendon may move freely; however, progressively, adhesions tethering and restricting movement of the flexor tendon are observed.[21]

released during extension, caused by narrowing of the pulley system of the finger. This may be due to inflammatory tenosynovitis resulting in tendon/sheath thickening or focal thickening of the pulley with a normal tendon/sheath. Pulley thickening can be due to mechanical overuse or systemic conditions such as diabetes where it is thought that chronically elevated blood glucose levels may damage connective tissue.

On ultrasound the pulley appears thickened (± neovascularity) and compresses the flexor tendon, and/or the tendon and sheath appear thickened, compromising sliding of the tendon through the pulley on dynamic examination (Fig. 5.45).[7,17] Trigger finger is also a common complication of long-standing rheumatoid arthritis.

REPORT—DUPUYTREN'S CONTRACTURE FIG. 5.46

Clinical History: Firm tender lump in left palm, not inflamed or infected, no FB ? ganglion ? nodule attached to tendon

Ultrasound Report: The clinically evident mass in the left palm (MCP joint level) corresponds to a 1 cm superficial, indistinct, nodular lesion superficial to the ring finger flexor tendon. No vascularity demonstrated. On dynamic assessment, the flexor tendon moves freely and I note from the patient that he has no movement issues. This lesion is not a ganglion and considering its location, is likely to be Dupuytren's contracture.

REPORT—TRIGGER FINGER (FIG. 5.45)

Clinical History: Inability to flex right middle finger, ? rupture of flexor digitorum superficialis ? trigger finger.

Ultrasound Report: There is no evidence of a tear of the flexor tendons (superficialis and profundus) of the right middle finger. However, at the A1 pulley, the tendons do not move smoothly due to thickening of the pulley, tendon sheath, and tendons in keeping with trigger finger with tendinopathy.

Nerve Entrapment

Nerve entrapment pathologies are usually a clinical diagnosis with the location of symptoms assisting the identification of the affected nerve (Fig. 5.47), with electrodiagnostic testing used for confirmation.

Ultrasound does not usually play a routine role in diagnosis or management; however, it can be useful in demonstrating the compressive cause of the entrapment. Within the carpal tunnel, this may include pathologies such as a ganglion or tenosynovitis[5,13,14] causing carpal tunnel syndrome. Patients usually present initially with strong tingling sensation on the palmar surface of the thumb, index, middle, and half the ring finger. The

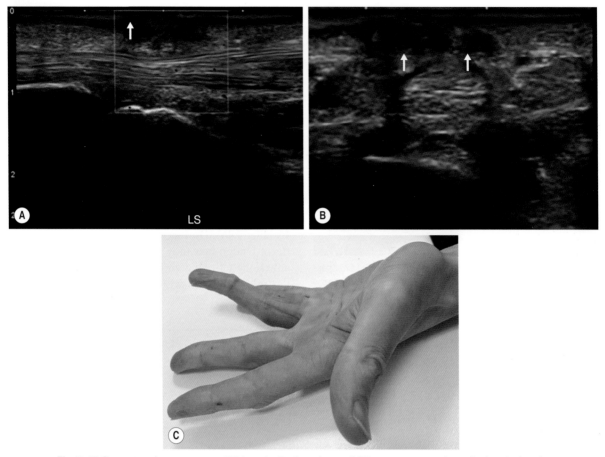

Fig. 5.46 Dupuytren's contracture. **(A)** Longitudinal section and **(B)** transverse section volar hand, showing an ill-defined nodule *(arrows)* superficial to the flexor tendon of the ring finger. **(C)** Photo of advanced disease where the patient is unable to extend the ring finger.

clinical tests used to determine the presence of carpal tunnel syndrome are Phalen's test and Tinel's sign (Fig. 5.48).

Tinel's sign is not specific to carpal tunnel syndrome and can be applied to any nerve entrapment. Phalen's test compresses the nerve in the tunnel to recreate the symptoms.[24]

Within Guyon's canal, nerve entrapment symptoms can be caused by an accessory abductor digit minimi muscle, a ganglion, or an ulnar artery thrombus or pseudoaneurysm following repetitive "trauma."

Ultrasound scanning can offer some important information for carpal tunnel release surgery, such as the presence of a bifid median nerve and persistent median artery. These may affect the surgical planning but may

also be a cause of symptoms. As well as compressive pathologies, it can be possible to observe secondary nerve changes as a result of the entrapment on ultrasound such as loss of normal fascicular pattern, swelling of the nerve outside the carpel tunnel/Guyon's canal, and flattening/compression of the nerve as it enters the tunnel/canal. Although these findings are of limited value, they support the diagnosis of nerve entrapment (Fig. 5.49).[13,14] After carpal tunnel release surgery, the flexor retinaculum may appear thickened and anteriorly displaced, which makes it difficult to assess. Although it is common practice to measure the nerve volume (see Fig. 5.49C), normal median nerve size can vary. Ultrasound does not correlate with clinical outcome after surgery and therefore is of limited value.[10]

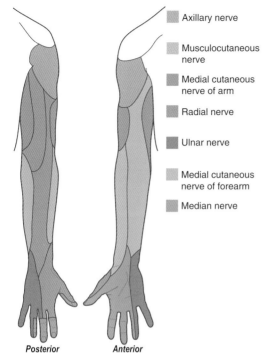

- Axillary nerve
- Musculocutaneous nerve
- Medial cutaneous nerve of arm
- Radial nerve
- Ulnar nerve
- Medial cutaneous nerve of forearm
- Median nerve

Posterior   Anterior

Fig. 5.47 Cutaneous nerve supply of the upper limb.

Ganglia

Ganglia are cystic lesions which arise from a tendon sheath or joint capsule, commonly seen on the dorsal surface of the hand or wrist. Clinically, they often feel hard, can be stable but may go up and down in size and are not always symptomatic. On ultrasound they appear as a cystic lesion with posterior acoustic enhancement. They are typically well-defined with regular smooth margins, although they can be lobulated with a neck distant to the main lesion, with no increased peripheral vascularity on Doppler assessment (Fig. 5.50).

REPORT—GANGLION (FIG. 5.50)
Clinical History: Lump dorsal aspect of right wrist ? ganglion ? nodule
Ultrasound Report: Scanning over the area of concern (as indicated by the patient) reveals an 18 mm lobulated ganglion which is arising via a short neck from the scapholunate ligament. No direct association with the neurovascular structures.

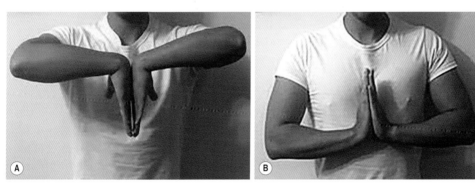

Tinel's Sign

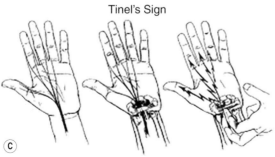

Fig. 5.48 Clinical tests for carpal tunnel syndrome. **(A)** Phalen's manoeuver; **(B)** Reverse Phalen's test; **(C)** Tinel's sign.

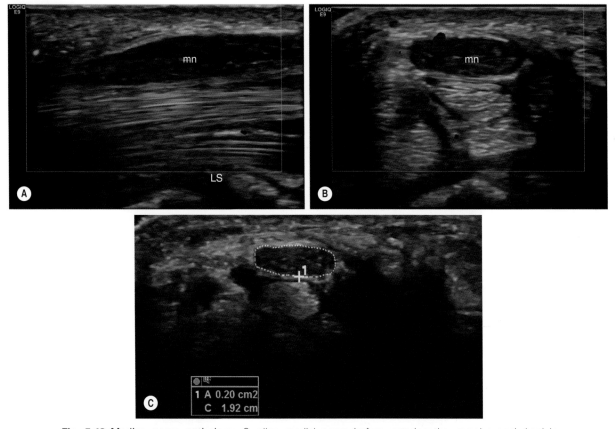

Fig. 5.49 Median nerve pathology. Swollen medial nerve before entering the carpal tunnel *(mn)* in **(A)** longitudinal section and **(B)** transverse section, with internal vascularity demonstrated on power Doppler. **(C)** Volume measurement of the median nerve.

Treatment includes aspiration or surgery, neither always successful, with a significant chance of recurrence. Information that is useful for referrers is the size and site of the lesion with its origin if possible and the proximity of any neurovascular structures in case of surgical intervention. Although ganglia with a typical history can be diagnosed on ultrasound alone, it is worth noting that synovial sarcomas can have a similar appearance and clinical history is key. Any lesion which is painful and reported to be growing should be treated with caution and depending on departmental protocols, should be considered for further investigations (see chapter 11).[7,8]

Giant Cell Tumours synovitis

Giant cell tumour (GCT) of the tendon sheath is the second most common tumour of the hand after ganglia.[25]

They are usually painless, slow growing, benign soft tissue lesions on the palmar/volar aspect of the distal finger affecting individuals between the age of 30 and 50 years; more common in women than men. Despite its benign character, local recurrence after excision has been reported in up to 45% of cases. There is no defined treatment protocol and local excision with or without radiotherapy is the treatment of choice to date. On ultrasound they appear as a hypoechoic, predominantly homogeneous, well-defined, solid lesion with or without internal vascularity on the tendon sheath (Fig. 5.51). GCT's can cause underlying pressure bone erosions which can help in the diagnosis. Whilst these appearances are typical, other more suspicious lesions may also demonstrate these features; therefore, histology is usually required for confirmation.

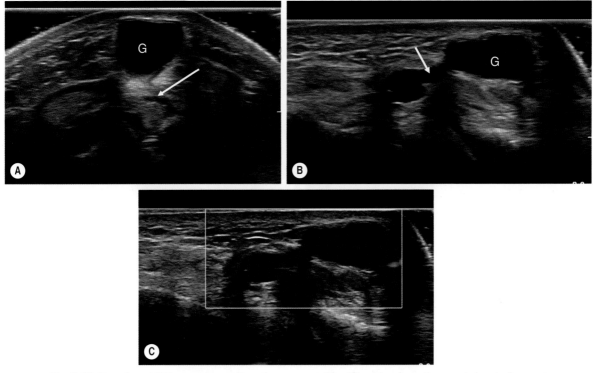

Fig. 5.50 Ganglion. **(A)** Transverse section shows a ganglion *(G)* arising from the scapholunate ligament (SLL) *(arrow)*. **(B)** Longitudinal section shows the neck *(arrow)* extending towards the SLL. **(C)** No vascularity within the ganglion.

REPORT—GCT (FIG. 5.51)
Clinical History: Lump on the volar aspect of the middle finger ? ganglion.
Ultrasound Report: scanning over the area of concern (as indicated by the patient) reveals a well-defined, solid lesion measuring 17 mm on the volar aspect of the middle finger flexor tendon sheath. No internal vascularity demonstrated. The tendon appears to move freely on dynamic assessment. Appearances are suggestive of a giant cell tumour rather than a ganglion. Pease note that this is not a histological diagnosis. Plastics referral for excision and biopsy is advised.

Foreign Bodies

Ultrasound referrals for confirmation and localisation of foreign bodies in the hand and wrist are common, certainly in the presence of radiolucent foreign bodies such as wood. It is not uncommon to be requested to mark the location of a foreign body (using a pen on the patient's skin) to assist surgical removal. Usually, patients present with an appropriate history of a penetrating wound with pain and swelling during the acute/subacute phase of the injury. It can be useful if the patient is able to state the direction of the penetration as a foreign object is easier to locate in its longest plane. On ultrasound the foreign body appears as a hyperechoic structure with posterior acoustic shadowing if it is a bone or vegetation fragment, or posterior comet tail artefact if it is a glass or metal fragment. During the subacute phase, there can be peripheral oedema and granuloma formation surrounding the foreign body creating a hypoechoic halo, with or without vascularity. If the foreign body has penetrated a tendon sheath, infective tenosynovitis can also be present. Chronically, a foreign body is much more difficult to identify on ultrasound as the hypoechoic halo of oedema and granuloma is usually gone (Fig. 5.52), unless a sterile granuloma has formed around the foreign body.

Joint, Bony Pathology

When assessing the hand and wrist with ultrasound, it is important not to overlook the bony anatomy. It is

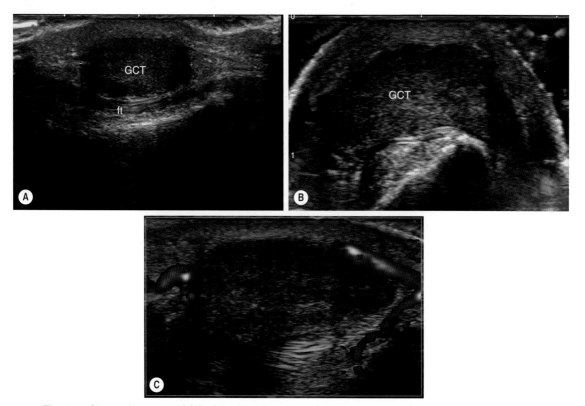

Fig. 5.51 Giant cell tumour *(GCT)* of the flexor tendon sheath. **(A)** Longitudinal section and **(B)** transverse section of the GCT with the flexor tendon *(ft)* on the deep aspect of the tumour. **(C)** Only peripheral vascularity is seen on power Doppler.

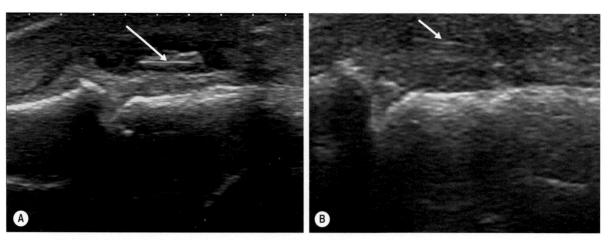

Fig. 5.52 Foreign body (FB). Thorn in the hand *(arrow)*. **(A)** Acute phase with surrounding granuloma. **(B)** Two years later (as the FB was not removed), it is much more difficult see.

possible for displaced fractures or dislocations, invisible on X-ray, to be incidentally found on ultrasound. Synovitis and erosions can be incidental findings in patients with an undiagnosed inflammatory arthropathy. Joint pathology is discussed in detail in Chapter 10.

TIP

- When describing location of pathology in written reports, try to avoid conventional ultrasound terms (e.g., medial, lateral, anterior, posterior) choosing descriptors such as radial, ulna, dorsal, and volar instead.

MULTIPLE CHOICE QUESTIONS

1. Which two tendons lie within extensor compartment II?
   a. Extensor pollicis longus
   b. Extensor pollicis brevis
   c. Extensor carpi radialis brevis
   d. Abductor pollicis longus tendons
   e. Extensor carpi radialis longus
   f. Extensor carpi ulnaris
   g. Extensor digiti minimi
   h. Extensor indicis proprius
2. Which three tendons lie outside of the carpel tunnel?
   a. Flexor carpi radialis
   b. Palmaris longus
   c. Flexor pollicis longus
   d. Flexor digitorum superficialis
   e. Flexor carpi ulnaris
   f. Flexor digitorum profundus
3. If you flex the PIP joint of the fingers, whilst keeping the DIP joints extended, which tendons will be seen to move dynamically on ultrasound?
   a. Flexor digitorum superficialis
   b. Flexor digitorum profundus

4. Carpal tunnel syndrome is a compression neuropathy that effects the:
   a. median nerve.
   b. ulna nerve.
   c. radial nerve.
5. A Stener lesion is:
   a. a type of joint cyst associated with the metacarpal phalangeal joint.
   b. a vascular lesion associated with the small vessels of the thumb pulp.
   c. Associated with a rupture of the ulna collateral ligament of the thumb.
   d. a ligamentous injury to the radial collateral ligament of the thumb.

REFERENCES

1. Introcaso J, Van Holsbeeck M. Musculoskeletal ultrasound. 3rd ed. London: The Health Sciences Publisher; 2016.
2. Newton A, Hawkes D, Bhalaik V. Clinical examination of the wrist. Orthop Trauma. 2017;31(4):237–247.
3. Soames R, Palstanga N. Anatomy and human movements structure and function. 7th ed. London: Elsevier; 2019.
4. Keogh CF, Wong AD, Wells NJ, Barbarie JE, Cooperberg PL. High-resolution sonography of the triangular fibrocartilage: initial experience and correlation with MRI and arthroscopic findings. AJR Am J Roentgenol. 2004;182(2):333–336.
5. Beggs I. Musculoskeletal ultrasound. Philadelphia: Wolters Kluwer, Lippincott Williams & Wilkins; 2013:73–101.
6. Bianchi S, Martinoli C, Sureda D, Rizzatto G. Ultrasound of the Hand. Eur J Ultrasound. 2001;14:29–34.
7. Lee S, Hyun Kim B, Kim S, Kim J, Park S, Choi K. Current status of ultrasonography of the finger. Ultrasonography. 2016;35(2):110–123.
8. McNally E. Ultrasound of the small joints of the hands and feet: current status. Skeletal Radiol. 2008;37(2):99–113.
9. Lee J, Healy J. Normal sonographic anatomy of the wrist and hand. Radiographics. 2005;25:1577–1590.
10. Chiavaras MM, Jacobson JA, Yablon CM, Brigido MK, Girish G. Pitfalls in wrist and hand ultrasound. Am J Roentgenol. 2014;203(3):531–540.

11. European Society of Musculoskeletal Radiology (ESSR). Musculoskeletal ultrasound technical guidelines III. Wrist. 2010. Available at: www.essr.org.

12. Grandizio L, Klena J. Sagittal band, boutonniere, and pulley injuries in the athlete. Curr Rev Musculoskelet Med. 2017;10(1):17–22.

13. Salvatore G, Ferdinando D. Normal sonographic anatomy of the wrist with emphasis on assessment of tendons, nerves and ligaments. J Ultrasound Med. 2016;35:1081–1094.

14. Presazzi A, Bortolotto C, Zacchino M, Madonia L, Draghi F. Carpal tunnel: normal anatomy, anatomical variants and ultrasound technique. J Ultrasound. 2011;14(1):40–46.

15. Thompson N, Mockford B, Cran G. Absence of the palmaris longus muscle: a population study. Ulster Med J. 2001;70(1):22–24.

16. Chatterjee R, Vyas J. Diagnosis and management of intersection syndrome as a cause of overuse wrist pain. BMJ Case Rep 2016;2016:bcr2016216988.

17. Boutry N, Titécat M, Demondion X, Glaude E, Fontaine C, Cotton A. High-frequency ultrasonographic examination of the finger pulley system. J Ultrasound Med. 2005; 24:1333–1339.

18. Schöffl V, Heid A, Küpper T. Tendon Injuries of the hand. World J Orthop. 2012;3(6):62–69.

19. Goubau J, Goubau L, Van Tongel A, Van Hoonacker P, Kerckhove D, Berghs B. The wrist hyperflexion and abduction of the thumb (WHAT) test: a more specific and sensitive test to diagnose de Quervain tenosynovitis than the Eichhoff's Test. J Hand Surg Eur Vol. 2013;39(3):286–292.

20. Mattox R, Battaglia PJ, Scali F, Ottolini K, Kettner NW. Distal intersection syndrome progressing to extensor pollicis longus tendon rupture: a case report with sonographic findings. J Ultrasound. 2016;20(3):237–241.

21. Morris G, Jacobcon J, Brigido M, Gaetke-Udager K, Yabolon C, Ding Q. Ultrasound features of palmar fibromatosis or Dupuytren contracture. J Ultrasound Med. 2018;38(2):387–392.

22. Tsiouri C, Haton M, Baratz M. Injury to the ulnar collateral ligament of the thumb. Hand. 2008;4(1):12–18.

23. Andersson J. Treatment of scapholunate ligament injury. EFORT Open Rev. 2017;2(9):382–393.

24. Seror P. Phalen's test in the diagnosis of carpal tunnel syndrome. J Hand Surg Br. 1988;13(4):383–385.

25. Darwish FM, Haddad WH. Giant cell tumour of tendon sheath: experience with 52 cases. Singapore Med J. 2008;49(11):879–882.

Ultrasound of the Anterior Abdominal Wall and Groin

Andrew Longmead and Richard Brindley

CHAPTER OUTLINE

LEARNING OBJECTIVES

- Recognise normal abdominal wall and groin anatomy and be able to assess this on ultrasound.
- Develop an understanding of pathology diagnosed on ultrasound including abdominal wall and groin herniae.
- Increase the reader's knowledge of management of pathology.
- Give examples of reports to help with future reporting skills.

INTRODUCTION

The structures of the abdominal wall and groin are investigated on ultrasound as potential sites of herniae. They are also commonly examined to assess muscle injury, the nature of soft tissue masses, and postoperative complications following hernia repair, vasectomy, and vascular intervention.

It should be remembered than groin symptoms may originate from pathology in the hip, pubic symphysis, or spine because of the relationship of the structures and complex nerve pathways. This chapter will concentrate on the inguinal and femoral canals in the groin rather than duplicate material covered in Chapter 7.

EQUIPMENT AND PATIENT POSITIONING

For optimal ultrasound assessment of the anterior abdominal wall anatomy, a high frequency ultrasound probe is the primary choice. Lower frequency and curvilinear probes may be required for patients with increased body habitus where tissue thickness is deeper and greater signal penetration is required to visualise the anatomy.

Most modern ultrasound scanners offer functions that can be utilised to help interpretation of a mass and hernia. These include extended field of view and panoramic imaging. Doppler imaging can be used to identify and evaluate key vascular anatomy, for example, visualisation of the inferior epigastric vessels in the search to find the deep inguinal ring or to ensure the femoral vein is patent when assessing for a potential femoral hernia.

A flexible approach to using a range of technical manoeuvres is often required to aid ultrasound visualisation of a hernia, including intermittent increased intraabdominal pressure, obtained through instructing the patient to strain, cough, raise their head or legs or perform Valsalva manoeuvre. Although coughing is useful at times, it is often too quick and varied in its pressure to visualise a potential hernia adequately. Valsalva can be achieved by asking the patient to forcibly exhale through a closed mouth. Alternately, you can ask the patient to strain into their lower abdomen. These methods can provide sustained lower abdominal pressure to visualise movement/distension within the inguinal canal.

Careful use of sonopalpation can be effectively employed to encourage herniated tissue to move in and out of a defect. Conversely, attention must be given to the use of light pressure on the probe to avoid obscuring or reducing any hernia contents, particularly at the start of the examination or when asking the patient to strain.

From a patient positional aspect, most examinations are initially performed supine; however, some studies have shown that gravity may keep the hernia sac in the abdominal cavity and counteract the increased abdominal pressure developed by the Valsalva manoeuvre. In contrast, a standing posture can generate a constant outward and downward force, thus optimally demonstrating a hernia.[1] If a hernia cannot be demonstrated with the patient supine, rescanning with the patient erect is suggested.

> ◎ **TOP TIP**
>
> Having a flexible approach to the use of a variety of Valsalva or straining techniques, combined with scanning patients erect or supine, can help visualise small/reducible herniae. If you cannot see a hernia with the patient supine, rescan with the patient erect.

ANATOMY OF THE ANTERIOR ABDOMINAL WALL

The abdominal wall provides an important role in forming a firm but flexible cavity for the internal abdominal organs, ensuring protection against injury and assisting in both the ability to create forceful expiration and increasing intraabdominal pressure for actions such as coughing, vomiting, and defecation.[2] The layers constituting the abdominal wall from the superficial aspect include the skin, subcutaneous fat/superficial fascia, muscle, deep fascia, and parietal peritoneum.

The muscles of the abdominal wall that are readily visualised on ultrasound are the rectus abdominis, the external obliques, the internal obliques and the transverse abdominis (Fig. 6.1). Fibres from these muscles form an aponeurosis—the rectus sheath or rectus fascia.

Described in more detail later, the anterior and posterior layers of the sheath fuse laterally at the linea semilunaris (semilunaris fascia, Spigelian line) and in the midline at the linea alba. The fibres of the musculature also contribute to the inguinal ligament and conjoint inguinal tendon in the groin.

The vertical muscle—rectus abdominis—is a long paired vertical muscle situated either side of the midline running from the lower portion of the ribcage and xiphisternum, inferiorly to the symphysis pubis, pubic crest, and pubic tubercle. It is divided in the midline by the connective tissue of the linea alba. At several locations, the muscle is intersected by fibrous intersections which are visible in athletes as a "six-pack." The rectus abdominis compresses the abdominal viscera, prevents herniation, and stabilises the pelvis during walking.

The three flat muscles, on either side of the body, are external oblique, internal oblique, and transversus abdominis. External oblique is the largest and most superficial flat muscle of the abdominal wall and its function is to pull the chest downwards, compress the abdominal cavity to increase intraabdominal pressure, and allow side bending and rotational movements. It is situated on the lateral and anterior abdomen, arising from the lower eight ribs. The lower fibres run downwards with attachments to the iliac crest. The middle and upper fibres are directed downwards in an oblique direction, becoming aponeurotic at the midclavicular line forming the anterior layer of the rectus sheath. Fibres from the aponeurosis of both external oblique muscles cross over in the midline as part of the linea alba. Inferiorly, the aponeurosis of the external oblique forms the inguinal ligament.

Internal oblique is located deep to the external oblique and is much thinner and smaller. Its fibres run superomedial from the thoracolumbar fascia of the back, the iliac crest, and inguinal ligament/conjoint tendon to the lower three ribs. It becomes aponeurotic at the level of the ninth costal cartilage to fuse in the midline at the linea alba. Its functions are like those of the external oblique.

Transversus abdominis is the deepest of the flat muscles and has fibres that run transversely from the lateral aspect of the inguinal ligament, anterior inner lip of the iliac crest, cartilages of the lower six ribs (interdigitating with the diaphragm), and from the thoracolumbar fascia. It forms a broad aponeurosis (the Spigelian fascia), the lower fibres curving inferomedially to insert along with

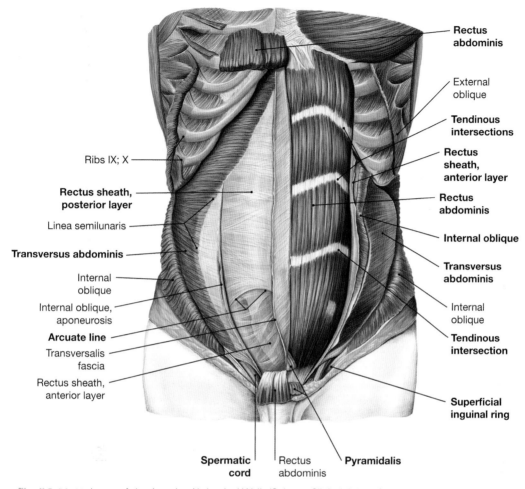

Fig. 6.1 Musculature of the Anterior Abdominal Wall. (Sobotta Clinical Atlas of Human Anatomy. Hombach-Klonisch, Sabine; Klonisch, Thomas; Peeler, Jason. Published January 1, 2019. Pages 39-82. © 2019.)

the internal oblique into the pubic crest to form the conjoint inguinal tendon. The other fibres pass horizontally to the midline to contribute to the linea alba. The transversus abdominis is an important muscle in providing thoracolumbar and pelvic stability as well as contributing to the other functions of the abdominal wall described previously.

Deep to the transversus abdominis muscle is the transversalis fascia which is the lining fascia between the abdominal wall musculature and the peritoneum. Below the level of the umbilicus, the rectus sheath runs anterior to the rectus abdominis muscle, which is covered only by the fascia posteriorly at this level. The deep inguinal ring is an opening in the transversalis fascia at

the midpoint of the inguinal ligament through which runs the spermatic cord in males and the round ligament in females.

Another important structure to consider and a potential site of a hernia is the umbilicus, which is the fibrous remnant of the umbilical cord. The layers of the anterior abdominal wall fuse at the umbilical ring-a small round defect in the linea alba-and the depression of the umbilicus is caused by adherent skin.

Vasculature of the abdominal wall is provided by the superficial epigastric, superficial circumflex iliac, and deep circumflex, superior, and inferior epigastric arteries and veins (Fig. 6.7). The inferior epigastric artery (IEA) and paired veins (IEV) are particularly important landmarks when assessing the inguinal region. The vessels originate from the external iliac artery (EIA) and vein (EIV), located immediately superior to the inguinal ligament and extend superiorly posterior to the rectus abdominis muscles. This level is also known as the arcuate line, where the rectus sheath is deficient as described previously.

> ## ◎ TOP TIP
>
> A good understanding of the anatomy is essential for optimum ultrasound assessment of herniae.

Ultrasound Technique and Normal Appearances

With increased competence, ultrasound operators may focus the scan over the area of interest, but for those with less experience, a good way to begin the assessment of the upper abdominal wall anatomy is to start with the probe held transversely over the epigastric region in the midline, scanning from the level of xiphisternum inferiorly to the level of umbilicus (Fig. 6.2A).

Deep to the layers of the skin and subcutaneous fatty tissue, the central portion of the anterior abdominal wall musculature will be seen (Fig. 6.2B), which consists of the rectus abdominis muscles located on either side of the midline[2].

Sliding the probe towards the umbilicus, following the linea alba, the full extent of the rectus abdominis muscles can be seen in transverse section (TS) (Fig. 6.3A,B).

Sliding the probe either side of the rectus abdominis muscles laterally (Fig. 6.4A) will allow visualisation of the flat oblique muscles (Fig. 6.4B,C), transversus abdominis, transversalis fascia, peritoneum, omental fat, and bowel[3](Fig. 6.4D).

At the lateral edge of the rectus abdominis muscles, the semilunaris fascia (Spigelian line) is identified at the medial aponeurosis of the oblique muscles (see Fig. 6.4C,D).[4]

The umbilicus can be a difficult area to assess and interpret with ultrasound (Fig. 6.5), and an additional amount of gel to fill the void is often required, along with the use of a lower frequency transducer. Alternatively, an endocavity probe may be inserted directly into the umbilicus to detect a potential defect and hernia contents.[5]

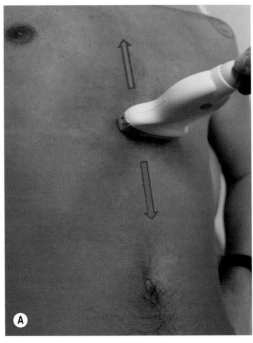

Fig. 6.2 (A) Probe position and movement to assess the rectus abdominis muscles TS. *Blue arrows* denote movement of probe.

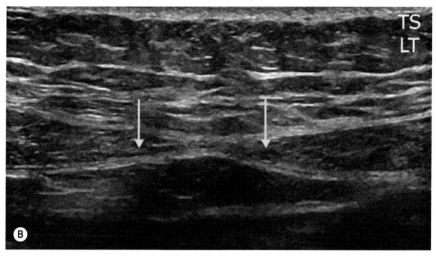

Fig. 6.2, cont **(B)** Rectus abdominis muscles. US image starting position epigastric area midline TS. Rectus abdominis *(yellow arrows)*. *TS,* Transverse section; *US,* ultrasound.

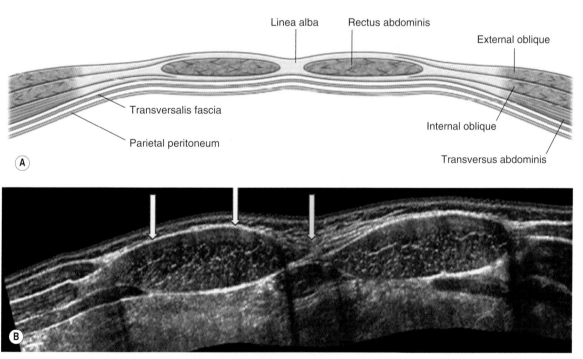

Fig. 6.3 **(A)** Transverse section midline rectus abdominis, rectus sheath, and linea alba. **(B)** Ultrasound image hyperechoic rectus sheath *(white arrows)* and linea alba *(yellow arrow)*.

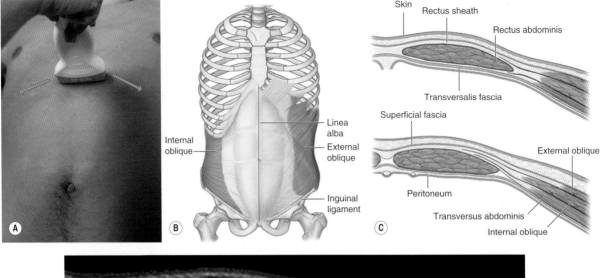

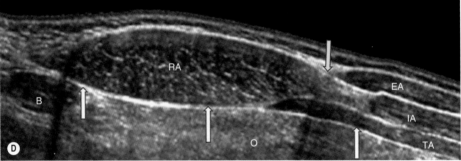

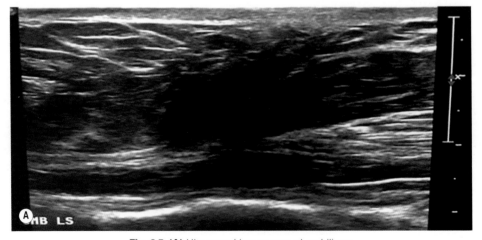

Fig. 6.4 (A) Probe position and movement to assess the oblique muscles. *Blue arrows* denote movement of probe. **(B)** Oblique muscles. **(C)** Left abdominal wall anatomy. **(D)** Ultrasound image left rectus abdominis *(RA)* and oblique muscles. *B,* Bowel; *EA,* external oblique; *IA,* internal oblique; *O,* omental fat; *TA,* transversus abdominis; *white arrows,* transversus fascia and peritoneum; *yellow arrow;* semilunaris fascia/spigelian line.

Fig. 6.5 (A) Ultrasound image normal umbilicus;

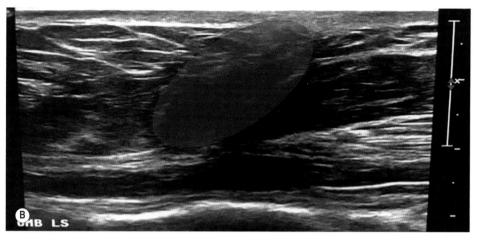

Fig. 6.5, cont   (B) green oval denotes umbilical tissue.

ANATOMY OF THE INGUINAL AND FEMORAL CANALS

The inguinal ligament is a continuation of the aponeuroses of the oblique muscles and extends medially, inferiorly, and obliquely from the anterior superior iliac spine (ASIS) to the pubic tubercle[6] (Fig. 6.6).

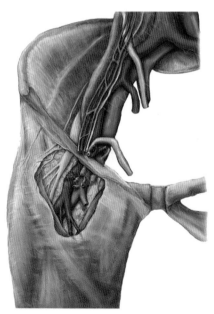

Fig. 6.6 Inguinal Ligament *(green line)* (From https://www. kenhub.com/en/library/anatomy/inguinal-canal.)

Located deep and just superior to the medial portion of the inguinal ligament is the inguinal canal, a short tunnel measuring approximately 4 cm in length in the inferior abdominal wall.[6] The roof of the canal is formed by the internal oblique and transverse abdominis muscles, the anterior wall by the aponeurosis of the external and internal oblique muscles, the floor by the inguinal and lacunar ligament, and the posterior wall by the transverse fascia and conjoint tendon (Fig. 6.7).[7]

During fetal development, the inguinal canal is created by an outpouching of the peritoneum, a peritoneal diverticulum described as the processes vaginalis. The gonads in both sexes must descend through this canal into the pelvic cavity from the superior lumbar region of the posterior abdominal wall where they originated. The canal courses obliquely, lateral to medial and superior to inferior, transmitting the spermatic cord and ilioinguinal nerves in males and the round ligament of the uterus and ilioinguinal nerve in females. When the inguinal canal fails to completely close during fetal development, an opening is left patent for abdominal contents to protrude through, potentially resulting in herniae seen in babies and young children.[8]

The inguinal canal has two openings, the deep and superficial rings. The deep ring is formed by the transversalis fascia and located above the midpoint of the inguinal ligament.[9] The superficial ring is located more distally, superior and medial to the pubic tubercle (see Fig. 6.7). Identifying the deep ring is essential and the IEA and IEVs provide a key landmark to identify the

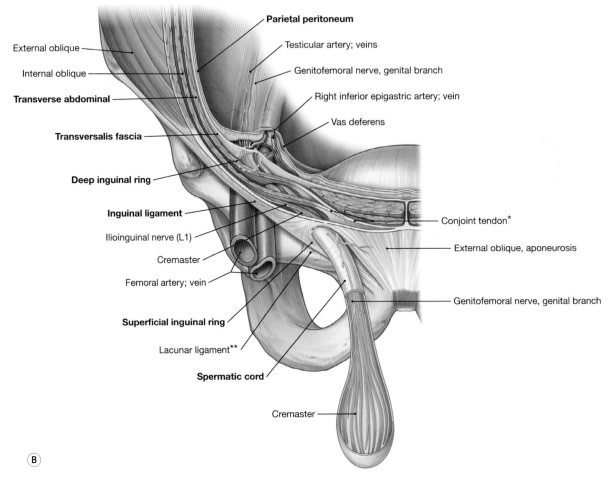

Fig. 6.7 Anatomy of the inguinal canal. (Sobotta Clinical Atlas of Human Anatomy. Hombach-Klonisch, Sabine; Klonisch, Thomas; Peeler, Jason. Published January 1, 2019. Pages 281-361. © 2019.)

deep ring as they course immediately posterior to it (Fig. 6.7).

The femoral canal is another important structure in the groin and a potential site of a hernia. This is the smallest, most medial component of the femoral sheath which contains the femoral artery and vein, lymph nodes, and nerves. Positioned in the leg crease, it is inferior to the inguinal ligament and medial to the femoral vein (Fig. 6.8). Its clinical significance is that the entrance to the femoral canal is the femoral ring through which peritoneal fat and/or bowel can enter as a femoral hernia. It can result in a surgical emergency if the bowel becomes strangulated.

Ultrasound Technique and Normal Appearances of the Inguinal Canal

The external oblique muscle forms the inguinal ligament, seen on ultrasound as a thick hyperechoic linear structure (Fig. 6.9). To guide probe placement and orientation, the surface landmarks of the ASIS and pubic tubercle can be palpated to help locate the inguinal ligament which runs between the two. It is a useful structure to locate as it is a reminder of the orientation of the inguinal canal of which it forms the floor.

The inguinal canal itself is a subtle structure to visualise on ultrasound. The following steps describe how to locate the inguinal canal structures[10]:

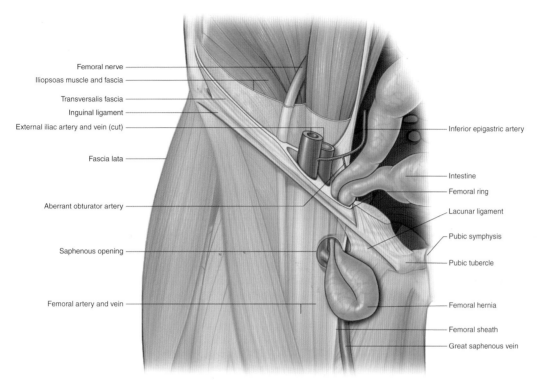

Fig. 6.8 Anatomy of the Femoral Canal. (Gray's Surgical Anatomy. Brennan, Peter A, MD, PhD, FRCS (Eng), FRCSI, . . . Show all. Published January 1, 2020. Pages 393-413.e2. © 2020.)

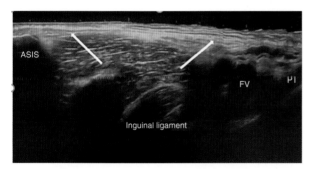

Fig. 6.9 Ultrasound image, panoramic longitudinal view of the inguinal ligament (*white arrows*) extending from the anterior superior iliac spine *(ASIS)* to the pelvic tubercle *(PT)*. Note the hypoechoic round femoral vessels *(FV)* on the right.

Step 1:

Begin with the probe positioned centrally and transversely over the rectus abdominis muscles, just proximal to the umbilicus and move laterally depending on which side is to be assessed. The left side is shown in the image in Fig. 6.10A.

Slide the transducer inferiorly until the inferior epigastric vessels (IEV) are seen as three hypoechoic oval structures (Fig. 6.10B). Anatomical knowledge of the course of these vessels helps with Step 2,[11] and Doppler can be used to help identify them.

Step 2:

Once the IEV are identified, with the probe held transversely, scan inferiorly and laterally (Fig. 6.11A,B), carefully tracking the course of the vessels as they diverge laterally to join the EIV.

Step 3:

At this point, as the IEV pass directly under the inguinal canal, the probe is rotated into an oblique orientation and positioned medially so that the canal is now being visualised in TS (Fig. 6.12). The deep ring appears as a subtle ovoid shaped structure containing hypoechoic vessels.

The inguinal canal should then be assessed at the level of the deep ring using an appropriate technique such as Valsalva or other method to increase intraabdominal

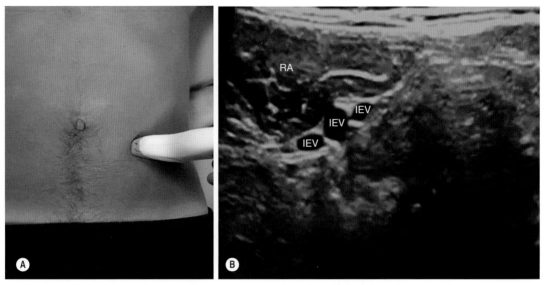

Fig. 6.10 (A) Probe position to locate the emergence of the left inferior epigastric vessels from the rectus sheath. **(B)** Ultrasound image, transverse section of the three hypoechoic inferior epigastric vessels *(IEV)*. *RA,* Rectus abdominis muscle.

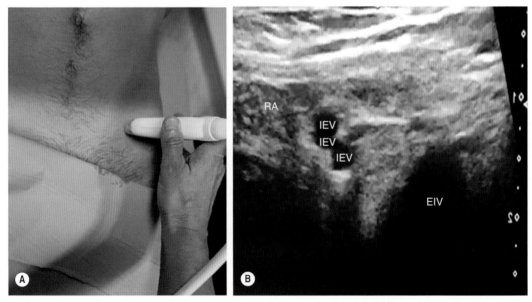

Fig. 6.11 (A) Probe position tracking the inferior epigastric vessels laterally and obliquely and **(B)** ultrasound image inferior epigastric vessels *(IEV)*. *EIV,* External iliac vessels; *RA,* rectus abdominis muscle.

pressure to push any hernia contents into the canal (Fig. 6.13). This should be repeated along the length of the canal at regular intervals until the superficial ring is reached in order to exclude a direct inguinal hernia which would enter through a defect in the transversalis fascia, the posterior wall of the canal.[12] This would be

medial to the IEV in a region known as Hesselbach's or medial inguinal triangle.

In addition, longitudinal section (LS) views of the inguinal canal should be obtained by rotating the ultrasound transducer 90 degrees so that it is aligned with the oblique course of the canal (Fig. 6.14).

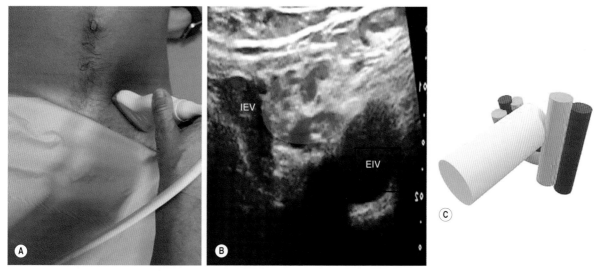

Fig. 6.12 (A) Probe orientated to show the deep ring in transverse. **(B)** Ultrasound image deep ring inguinal canal *(highlighted)*. *EIV,* External iliac vessels; *IEV,* inferior epigastric vessels. **(C)** Diagram showing the inferior epigastric vessels passing underneath the inguinal canal to join the external iliac vessels.

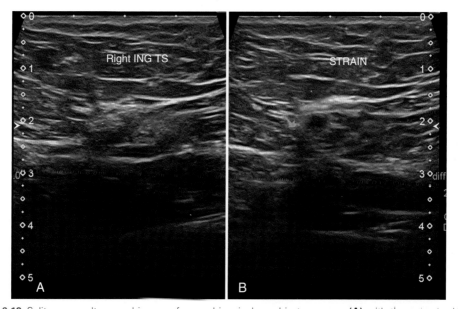

Fig. 6.13 Split screen ultrasound image of normal inguinal canal in transverse **(A)** with the patient relaxed and **(B)** patient asked to strain showing normal distention of vessels within the canal *(orange arrow)* but no canal disruption from a hernia.

In patients of a larger body habitus, the IEVs can be difficult to visualise. The reverse technique can be used in combination with a lower frequency probe to identify the external iliac vein, tracking proximally to visualise the inferior epigastric vessels.

Ultrasound Technique and Normal Appearances of the Femoral Canal

The pubic tubercle is located in the medial portion of the superior pubic ramus (Fig. 6.15) and is a key bony landmark for differentiating between inguinal and femoral

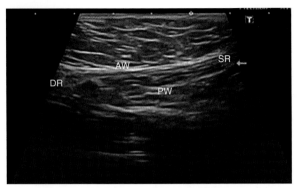

Fig. 6.14 Longitudinal Ultrasound Image of the Inguinal Canal. *AW,* Anterior wall of inguinal canal; *DR,* deep ring; *PW,* posterior wall; *SR,* superficial ring.

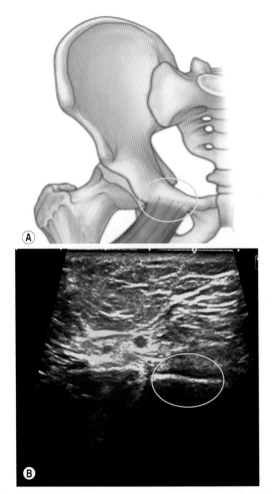

Fig. 6.15 (A) Diagram highlighting pubic tubercle *(yellow circle)* and **(B)** the same on ultrasound, a pink highlighted inguinal canal.

herniae. Both the rectus abdominis muscles and the distal portion of the inguinal ligament insert onto the pubic tubercle and can therefore be used to identify it. Inguinal herniae are located superior and medial to the pubic tubercle, whereas a femoral hernia will originate lateral and inferior to it.[13]

The femoral canal is located inferior to the inguinal ligament. Demarcating the inferior aspect of the femoral canal is the saphenofemoral junction, located at the saphenous opening (Fig. 6.8) where the great saphenous vein originates from the common femoral vein, and a useful landmark to identify as below this a femoral hernia will not be visualised. Scanning just proximal to the saphenofemoral junction[14] is therefore advised, with the femoral artery and vein to the far side of the screen and femoral canal central (Fig. 6.16).[14] As with all herniae, this should be assessed by instructing the patient to increase their intraabdominal pressure through means of cough, strain, or Valsalva. The femoral canal should also be assessed in LS by rotating the probe 90 degrees.

PATHOLOGY

Herniae Overview

A hernia can be defined as a defect (hole) within the muscle wall or surrounding fascia allowing underlying internal body tissue, most commonly fatty peritoneal tissue but potentially bowel, to protrude through the defect.[15] Often, peritoneum drawn through the hernial defect forms a sac-like structure around the other contents. Although a hernia may cause no or very few symptoms, they can be painful and may be associated with a swelling that may, or may not be reducible.

More serious complications of a hernia include incarceration and strangulation. Incarceration occurs when herniated contents become irreducible, either due to a narrow defect in the abdominal wall or due to adhesions. An important sign of incarceration involving bowel which has high specificity but limited sensitivity is fluid in the herniated bowel loop with bowel wall thickening and free fluid in the hernial sac.[15]

A strangulated hernia occurs when the blood supply to the herniated bowel is compromised, resulting in potential death of tissue, and is classed as a surgical emergency as is it can be fatal.[16] Ultrasound appearances may include reduced vascularity, oedema, and free fluid around a strangulated hernia, although these are

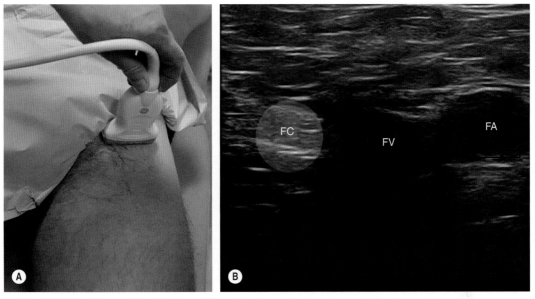

Fig. 6.16 (A) Probe position inferior and lateral to the pelvic tubercle and **(B)** ultrasound image transverse section of the femoral canal *(FC)*, femoral artery *(FA)*, and femoral vein *(FV)*.

not specific as they may also be seen in nonstrangulated herniae.[15,16]

Herniae are usually termed by the location of their occurrence within the upper abdominal wall or groin with the common terms being epigastric, umbilical, paraumbilical, inguinal, Spigelian, femoral, and incisional.

📍 **TOP TIP**

Be mindful of the pressure placed on the ultrasound probe as some hernia sacs can easily be reduced and therefore not visualised.

Hernia of the Upper Anterior Abdominal Wall

Epigastric, paraumbilical, and umbilical hernia. Ten percent of herniae occur in the midline between the xiphisternum and umbilicus and are often termed epigastric (Fig. 6.17). Those developing around the umbilicus are known as paraumbilical (Fig. 6.18) or within it, umbilical (Fig. 6.19). Accounting for 6% to 14% of all abdominal wall herniae, umbilical herniae are the second most common type of hernia and 90% of them are acquired, often due to factors that increase intraabdominal pressure such as obesity or ascites.[17] For patients presenting with a history of malignancy, particularly of gastrointestinal and gynaecological origins, umbilical hernia should be differentiated from metastatic umbilical nodules known as Sister Mary Joseph nodules, which are static and mostly solid in nature.[18]

REPORT—PARAUMBILICAL HERNIA

There is a mid-line supra paraumbilical hernia with a moderate sized hernia sac containing both fatty tissue and a small amount of fluid. This hernia is partially reducible under probe pressure and has a fascia neck defect measuring 20 mm wide.

Spigelian hernia. Spigelian herniae occur through a weakness in the semilunaris fascia between the lateral edge of the rectus abdominis muscle and the oblique muscles called the Spigelian line (Fig. 6.20). Most of these herniae occur in the lower abdomen where the posterior rectus sheath is deficient, an area known as the arcuate line. Although they are rare, making up only 1% to 2% of all abdominal wall herniae, they can be difficult to detect clinically and around 20% of them become incarcerated. Ultrasound can therefore be very useful in establishing the diagnosis.[19]

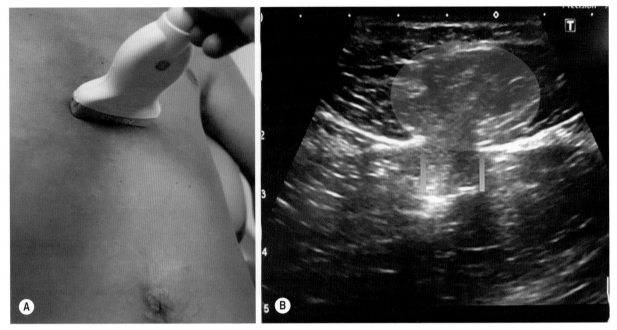

Fig. 6.17 (A) Transverse position over the epigastric region. **(B)** Ultrasound image, epigastric hernia. Note the defect of the linea alba *(yellow arrows)* with a hernia sac *(highlighted yellow)* containing fatty tissue.

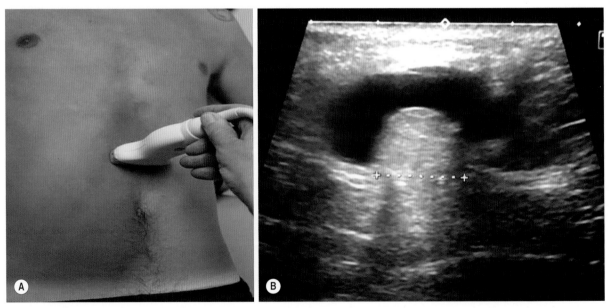

Fig. 6.18 (A) Transverse position over the region immediately superior to the umbilicus and **(B)** ultrasound image of a midline supra paraumbilical hernia.

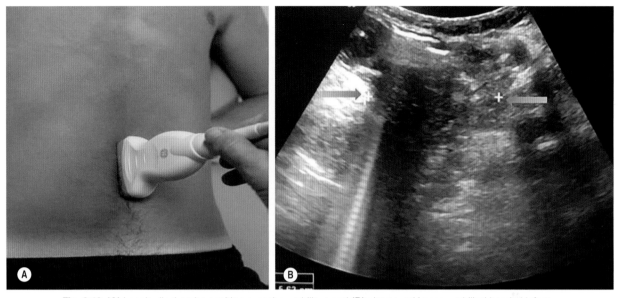

Fig. 6.19 (A) Longitudinal probe position over the umbilicus and (B) ultrasound image umbilical hernia (defect – *yellow arrows*) which contains both fatty tissue and a small amount of bowel. Notice the artefact from the bowel gas within the hernia. Peristalsis was observed.

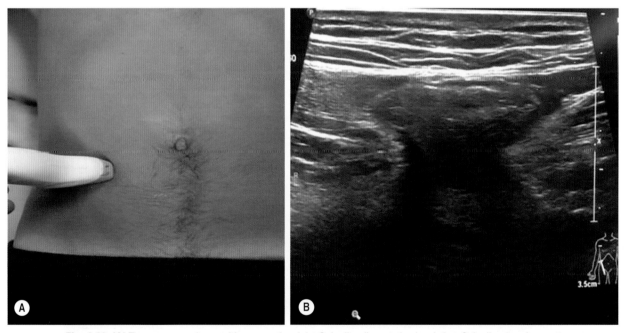

Fig. 6.20 (A) Transverse probe position over the right Spigelian line at the level that Spigelian hernia most commonly occur within the lower abdominal wall. (B) Ultrasound image showing a defect in the semilunaris fascia.

REPORT—SPIGELIAN HERNIA

In the right lower abdominal wall at the site of the patient's discomfort, there is a 20-mm defect within the right semi lunaris fascia with a small sac of fatty tissue that has herniated through. This sac is reducible under the pressure of the ultrasound probe and the ultrasound appearances are consistent with a Spigelian hernia.

Hernia of the Groin

Inguinal hernia. Inguinal herniae are the most common groin hernia, accounting for 75% of all herniae and as mentioned, there are two types, indirect and direct, with the former being the most common and affecting men more than women.[20]

An indirect hernia involves a protrusion of peritoneal fat/bowel entering the inguinal canal through a defect in the deep ring, emerging on the ultrasound image lateral to the inferior epigastric vessels (Figs. 6.21 and 6.22). Due to the movement of the hernia down the canal, they are also sometimes known as a "sliding" hernia. Large, indirect inguinal hernia can extend distally into the scrotum in males to form an inguinoscrotal hernia.

REPORT—INDIRECT INGUINAL HERNIA

There is a small- to moderate-sized, partially reducible, indirect inguinal hernia seen within the right groin which appears to contain fatty tissue and a small amount of bowel.

Direct inguinal herniae occur as a result of a defect in the posterior wall of the inguinal canal and enter the canal through a defect in the transversalis fascia.[21] This would be medial to the IE in a region known as Hesselbach's or medial inguinal triangle. Herniated tissues enter the canal in a localised fashion similar to the "mushroom effect" seen in epigastric herniae[22] (Fig. 6.23).

SAMPLE REPORT—DIRECT INGUINAL HERNIA

Fatty tissue is seen to protrude anteriorly through a 15-mm wide defect in the transversalis fascia, medial to the inferior epigastric vessels on Valsalva. This reduces fully on Valsalva and under the pressure of the ultrasound probe. Appearances are consistent with a direct inguinal hernia.

Femoral hernia. Accounting for just under 3% of all herniae, femoral herniae are most commonly seen in women of 40 to 70 years of age, although inguinal surgery can increase the chances of them occurring in men.[23]

A femoral hernia develops when a hernia sac—usually involving peritoneal fat but potentially bowel—passes into the femoral canal. In normal circumstances, asking the patient to strain will result in normal expansion of the femoral vein; however, in the presence of a femoral hernia (depending on its size and irreducibility), the expandability of the femoral vein may be inhibited. Scanning over the canal both transversely (Fig. 6.24) and longitudinally

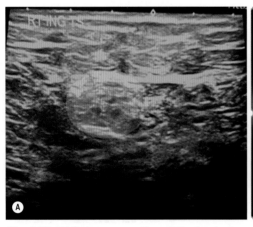 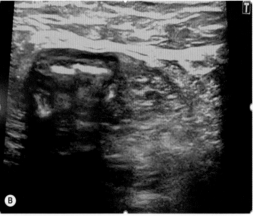

Fig. 6.21 (A) Transverse section of the inguinal canal without Valsalva, showing only the spermatic cord within the canal (highlighted in yellow) **(B)** The patient has been asked to strain and both fatty tissue and bowel are seen to enter the canal via the deep ring, causing canal disruption.

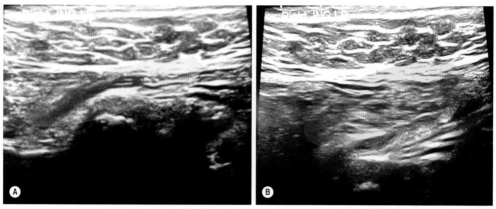

Fig. 6.22 (A) Ultrasound probe rotated 90 degrees and aligned to the longitudinal aspect of the inguinal canal. The ultrasound image shows the inguinal canal *(highlighted yellow)* with the patient in a relaxed state with vessels and a small amount of fatty tissue within the canal at the deep ring. **(B)** The patient has been asked to strain and both fatty tissue and a small amount of bowel are seen to migrate into the canal distally *(highlighted pink)*.

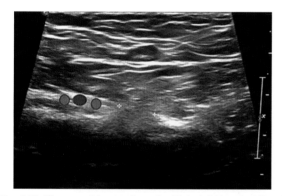

Fig. 6.23 Ultrasound Image Over the Right Mid-Inguinal Canal. Notice the defect with *calipers* across the posterior inguinal canal wall which has allowed a sac of fatty tissue to enter focally into the canal. The hernia originates medial to inferior epigastric vessel (highlighted as *red and blue*).

(Fig. 6.25) and comparison with the asymptomatic side may help in cases that are difficult to interpret.

SAMPLE REPORT—FEMORAL HERNIA

Within the proximal right femoral canal, there is evidence of a hernia sac containing fatty tissue and a small amount of fluid. This sac did not reduce on Valsalva and under the pressure of the ultrasound probe. Appearances are consistent with a non-reducible femoral hernia. The femoral vessels appear patent and compressible. Urgent onward specialist referral is advised in view of the findings.

Femoral hernia necks are usually small, and this increases the chance of strangulation. If strangulation is suspected during the scan and the hernia contents include bowel, it is a surgical emergency and requires immediate attention.[23]

Other Types of Hernia

Incisional hernia. An incisional hernia may occur at the site of previous surgery due to muscular weakness and the presence of scar tissue, although obesity and infection at the wound site are also predisposing factors (Fig. 6.26). It is estimated that 10% of all hernia operations are carried out to repair this type of defect.[24]

◎ TOP TIP

- Large abdominal wall herniae can be difficult to evaluate and even visualise due to the small foot plate of the ultrasound probe. Changing probes and depths can help, dependent on the habitus of the patient.
- Be mindful of the pressure placed on the ultrasound probe as some hernia sacs can easily be reduced and therefore not visualised.

Posterior abdominal wall hernia. Posterior abdominal wall or lumbar herniae are very rare. They occur through the superior or inferior lumbar triangle of the main muscle of the posterior wall—the quadratus lumborum[25] (Fig. 6.27). Although the most common

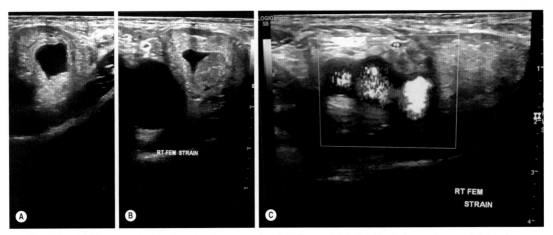

Fig. 6.24 (A) Ultrasound probe in transverse over the right femoral canal shows a hernia sac containing fatty tissue and a small amount of fluid. **(B)** The patient has been asked to strain and both fatty tissue and a small amount of fluid are seen to migrate into the canal distally. **(C)** Power Doppler is used to show the femoral vessels are patent.

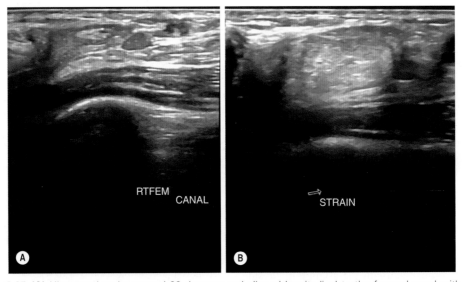

Fig. 6.25 (A) Ultrasound probe rotated 90 degrees and aligned longitudinal to the femoral canal with the patient relaxed. **(B)** Femoral canal with the patient having been asked to strain. The comparison of the two images shows an obvious area of fatty tissue in the right-sided image that has protruded into the canal with the patient straining.

content of this type of hernia is retroperitoneal fatty tissue, other herniated tissues may include kidney, colon, or less commonly, small bowel, omentum, ovary, spleen, or appendix.[25]

Sportsman's hernia (Gilmore's groin/incipient hernia). These terms are often used to describe nonspecific, inguinal-related, regional pain associated with sporting activities. One proposed theory of a cause of this pain is posterior abdominal wall weakness leading to bulging of abdominal structures compressing the genital branch of the genitofemoral nerve which passes through the inguinal canal. On dynamic ultrasound assessment,

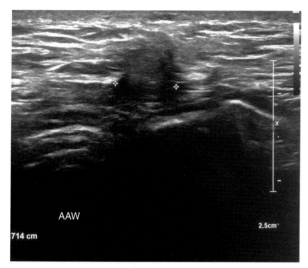

Fig. 6.26 Small incisional hernia located in the midline, midway between the xiphisternum and umbilicus located along the scar line of previous bowel surgery. *AAW*, Anterior abdominal wall.

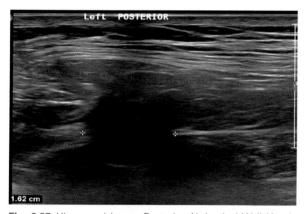

Fig. 6.27 Ultrasound Image Posterior Abdominal Wall Hernia with a 16-mm Wide Defect.

with straining, this bulging can often be seen against the posterior wall of the inguinal canal; however, it is equally visualised in asymptomatic patients (Fig. 6.28). The validity of this feature is therefore contentious and should be reported with caution.[26,27]

Alternative Common Pathologies

Although not an exhaustive list, common pathologies that may present as a lump in the abdominal wall or groin are lipomata (Fig. 6.29), divarication of the rectus abdominis muscles, prominent/everted xiphisternum,

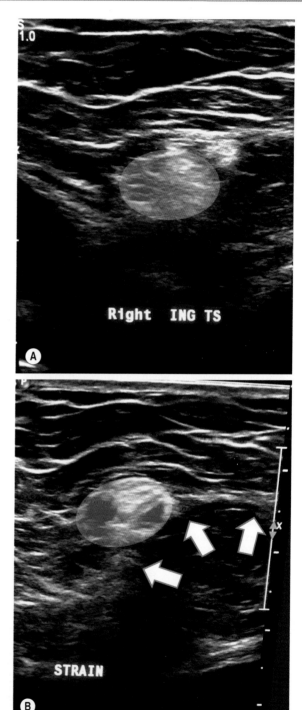

Fig. 6.28 (A) Ultrasound of the right inguinal canal in transverse *(highlighted)* with the patient in a relaxed state and **(B)** with the patient straining. *White arrows* showing bulging of the underlying peritoneum/bowel due to weakness of the posterior inguinal wall.

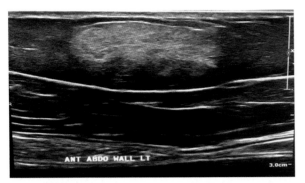

Fig. 6.29 Benign Lipoma Located Within the Subcutaneous Tissue Layer.

and lymph nodes. Haematomas and seromas are often visualised as postoperative hernia findings and are discussed further in chapter 11.

Lipomas, or spermatic cord lipomas as they are termed, can occur within the inguinal canal and these may produce similar symptoms to that of a hernia (Fig. 6.30). They can be difficult to distinguish on ultrasound from the fatty contents of a hernia sac and this should be acknowledged when reporting as it may influence surgical management.

Most spermatic cord lipomas are found incidentally during hernia surgery and recent studies have shown them to be more prevalent than originally thought, although actual discrete lipomas are rare as there is usually some connection to a protrusion of peritoneal fatty tissue. If a cord lipoma is suspected but the ultrasound finding remain inconclusive, consideration of alternative cross-sectional imaging is advised.[28]

Interestingly, anterior abdominal wall herniae containing fat can sometimes be mistaken for lipomas by inexperienced operators. Probe compression can often help distinguish one from the other.

Divarication/Diastasis Recti

Divarication or diastasis recti is seen clinically as a visible midline swelling, predominantly in the upper abdomen. This is exacerbated when there is increased abdominal pressure and occurs as a result of thinning and widening of the linea alba, in combination with laxity of the ventral abdominal musculature. This is often seen in post-partum females, young infants, and obese patients. Ultrasound has been described as the gold standard for measuring the increased distance between the rectus muscles, due to its excellent correlation with surgery, and intra observer reliability. The image is easily obtained by scanning the linea alba transversely. Normal appearances of the abdominal wall are shown in Fig. 6.31A.

A diagnosis of divarication can be made when the distance between the two medial aspects of rectus abdominis muscles measures 2.7 cm or over[29] (Fig. 6.31B). Asking the patient to strain will often demonstrate associated bulging of the abdominal contents against

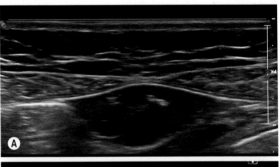

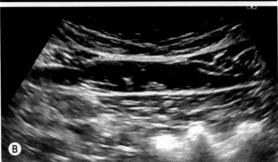

Fig. 6.31 (A) Ultrasound image normal appearances, transverse section linear alba/rectus abdominis muscles. **(B)** Divarication with a 35-mm wide measurement between the two medial borders of the rectus abdominis muscles.

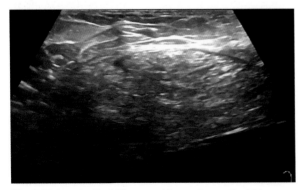

Fig. 6.30 Longitudinal Ultrasound Image Large Cord Lipoma.

the linea alba. It is important to scan along the linea alba to exclude small co-existent ventral herniae.[30,31]

Everted Xiphisternum

Arising from the inferior and posterior portion of the sternum is the xiphisternum, a small cartilaginous extension of the lower sternal body. Although it usually ossifies later in life, anomalies in the xiphoid process are common, and significant interindividual variations are seen in their orientation. In some cases, it may be flat and in others, it may be protruding at the distal end of the sternum. Eversion or anterior deflection of the xiphisternum can be clinically mistaken for an epigastric lesion or hernia and ultrasound can be useful to provide diagnostic differentiation. Patients often present with a painless hard lesion.[32]

Ultrasound appearances commonly show an anterior angulated bony structure with distal acoustic shadowing evident (Fig. 6.32).

Lymph Nodes

When assessing the groin, the palpable swelling presenting as a clinically suspected hernia may actually represent a superficially located lymph node on ultrasound. A benign lymph node will demonstrate an oval shaped hypoechoic solid structure with an internal fatty hilum and normal vasculature entering the hilum on Colour Doppler assessment. (Fig. 6.33A). Conversely, a pathological lymph node will have a typically round shape, be markedly hypoechoic with loss of the internal hilar component, and may show unorganised internal vascularity on Doppler assessment (Fig. 6.33B). This finding would require prompt appropriate onward referral for further assessment and management.

Fig. 6.34 lists other potential pathologies and their ultrasound features which may be alternatively discovered when assessing for a groin hernia.

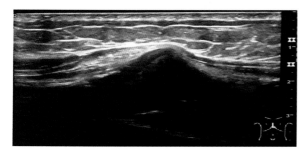

Fig. 6.32 Longitudinal Ultrasound Image Everted Xiphisternum.

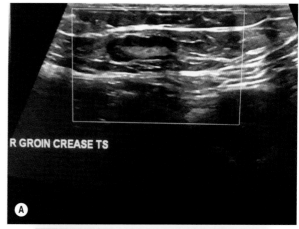

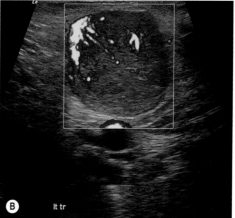

Fig. 6.33 (A) Ultrasound image normal, benign-looking lymph node and **(B)** abnormal-looking lymph node.

MANAGEMENT OF HERNIAE

As mentioned previously, patients with herniae typically present with a lump, pain, or both. Most herniae occur in the groin and more often in men than in women.[33] Current guidelines suggest patients with clinical suspicion of a symptomatic groin hernia are referred to secondary care for a specialist/surgical opinion first, which then may lead to a request for ultrasound assessment when clinical examination is equivocal (Fig. 6.35).

The main role of ultrasound is to help confirm the presence of a hernia, assess the contents and reducibility of the sac, and size of the fascial defect which can impact treatment options. Studies have reported high levels of sensitivity and specificity for hernia detection with ultrasound but this is highly dependent upon the

Differential hernia diagnosis table	Brief ultrasound description
Lymph nodes	Oval hypoechoic lesion with central echogenic hilum
Femoral aneurysm	Focal dilatation of the femoral artery greater than 1.5 cm.
Saphena varix	Tortuous tubular anechoic channels, low venous blood flow seen within on colour Doppler.
Spermatic cord lipoma	Echogenic/hypoechoic soft tissue lesion in the spermatic cord.
Encysted spermatic cord hydrocele	Well-defined cystic structure within/along the spermatic cord, can be septated.
Psoas abscess	Heterogeneous collection within the Psoas, (note the affected leg will be bent up and difficult to straighten).
Hydrocele in the canal of Nuck (female)	Anechoic fluid extending into the labia majora adjacent to the round ligament.

Fig. 6.34 Table of Alternative Pathologies. (From Keshwani N, Hills N, McLean L. Inter-rectus distance measurement using ultrasound imaging: Does the rater matter? Physiother Can. 2016;68(3):223-229.)

experience and competence of the operator.[34] Following ultrasound assessment, if diagnostic uncertainty remains, other imagining modalities may be utilised. Magnetic resonance imaging (MRI) may be useful for patients with recalcitrant groin pain, not due to an obvious hernia, and to look for alternative musculoskeletal pathology (Fig. 6.36). Computed tomography (CT) also has a key role in surgical planning for large ventral herniae where the defect is too extensive to quantify with ultrasound, particularly in those patients who have had previous surgery and have comorbidities.

Approximately one-third of inguinal herniae are asymptomatic and if detected, current advice for men in this group is to use a "watch and wait" strategy. If they become larger and more painful, most will then require surgery to avoid the risk of strangulation. In symptomatic male patients over the age of 30, current European guidelines determine this group should undergo mesh-based hernia repair due to its reduced rate of recurrence and complications in comparison with suture repair.[35] Conversely, surgical repair (herniorrhaphy) of inguinal and femoral herniae in female patients is often carried out electively regardless of symptoms due to the increased risk of serious complications compared with men.

A laparoscopic rather than an open approach is preferred due to a shorter convalescence, reduced complications, and acceptable recurrence rates.

The mesh used to repair hernia defects is sutured into the adjacent tissues. The aim is to restore structure and function of the abdominal wall. Mesh commonly appears as a linear hyper reflective interface on ultrasound, demonstrating posterior acoustic shadowing, although the echogenicity of the mesh can vary (Fig. 6.37). Scanning the periphery of the mesh under increased abdominal pressure is paramount to ensuring reducible herniae are not missed.[35,36]

COMPLICATIONS OF HERNIA REPAIR

Although prognosis following surgical repair is excellent, postoperative complications that can arise include haematoma, abscess, and seroma, as well as paresthesia/numbness in the groin that usually dissipates over time.

Haematomas following surgery are relatively common. They demonstrate variable appearances on ultrasound dependent on their age. Initial ultrasound appearances may be complex and heterogeneous, becoming relatively anechoic over time as they begin to resolve (Fig. 6.38A).

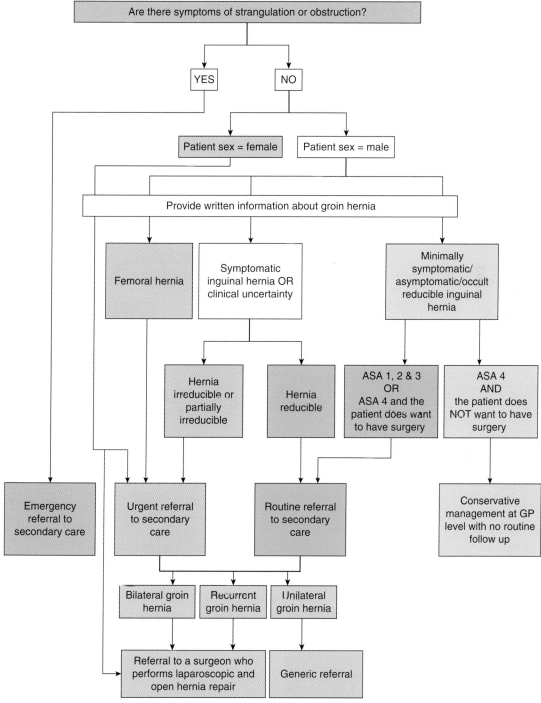

Fig. 6.35 Flow Diagram Showing the Recommended Management of Suspected Herniae in a Primary Care Setting by the British Hernia Society. (From HerniaSurge Group. International guidelines for groin hernia management. Hernia. 2018;22(1):1-165.)

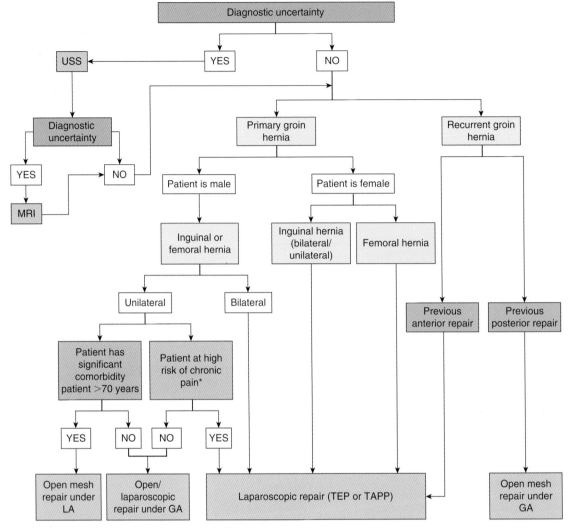

Fig. 6.36 Table Published by the British Hernia Society Showing the Role of Ultrasound in the Diagnostic Pathway. (From HerniaSurge Group. International guidelines for groin hernia management. Hernia. 2018;22(1):1-165.)

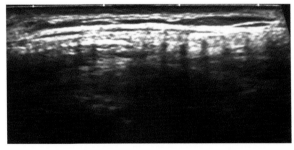

Fig. 6.37 Ultrasound Appearances of Mesh.

They are often subcutaneous but can be intramuscular or within the peritoneal planes and can be difficult to differentiate from more sinister pathologies.

An abscess may develop during the late postoperative period as a result of infection; this can be several weeks after surgery, although they can develop much earlier. It can be difficult to diagnose infection in a post-operative collection/haematoma on ultrasound and clinical correlation is vital as the patient would usually present with symptoms of fever, rigors, and raised inflammatory markers. Aspiration may be utilised to give a definitive diagnosis (Fig. 6.38B).

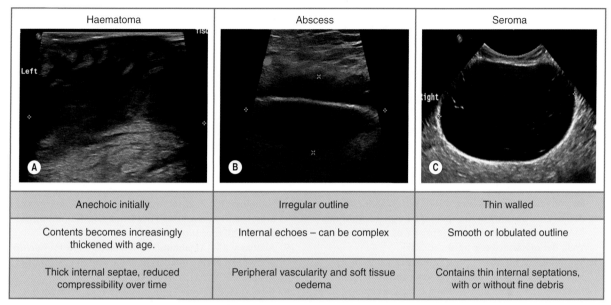

Haematoma	Abscess	Seroma
Anechoic initially	Irregular outline	Thin walled
Contents becomes increasingly thickened with age.	Internal echoes – can be complex	Smooth or lobulated outline
Thick internal septae, reduced compressibility over time	Peripheral vascularity and soft tissue oedema	Contains thin internal septations, with or without fine debris

Fig. 6.38 (A–C) Possible complications following hernia repair.

A seroma is a collection of proteinaceous serous fluid thought to arise from a disruption of lymphatic and vascular channels. Ultrasound appearances are of a thin-walled clear fluid collection (Fig. 6.38C) commonly occurring adjacent to the postoperative wound. Clinically there is focal swelling accompanied by pain or discomfort which often resolves within 6 to 8 weeks. Chapter 11 discusses the appearances of seroma and haematoma in more detail.

Other complications include urinary retention and bladder damage, bowel obstruction, mesh rejection and migration, enterocutaneous fistula and hernia recurrence. Testicular complications of inguinal hernia repair are rare, although one possible complication is ischemic orchitis which presents between 24 and 72 hours after surgery and occurs when blood flow to the testes is compromised.[37–39]

MULTIPLE CHOICE QUESTIONS

1. What is the name of the bright connective tissue seen between the rectus abdominis muscles?
   a) Semilunar line
   b) Spigelian line
   c) Linea alba
2. What are the names of the vessels used to locate the deep ring of the inguinal canal?
   a) Inferior epigastric vessels
   b) Superior epigastric vessels
   c) Inferior oblique vessels
3. What is the most common type of hernia?
   a) Spigelian hernia
   b) Indirect inguinal herniae
   c) Direct inguinal hernia
4. What is an incarcerated hernia?
   a) An irreducible hernia due to a narrow neck
   b) A hernia that is fully reducible
   c) A hernia only located in the groin
5. Where is the femoral canal?
   a) Paraumbilical region
   b) Potential space medial and adjacent to the femoral vein.
   c) A region superior to the inguinal ligament

REFERENCES

1. Wongsithichai P, Chang KV, Hung CY, Wang TG. Dynamic ultrasound with postural change facilitated the detection of an incisional hernia in a case with negative MRI findings. J Ultrasound. 2014;18(3):279–281.
2. Varacallo M, Scharbach S, Al-Dhahir MA. Anatomy, anterolateral abdominal wall muscles. [Updated 2019 Apr 6]. In: StatPearls [Internet]. Treasure Island, FL: StatPearls Publishing; 2020. Available at: https://www.ncbi.nlm.nih.gov/books/NBK470334/.
3. Parker SG, Wood CPJ, Sanders DL, Windsor ACJ. Nomenclature in abdominal wall hernias: Is it time for consensus? World J Surg. 2017;41(10):2488–2491.
4. Arslan OE. Anatomy of the abdominal wall. In: Shiffman MA, Mirrafati S, eds. Aesthetic Surgery of the Abdominal Wall. Berlin, Heidelberg: Springer; 2005.
5. Van Wingerden JP, Ronchetti I, Sneiders D, Lange JF, Kleinrensink GJ. Anterior and posterior rectus abdominis sheath stiffness in relation to diastasis recti: abdominal wall training or not? J Bodyw Mov Ther. 2020;24(1):147–153.
6. Revzin MV, Ersahin D, Israel GM, et al. US of the inguinal canal: comprehensive review of pathologic processes with CT and MR imaging correlation. Radiographics. 2016;36:2028–2048.
7. Jacobson J, Khoury V, Brandon C. Ultrasound of the groin: techniques, pathology, and pitfalls. Am J Roentgenol. 2015;205(3):513–523.
8. Tuma F, Lopez RA, Varacallo M. Anatomy, abdomen and pelvis, inguinal region (inguinal canal) [Updated 2019 Mar 21]. In: StatPearls [Internet]. Treasure Island, FL: StatPearls Publishing; 2020. Available at: https://www.ncbi.nlm.nih.gov/books/NBK470204/.
9. Kumar V, Patel J, Sharma C, Inkhiya S. Morphometric study of inguinal canal on cadaver. Int J Anat Res. 2018;6(2.1):5172–5175.
10. Vasileff W, Nekhline M, Kolowich P, Talpos GB, Eyler WR, van Holsbeeck M. Inguinal hernia in athletes: role of dynamic ultrasound. Sports Health. 2017;41(10):2488–2491.
11. Kandinata N, Van Fossen K. Anatomy, abdomen and pelvis, epigastric artery. [Updated 2018 Dec 30]. In: StatPearls [Internet]. Treasure Island, FL: StatPearls Publishing; 2020. Available at: https://www.ncbi.nlm.nih.gov/books/NBK537156/.
12. Jansen CJ, Yielder PC. Evaluation of hernia of the male inguinal canal; sonographic method. J Med Radiat. 2018;65:163–168.
13. Murphy KP, O'Connor OJ, Maher MM. Adult abdominal hernias. Am J Roentgenol. 2014;202:6: 506–511.
14. Campos NMF, Aguiar AI, Rodrigues CT, Curvo-Semedo L, Donato P. Dynamic ultrasound of abdominal wall hernias. European Society of Radiology. ECR 2019 EPOS; 2020 [cited 15 October 2020]. Available from: https://epos.myesr.org/poster/esr/ecr2019/C-3464
15. Lassandro F, Iasiello F, Pizza NL, et al. Abdominal hernias: radiological features. World J Gastrointest Endosc. 2011;3(6):110–117.
16. Earle D, Roth S, Saber A. SAGES guidelines for laparoscopic ventral hernia repair. Surg Endosc. 2016;30:3163–3183.
17. Mittal T, Kumar V, Khullar R, et al. Diagnosis and management of Spigelian hernia: a review of literature and our experience. J Minim Access Surg. 2008;4(4):95–98.
18. Chong WH, Chan CX, Tsang JPK, Yuen MKE. Approach to ultrasound evaluation of common abdominal wall pathology. ESSR; 2016. Available at: https://epos.myesr.org/poster/esr/essr2016/P-0049/Imaging%20findings%20OR%20Procedure#poster.
19. Aljubairy AM, Alqahtani MAM, Hakeem HF. Prevalence of inguinal hernia in relation to various risk factors. EC Microbiol. 2017;9(5):182–192.
20. Jenkins JT, O'Dwyer PJ. Inguinal hernias. BMJ. 2008;336(7638):269–272.
21. Jansen CJ, Yielder PC. Evaluation of hernia of the male inguinal canal; sonographic method. J Med Radiat. 2018;65:163–168.
22. Köckerling F, Koch, A, Lorenz R. Groin hernias in women—a review of the literature. Front Surg. 2019;6(4):1–8.
23. Goethals A, Azmat CE, Adams CT. Femoral hernia. [Updated 2019 Dec 18]. In: StatPearls [Internet]. Treasure Island, FL: StatPearls Publishing; 2020. Available at: https://www.ncbi.nlm.nih.gov/books/NBK535449/.
24. Basta MN, Kozak GM, Broach RB, et al. Can we predict incisional hernia? Ann Surg. 2019;270(3):544–553.
25. Sundaramurthy S, Suresh HB, Anirudh AV, Prakash Rozario A. Primary lumbar hernia: a rarely encountered hernia. Int J Surg Case Rep. 2016;20:53–56.
26. Dimitrakopoulou A, Schilders E. Sportsman's hernia? An ambiguous term. J Hip Preserv Surg. 2016;3(1):16–22.
27. McNally E. Practical Musculoskeletal Ultrasound. 2nd ed. Oxford: Churchill Livingstone; 2014.
28. Lilly MC, Arregui ME. Lipomas of the cord and round ligament. Ann Surg. 2002;235(4):586–590.
29. Benjamin DR, Van de Water AT, Peiris CL. Effects of exercise on diastasis of the rectus abdominis muscle in the antenatal and postnatal periods: a systematic review. Physiotherapy.2014 Mar;100(1):1-8
30. Keshwani N, Hills N, McLean L. Inter-rectus distance measurement using ultrasound imaging: Does the rater matter? Physiother Can. 2016;68(3):223–229.
31. Liaw LJ, Hsu MJ, Liao CF, Liu MF, Hsu AT. The relationships between inter-recti distance measured by ultrasound imaging and abdominal muscle function

in postpartum women: a 6-month follow-up study. J Orthop Sports Phys Ther. 2011;41(6):435–443.

32. Mashriqi F, D'Antoni AV, Tubbs RS. Xiphoid process variations: a review with an extremely unusual case report. Cureus. 2017;9(9):e1725. Available at: https://www.ncbi.nlm.nih.gov/pmc/articles/PMC5659327/.

33. HerniaSurge Group. International guidelines for groin hernia management. Hernia. 2018;22(1):1–165.

34. Zwaans WAR, Koning GG, Gurusamy KS, van Kleef M, Scheltinga MRM, Roumen RMH. Surgical interventions for the management of chronic groin pain after hernia repair (postherniorrhaphy inguinodynia) in adults. Cochrane Database Syst Rev. 2017;4:CD012630.

35. Elango S, Perumalsamy S, Ramachandran K, Vadodaria K. Mesh materials and hernia repair. Biomedicine (Taipei). 2017;7(3):16.

36. Wake BL, McCormack K, Fraser C, Vale L, Perez J, Grant AM. Transabdominal pre-peritoneal (TAPP) vs totally extraperitoneal (TEP) laparoscopic techniques for inguinal hernia repair. Cochrane Database Syst Rev. 2005;1:CD004703.

37. Halligan S, Parker SG, Plumb AA, et al. Imaging complex ventral hernias, their surgical repair, and their complications. Eur Radiol. 2018;28:3560–3569.

38. Royal College of Surgeons. Commissioning guide: groin hernia. Royal College of Surgeons of England (RCS); 2016.

39. Furtschegger A, Sandbichler P, Judmaier W, Gstir H, Steiner E, Egender G. Sonography in the postoperative evaluation of laparoscopic inguinal hernia repair. J Ultrasound Med. 1995;14(9):679–684.

Ultrasound of the Hip and Thigh

Sara Riley

LEARNING OBJECTIVES

After reading the chapter you will have a good understanding of:
- The relevant anatomical structures of the hip/thigh
- Ultrasound technique and normal appearances of the hip/thigh, including tips and pitfalls
- Common pathologies of the hip/thigh, including clinical presentation, management of the conditions, and report writing
- The value of other imaging modalities

INTRODUCTION

Clinical evaluation of hip and thigh can be challenging, making it difficult to isolate the cause of symptoms. Although there are limitations, because the structures are deep, ultrasound has a role in the diagnosis of disorders involving the muscles, tendons, and soft tissues, as well as the joint for effusion/synovitis.

Plain radiography is often the primary imaging modality, especially where arthritis or bony injury/dislocation are suspected. Computed tomography (CT) and magnetic resonance imaging (MRI) are important for the detection of occult traumatic/stress fractures and osteonecrosis of the femoral head. MRI is particularly good at assessing bone oedema and intra-articular pathology including complex ligamentous injury.[1,2]

A lower frequency linear or curvilinear ultrasound transducer is needed to obtain the penetration required to image the hip and thigh in an adult or large child. A higher frequency transducer may be used in ultrasound of the peadiatric hip and superficial musculature.

ANATOMY

The X-ray in Fig. 7.1 shows the bony landmarks of the hip which are important for muscle/ligament attachments and joint anatomy and will be mentioned throughout this chapter.

Hip Joint

The hip joint is a synovial articulation between the acetabulum of the pelvis and the proximal femur. The acetabulum is a cup-like depression which is deepened by the presence of a fibrocartilaginous collar, the acetabular labrum. Only part of the labrum is visible on ultrasound, therefore MRI is the modality of choice for labral injury and femoroacetabular impingement. The joint surface is lined by hyaline cartilage which is covered by a thin layer of lubricating synovium. The capsule is strongly reinforced by intra/extracapsular

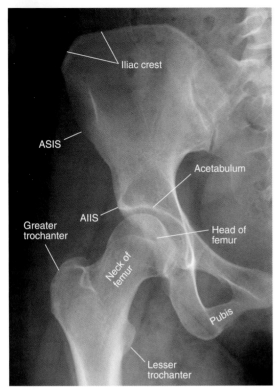

Fig. 7.1 X-Ray of the right hip shows important bony landmarks. *AIIS,* Anterior inferior iliac spine; *ASIS,* anterior superior iliac spine.

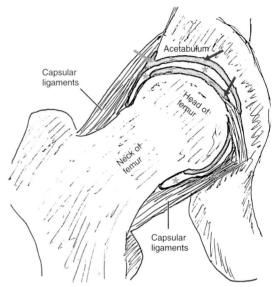

Fig. 7.2 Coronal section of the articular hip structures. *Blue arrow,* labrum; *green asterisks,* synovial lined recess; *red arrows,* hyaline cartilage. (Line drawing courtesy of Sara Riley).

ligaments and musculature, providing a stable joint (Fig. 7.2).[3,4]

Musculature of the Hip and Thigh

Anterior

Iliopsoas is a combination of the psoas major and iliacus muscles and is the strongest flexor of the hip. The psoas major and iliacus muscles are separate muscle bellies in the posterior abdominal wall. They merge as they pass deep to the inguinal ligament into the anterior compartment of the thigh where they insert into the lesser trochanter of the femur (Fig. 7.4).

The synovial lined iliopsoas bursa is positioned between the iliopsoas myotendinous junction and the hip joint capsule. It communicates with the joint in 15% of cases via a foramen in the capsular ligaments, see pathology section Fig. 7.31. This percentage increases in the presence of inflammatory arthritis and following arthroplasty. The bursa is not visible on ultrasound unless distended with fluid.

Rectus femoris crosses both the hip and knee joints, is a flexor of the hip, and an extensor of the knee. The anatomy is complicated, arising by a short strong tendon from the anterior inferior iliac spine (AIIS) (direct head) and by an indirect tendon from the superolateral margin of the acetabulum. The tendons merge to form a conjoined tendon 1 cm distal to the origin with two components, a superficial component which blends with the anterior muscle fascia and a deep component which forms the central tendon with a long myotendinous junction. There is an intermingling of muscle fibres related to each origin.

In the distal third of the thigh, the muscle belly of rectus femoris stops and forms the superficial tendinous lamina of the conjoint quadriceps tendon which inserts onto the patella.

The other quadriceps muscles (vastus lateralis, vastus intermedius, and vastus medialis) have origins arising directly from the superior femur. They have shorter tendinous components to the quadriceps tendon (see Chapter 8).

Sartorius is the longest muscle in the body. It arises from the anterior superior iliac spine (ASIS) and courses down, crossing rectus femoris along the inner thigh to join gracilis and semitendinosus (ST) to form a conjoined pes anserine (goose's foot) tendon inserting on the tibia[5] (see Chapter 8) (Fig. 7.4).

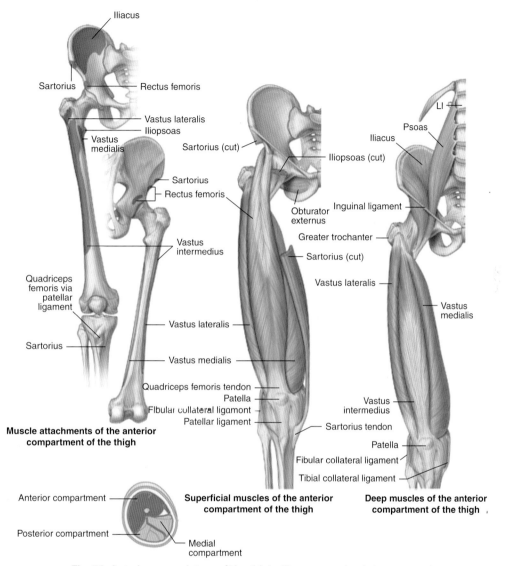

Fig. 7.3 Anterior musculature of the thigh. (From www.elsevierimages.com)

Fig. 7.3 is an illustration showing the deep/superficial compartments and muscle attachments of the anterior hip and thigh.

Medial

As a group, the adductor muscles are responsible for adduction of the thigh and individually for flexion, medial/lateral rotation, and extension of the hip. The muscles are pectineus, adductor longus, adductor brevis, adductor magnus, and gracilis (Fig. 7.4).

Pectineus originates from the pectineal line on the anterior surface of the pubis and inserts onto the pectineal line on the posterior surface of the femur, inferior to the lesser trochanter.

Adductor longus arises from the anterior surface of the pubis, just lateral to pubic symphysis, and inserts on the middle third of the linea aspera of the femur.

Adductor brevis arises from the anterior surface of the inferior pubic ramus, inferior to the origin of adductor longus, and inserts onto the pectineal line

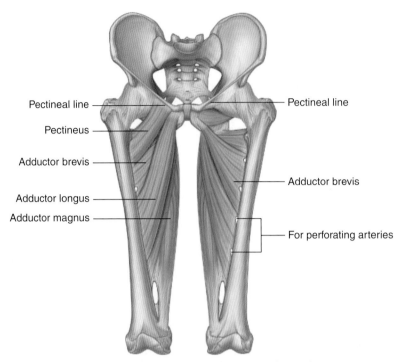

Fig. 7.4 Medial thigh showing the adductor and pectineus muscle anatomy.

and superior part of the medial lip of linea aspera of the femur.

Adductor magnus, the largest and deepest of the adductor group, arises from the inferior pubic ramus, ischial ramus, and inferolateral area of ischial tuberosity. It inserts on the gluteal tuberosity, medial lip of the linea aspera, medial supracondylar ridge, and adductor tubercle of the femur.

Lastly, gracilis originates from the inferior margin of pubic symphysis, inferior ramus of pubis, and adjacent ramus of ischium. Its insertion is the medial surface of the tibial shaft as a component of the pes anserine tendon[5] (see Chapter 8).

The origins of adductor longus, adductor brevis, and gracilis are via a fibrocartilaginous enthesis, which allows for increased strength, protects the tendons from compression, and the bone from excessive shear forces. It is important to consider this when assessing the adductors for tendinopathy and injury.

The origin of adductor longus also merges with the abdominal wall musculature and symphysis pubis via a common aponeurosis. This explains why pain in the pubic region, groin, and thigh can be difficult to assess clinically.[6]

Lateral

Also known as the greater trochanteric region, the main structures for evaluation with ultrasound are the gluteal muscles/tendons, and adjacent structures. Morphological similarities between the abductor mechanisms of the hip and shoulder have given rise to the term "rotator cuff of the hip."

The gluteus minimus muscle arises from the lateral surface of the iliac wing deep to the anterior portion of gluteus medius. It crosses the hip joint and the tendon inserts on to the anterior facet of the greater trochanter (GT). The gluteus medius muscle also arises from the lateral surface of the iliac wing, superficial and posterior to gluteus minimus. The anterior portion passes obliquely over gluteus minimus to insert in a broad attachment on the lateral facet of the GT, whereas the more posterior fibres insert into the superoposterior facet (Fig. 7.5).[7]

The gluteus maximus muscle is the most superficial and largest of the gluteal muscles. It arises from the

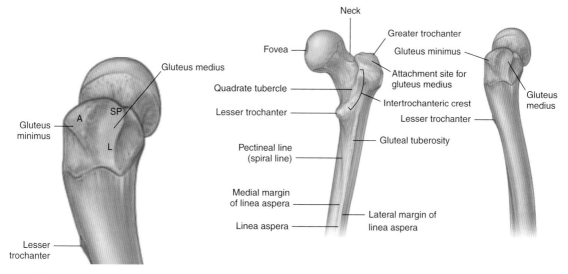

Fig. 7.5 Anatomy of the greater trochanter. The anterior facet *(A)* for gluteus minimus insertion and the lateral *(L)* and superoposterior *(SP)* facets for gluteus medius insertion. © Elsevier Ltd. Drake et al: gray's anatomy for students - www.studentconsult.com

posterior surface of the ilium, and slopes across the buttock to insert into the iliotibial tract and gluteal tuberosity of the femur.

Tensor fascia latae is a small muscle arising from the ASIS. It continues distally in the lateral thigh where it is enveloped by the iliotibial tract. This is a large sheet of aponeurotic fascia which also partially envelops gluteus maximus. The iliotibial tract originates from the iliac crest and continues distally in the lateral thigh to insert into the tibia (see Chapter 8).

There are numerous bursae in the greater trochanteric region which can vary in number. These include the trochanteric bursa (subgluteus maximus bursa) which is located between gluteus maximus, iliotibial tract, and gluteus medius tendons; the subgluteus medius bursa deep to the insertion of the gluteus medius on the lateral facet of the GT; and the subgluteus minimus bursa deep to the insertion of the gluteus minimus on the anterior facet. Like the iliopsoas bursa, the synovial peritrochanteric bursae are not visible on ultrasound in normal conditions.

Fig. 7.6 is an illustration which shows the gross musculature of the abductors, posterior hip, and thigh.

Posterior

The hamstring complex (HMC) (biceps femoris [BF], semitendinosus [ST] and semimembranosus [SM] muscles) is important anatomy in the posterior hip/thigh. The muscles span two joints and are hip extensors and knee flexors in the gait cycle. Their name (hamstring) is derived from the method of tying up and hanging legs of ham for curing (Fig. 7.6).

The easiest way to understand the gross anatomy of the HMC is to imagine a tuning fork lying lengthways in the thigh with the handle as the common tendinous origin on the ischial tuberosity and the muscles as the forks, on the lateral side BF and medial side ST and SM.

BF is a double-headed muscle, with the long head arising from the medial facet of the ischial tuberosity and the short head from the lateral linea aspera, lateral supracondylar line, and intermuscular septum. The myotendinous junctions span the length of the muscle bellies, the distal tendons inserting predominantly onto the fibula (see chapter 8). The muscle is innervated by the sciatic and peroneal nerves. The dual innervation may result in asynchrony in the coordination or intensity of stimulation of the two heads, a possible cause for this muscle having the highest frequency of tears of the HMC.

ST arises from the inferomedial impression of the upper portion of the ischial tuberosity by way of a conjoint tendon with the long head of the BF muscle.

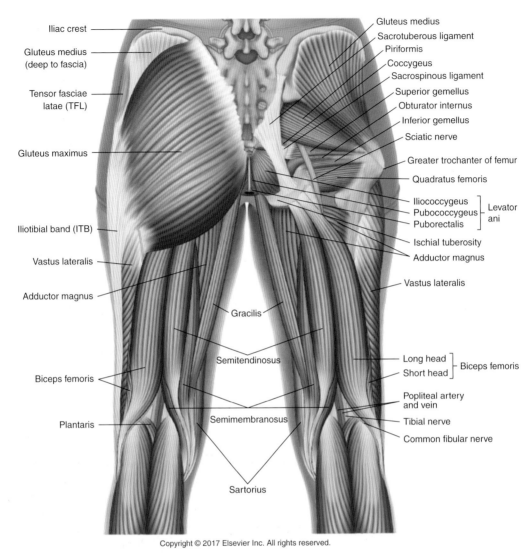

Fig. 7.6 Musculature of the abductors and posterior thigh. (From Musculino J. E; The muscular system manual – Th skeletal muscles of the human body, 4th ed. Elsevier 2017).

In the proximal thigh, the ST muscle is larger than the SM. In the distal thigh, the ST muscle forms a long tendon which lies anterior to the SM muscle, superior to the popliteal fossa, and travels to insert onto the tibia as one of the pes anserine tendons (see Chapter 8).

The SM muscle originates on the superolateral aspect of the ischial tuberosity, beneath the proximal half of the ST muscle. Distally, the SM muscle has multiple tendinous insertions to the medial tibial condyle (anterior, direct, and inferior arms), the posterior oblique ligament (capsular arm), and the posterior joint capsule and arcuate ligament (oblique popliteal ligament).

At the level of the ischial tuberosity, deep to the common insertion of the hamstrings, is the ischial bursa which is not visible unless pathology is present.

The sciatic nerve is worth considering due to its close relationship to the HMC and buttock muscles as it travels down the thigh (Fig. 7.6). The sciatic nerve is derived from the lumbosacral plexus. After its formation, it leaves the pelvis and enters the gluteal region via the greater sciatic foramen. The nerve courses through the gluteal region then enters the posterior thigh by passing deep to the long head of the BF.

Within the posterior thigh, the sciatic nerve gives rise to branches that innervate the hamstring muscles and adductor magnus. When the sciatic nerve reaches the superior popliteal fossa, it bifurcates into the tibial and common peroneal nerves.

ULTRASOUND TECHNIQUE AND NORMAL ULTRASOUND APPEARANCES

Ultrasound examination of the anterior hip/thigh is performed with the patient in the supine position. The hip should be in a neutral position in extension and slight external rotation.

Hip Joint, Iliopsoas Complex

For assessment of the joint and iliopsoas complex it is best to start at the level of the femoral head and acetabulum in longitudinal section (LS) (Fig. 7.7A) as these landmarks are easily recognisable (Fig. 7.7B). The transducer is then moved inferiorly to include the femoral neck and anterior recess. At this level the probe is aligned in an oblique orientation with the distal end of the probe rotated laterally (Fig. 7.7C). Wide field of view and panoramic ultrasound are useful for an overview of the joint; however, the individual joint structures are better demonstrated in detail separately.

A thin hypoechoic layer of hyaline cartilage is seen covering the femoral head and the acetabular labrum, a hyperechoic triangular structure, is seen superior to the

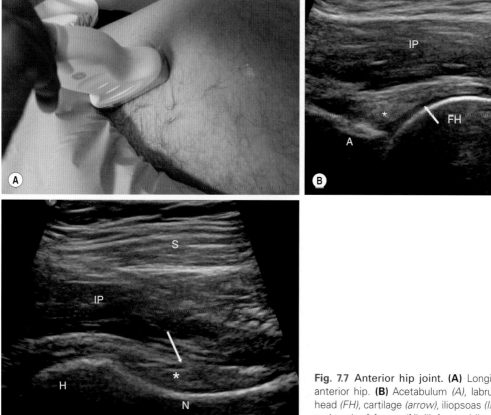

Fig. 7.7 Anterior hip joint. **(A)** Longitudinal section anterior hip. **(B)** Acetabulum *(A)*, labrum *(*)*, femoral head *(FH)*, cartilage *(arrow)*, iliopsoas *(IP)*. **(C)** Head *(H)* and neck of femur *(N)*, iliofemoral ligament/joint capsule *(arrow)*, joint recess/synovial layers *(*)*, iliopsoas *(IP)*, sartorius *(S)*.

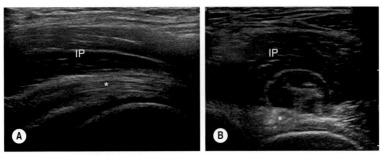

Fig. 7.8 Iliopsoas muscle and tendon. (A) Longitudinal and **(B)** transverse sections anterior hip demonstrating the iliopsoas tendon *(*)*, and the iliopsoas muscle *(IP)*.

synovial recess (see Fig. 7.7B). The iliofemoral ligament is superficial to the labrum and the iliopsoas muscle is situated in front of the femoral head and joint space (see Fig. 7.7C). Its tendon has a posteromedial position and therefore a minor medial adjustment of the transducer is required in sagittal section to visualise the tendon (Fig. 7.8A). The iliopsoas muscle and tendon are also assessed in transverse section (TS) where the posteromedial position of the tendon is apparent (Fig. 7.8B).

The anterior joint capsule appears as a slightly concave hyperechoic structure (see Fig. 7.7C) between the iliopsoas muscle and the joint recess. The joint recess is less echogenic anterior to the femoral neck and consists of two layers, anterior and posterior, which are together in normal physiological conditions (Fig. 7.9) but are separated when an effusion is present. A small sliver of physiological fluid may be present in normal conditions. Attempts should be made to heel the distal part of the probe into the thigh in order to avoid anisotropy

of the joint recess which can simulate an effusion. An additional pitfall relates to leg positioning: internal rotation of the hip may cause the anterior joint capsule to become convex anteriorly, simulating synovial hypertrophy.[8–11]

In the peadiatric patient, cartilage is present rather than mature bone at the ossification sites (see Fig. 7.9). This can be easily confused with fluid by the inexperienced practitioner as it is hypoechoic in appearance. By applying pressure with the probe, the cartilage will remain unchanged whereas fluid will move. Comparison with the contralateral side is also helpful.

> ◎ **TIPS**
>
> When examining the anterior joint recess, heel the transducer into the thigh to avoid anisotropy which can simulate an effusion.
>   Internal rotation of the hip may cause the anterior joint capsule to become convex anteriorly, simulating synovial hypertrophy.

Anterior Musculature (Quadriceps and Sartorius)

The musculature of the anterior thigh is normally scanned for injury or to locate the position of a mass. Using a systematic approach to identify the muscles and adjacent structures, start from the ASIS in TS. At this level the short tendons of sartorius medially and tensor fasciae latae (TFL) laterally are seen (Fig. 7.10). With a distal excursion of the transducer, sartorius travels medially crossing rectus femoris, whilst TFL remains lateral in front of vastus lateralis.

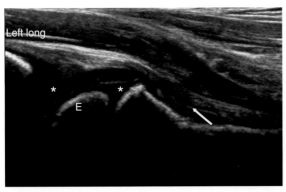

Fig. 7.9 Longitudinal section of a normal 3 year old hip joint. *Arrow* shows the echogenic joint recess between the synovial layers. Cartilage *(*)*, epiphysis ossification *(E)*.

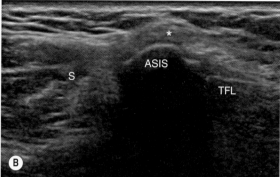

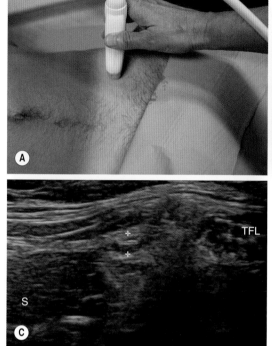

Fig. 7.10 Antero-superior hip structures. **(A)** Transverse section (TS) anterior superior iliac spine *(ASIS)*. **(B)** Sartorius *(S)* and tensor fasciae latae *(TFL)* muscles and the origin of their tendons *(*)*. **(C)** TS slightly inferior to ASIS. The lateral femoral cutaneous nerve is shown between the calipers.

The lateral femoral cutaneous nerve can be identified slightly inferior to ASIS as a small fascicular structure superficial to sartorius (see Fig. 7.10). The nerve supplies sensation to the anterolateral thigh. Compression of the nerve may cause a condition called meralgia paresthetica (numbness of the thigh). Tight clothing, obesity or weight gain, and pregnancy are common causes of meralgia paresthetica. Diagnostic and therapeutic injection of local anaesthetic around the nerve may be performed under ultrasound guidance.[12,13]

Placing the transducer in LS at the level of AIIS, superior to the acetabulum, the direct head of rectus femoris (RF) can be identified at its origin as an echogenic fibrillar structure (Fig. 7.11). Due to anisotropy, the indirect tendon of RF is poorly imaged in this position. To visualise the indirect tendon at its origin on the superolateral acetabulum, a modified technique is required with a lateral to medial angulation of the transducer in a transverse plane.

In TS, centrally in the proximal third of the thigh, the RF muscle is situated anterior to the vastus intermedius muscle which lies adjacent to the femur. The central deep and superficial myotendinous junctions of RF are shown in Fig. 7.12. The vastus lateralis and vastus medialis muscles are seen either side of RF (Fig. 7.12). By moving the probe laterally and medially these large muscles are imaged in their entirety.

In TS in the distal thigh, the superficial tendinous lamina of RF is seen overlying the muscle belly of the vastus intermedius muscle (Fig. 7.13). The quadriceps tendon will be further explained in Chapter 8.

Medial

To examine the adductors the patient is positioned with the thigh abducted and externally rotated and the knee flexed. Due to the intimate nature of the examination, a chaperone may be offered, and care should be taken to ensure that the patient's dignity is maintained with suitable cover of the pubic region.

The transducer is placed over the proximal medial thigh in TS. Fig. 7.14 shows the relationship between the anterior quadriceps compartment, femoral neurovascular bundle, and medial adductor compartment. Three adductor muscle layers are visualised from superficial to deep: adductor longus (lateral)/gracilis (medial), adductor brevis, and adductor magnus.

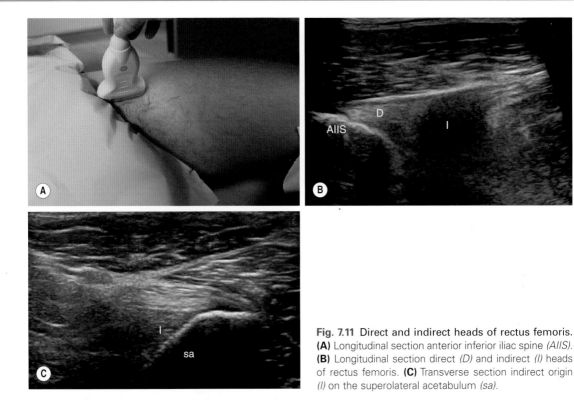

Fig. 7.11 Direct and indirect heads of rectus femoris.
(A) Longitudinal section anterior inferior iliac spine *(AIIS)*.
(B) Longitudinal section direct *(D)* and indirect *(I)* heads
of rectus femoris. **(C)** Transverse section indirect origin
(I) on the superolateral acetabulum *(sa)*.

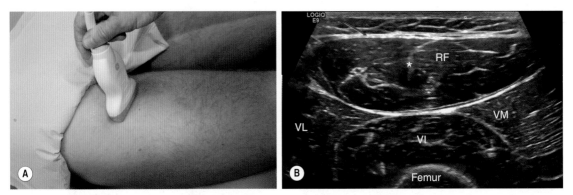

Fig. 7.12 Quadriceps musculature. (A) Transverse section anterior thigh. **(B)** Rectus femoris *(RF)*, vastus intermedius *(VI)*, vastus lateralis *(VL)*, and vastus medialis *(VM)*. Central tendon *(*)* and superficial tendon/aponeurosis *(red arrow)* of RF.

To image the adductors in LS, the transducer is rotated in an oblique section on the medial thigh (Fig. 7.15).

To include the origin of the tendinous and fibrocartilaginous attachments (Fig. 7.16), the transducer is moved until the pubic bone is included on the image. The fibrocartilage entheses have a triangular hypoechoic appearance which can be difficult to interrogate due to anisotropy. A small hockey stick transducer enables more dexterity which may help reduce the artefact. The superficial portion of the adductor longus origin can appear blurred due to the merging of fibres with the abdominal wall musculature.[8–11]

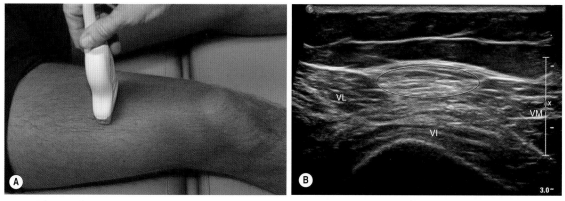

Fig. 7.13 Quadriceps musculature (mid/distal thigh). (A) Transverse section mid/distal anterior thigh. **(B)** The superficial tendinous lamina of rectus femoris is shown within the red outline anterior to the vastus intermedius muscle *(VI). VL,* Vastus lateralis; *VM,* vastus medialis.

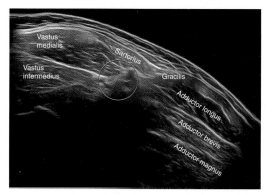

Fig. 7.14 Relationship of the anterior and medial thigh compartments. Transverse section of the proximal anteromedial thigh showing the relationship of the anterior and medial compartments and the femoral neurovascular bundle *(red outline).*

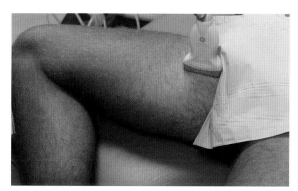

Fig. 7.15 Patient and probe position for assessment of the adductors in longitudinal section.

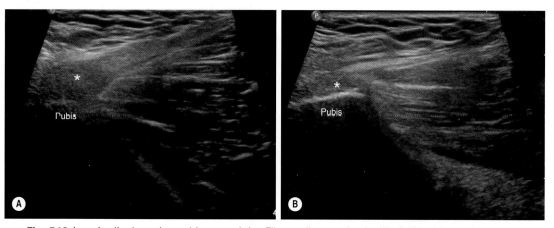

Fig. 7.16 Longitudinal section adductor origin. Fibrocartilage enthesis *(*)* of **(A)** adductor longus and **(B)** brevis.

Lateral Hip

The patient is positioned in a decubitus position. A pillow placed between the knees can make this position more comfortable for the patient and can help prevent compression of fluid filled bursae.

The transducer is placed in TS over the lateral hip. The key landmark is the apex of the GT between the anterior and lateral facets (Fig. 7.17). In slimmer patients, the bony protuberance of the GT can be palpated, whereas in larger patients, a tip is to start distally over the femur in TS and move proximally until the apex of the GT is visible. The gluteus minimus tendon is identified over the anterior facet, and the gluteus medius tendon over the lateral and superoposterior facets (see Fig. 7.17).

Each tendon insertion should be evaluated in both TS and LS. The transducer should be positioned so that the tendon is perpendicular to the beam to eliminate anisotropy, otherwise it is easy to misdiagnose tendinopathy and bursitis.

Fig. 7.18 shows the approximate transducer position over the different facets in LS.

Superficial to the gluteus minimus tendon in LS, the hypoechoic muscle of the gluteus medius and the echogenic iliotibial tract can be seen (Fig. 7.19). Superficial to the gluteus medius tendon over the lateral facet is the

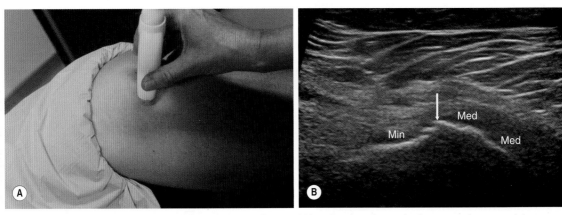

Fig. 7.17 Transverse section of the greater trochanter. **(A)** probe placed over the bony protuberance of the right greater trochanter (**B**, *arrow*). The gluteus minimus *(min)* and gluteus medius *(med)* tendons are seen overlying the individual facets.

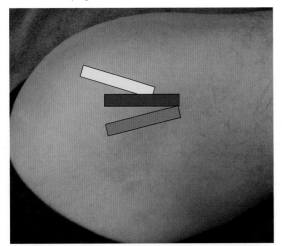

Fig. 7.18 Different transducer positions to demonstrate the gluteus tendons in longitudinal section. Gluteus minimus *(blue)*, lateral facet gluteus medius *(red)*, and superoposterior *(yellow)*.

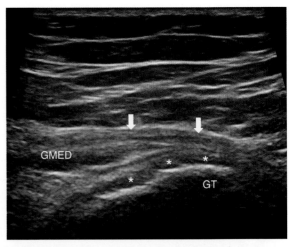

Fig. 7.19 Longitudinal section anterior facet of greater trochanter. Gluteus minimus tendon *(asterisks)*, and gluteus medius muscle *(GMED)*, and iliotibial band *(arrows)*.

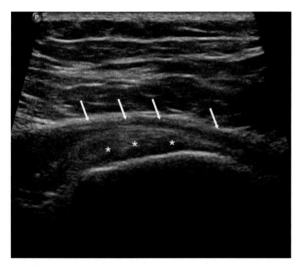

Fig. 7.20 Longitudinal section lateral facet of greater trochanter. Gluteus medius tendon *(asterisks)*, and iliotibial band *(arrows)*.

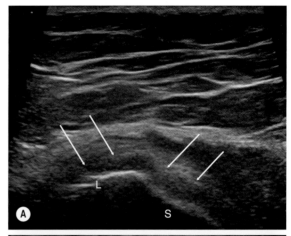

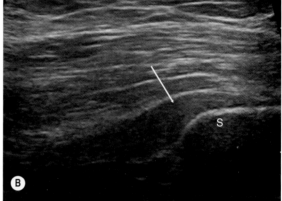

Fig. 7.21 Gluteus medius tendon *(arrows)*. **(A)** Transverse section of the lateral *(L)* and superoposterior *(S)* greater trochanter (GT) facets. **(B)** Longitudinal section superoposterior *(S)* facet of the GT.

iliotibial tract (Fig. 7.20). To fully assess the superoposterior portion of the gluteus medius tendon, the probe is moved posteriorly (Fig. 7.21).[8–11]

Whilst assessing the gluteal tendons, attention should be paid to the bursae, looking for fluid.

As mentioned, the iliotibial tract is seen as a ligamentous structure superficial to the gluteal tendons at the level of the GT. It can be seen at its origin on the iliac crest in sagittal section (Fig. 7.22) and can be followed in the distal thigh to its insertion (see Chapter 8).

◎ TIPS

To locate the greater trochanter, start distally over the femur in transverse section and move proximally until the apex of the greater trochanter is visible.

Ensure that the gluteal tendons are examined at their individual facets to avoid misinterpretation.

Posterior

Ultrasound of the posterior quadrant is less frequently requested as injury is less common in the general population. For examination of the posterior hip, the patient lies prone (Fig. 7.23) with the feet hanging off the couch.

The main landmark is the ischial tuberosity. This can be palpated in some individuals at the buttock crease. The HMC origin can be scanned in TS and LS (Fig. 7.24)

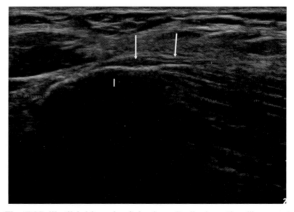

Fig. 7.22 Iliotibial band origin. Longitudinal section iliac crest *(I)*, origin of iliotibial band *(arrows)*.

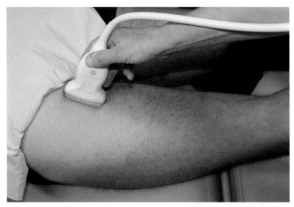

Fig. 7.23 Patient and probe position for assessing the common tendon origin of the hamstrings.

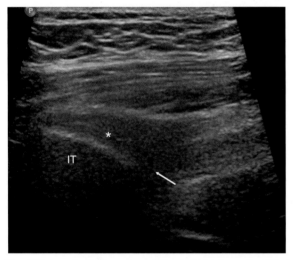

Fig. 7.24 Longitudinal section of the ischial tuberosity *(IT)* at the hamstring origin *(*)*; the position of the ischial bursa is shown by the arrow.

using toggling movements of the transducer to avoid anisotropy. As with the adductor attachment, this can be a difficult structure to interpret and often appears tendinopathic when asymptomatic. The ischial bursa is located deep to the common tendon origin but is not seen unless pathological.

It is useful to identify the separate hamstring muscles on ultrasound for injury assessment and masses. There are several ways to approach this. Starting at the proximal common tendon origin in TS, shifting the probe downward the muscle of SM is medial small, and

triangular. In the middle is ST, with BF laterally. At this level, the sciatic nerve is seen deep to the BF muscle. The hyperechoic "Mercedes Benz" sign is a recognised landmark demonstrating the fascial planes between the muscles and sciatic nerve (Fig. 7.25).[14]

The other approach involves starting in the distal thigh in TS, just above the popliteal fossa. The ST tendon is seen anterior to the SM muscle as the "cherry on the cake" sign (Fig. 7.26). By following these structures proximally, the hamstring muscles can be identified as separate muscle bellies in the order described previously.

◎ TIP

The "cherry on the cake sign" in the distal thigh, where the semitendinosus tendon lies superficial to semimembranosus muscle, and the "Mercedes Benz sign" representing the intermuscular fascial planes, are useful landmarks when trying to identify the individual hamstring muscles.

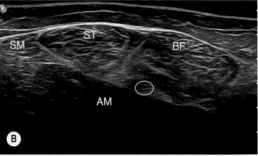

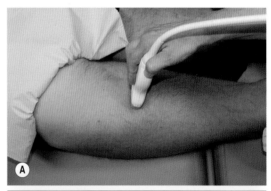

Fig. 7.25 Assessment of the hamstrings in transverse section. **(A)** Probe position posterior thigh. **(B)** Hamstring muscles: semimembranosus *(SM)*, semitendinosus *(ST)*, biceps femoris *(BF)*, sciatic nerve *(yellow outline)*, adductor magnus muscle *(AM)*. Red line is the "Mercedes-Benz sign" of the echogenic aponeuroses.

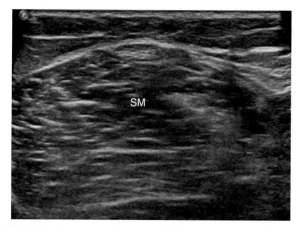

Fig. 7.26 Transverse section distal thigh. The "Cherry on the Cake" Sign. The semitendinosus tendon *(red outline)* is seen superficial to the semimembranosus muscle *(SM)*.

PATHOLOGY

Hip Joint Effusion

In the adult, joint effusion can be associated with osteo-arthritis, inflammatory arthritis, infection, and avascular necrosis of the femoral head. Patients exhibit decreased range of movement as well as pain.

In the child, especially those under 10 years of age, joint effusion causes an acutely painful hip with limping and inability to weight bear and is a common reason for referral to the emergency department. Children with juvenile idiopathic arthritis may also present with joint effusion and signs of active joint inflammation (see Chapter 10).

It may be possible to see abnormalities of the growth plates on ultrasound, such as slipped upper femoral epiphysis which usually affects older children, and Perthe's disease, a condition of the developing skeleton which causes disruption of the blood supply to the femoral head making it fragmented and distorted.

It is important in both adults and children to consider an X-ray for improved detection of osseous abnormalities.

Ultrasound is most often requested when clinicians are concerned that there is sepsis in the joint causing septic arthritis, which if left untreated, can cause destruction of the joint.

When a joint effusion is present on ultrasound, some degree of fluid is present anterior to the femoral neck causing outward displacement (convexity) of the joint capsule. As mentioned, a small amount of fluid is normal. To help assess the relevance of the joint fluid, the distance from the joint capsule to the femur can be measured. When comparison is made with the contralateral asymptomatic hip, there should be less than 2 mm difference in the distance. Fig. 7.27 shows a left hip effusion in a 6-year-old, compared with the normal right side. The depth of fluid within the joint recess may be helpful

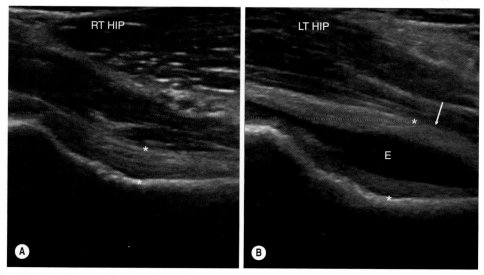

Fig. 7.27 Hip effusion. Normal right hip for comparison **(A)** and effusion *(E)* in the left hip **(B)**. Convexity of the left joint capsule *(arrow)*. Joint capsule to femoral neck diameter shown between the asterisks.

to include on the report to emphasise the size of the effusion and in case of future serial scans.

If an effusion is simple, the fluid should be anechoic. The presence of internal echoes is suggestive but not diagnostic for sepsis and in cases of trauma, blood has a similar appearance. Thickening of the synovium in osteo or inflammatory arthritis can also mimic a septic joint effusion. Tips to help differentiate between the two include; power Doppler ultrasound, which may show hyperaemia in actively inflamed synovium but not in septic fluid, although at this depth, Doppler interrogation is difficult. "Balloting" of the joint with the ultrasound probe may help by eliciting movement of turbid fluid.[15]

It is important to remember that ultrasound cannot exclude infection, and where there is clinical suspicion, joint aspiration and lavage may be required. Synovial biopsy should be considered in patients with uncertain diagnosis as other possible causes of synovial hypertrophy include pigmented villonodular synovitis, synovial chondromatosis, and amyloid deposition.[16]

REPORT—JOINT EFFUSION (FIG. 7.27) (A&E REFERRAL)

Clinical History: 6-year-boy with pain in the left hip and limping

Ultrasound Report: (Comparison with the normal right hip). There is a hip joint effusion in the left hip. The depth of fluid measures 5 mm.

Ultrasound is unable to exclude infection, this would require diagnostic aspiration.

Ultrasound is particularly helpful in patients who have had arthroplasty as it is able to detect periarticular collections and oedema associated with metalwork infection, which are not seen on radiography or may be obscured by artefact on MRI. However, small effusions are easily missed as they can be loculated and a more extensive assessment should include the lateral and posterior joint. Complications related to arthroplasty due to particle wear disease cause loosening of the prosthesis and granulomatous reactive pseudotumour formation, which has the appearance of thickened soft tissue adjacent to the prosthesis.

Ultrasound may be used to guide diagnostic and therapeutic procedures around the hip. Direct needle visualisation confirms needle and injectate position. Diagnostic injection procedures include intraarticular local anaesthetic to confirm joint based symptoms and gadolinium solution for MR arthrography. Therapeutic procedures include corticosteroid injection for arthritis, both degenerative and inflammatory, and the use of hyaluronic acid to support and maintain the normal joint fluid.[16]

 TIP

Remember: even when a joint effusion appears simple/anechoic on ultrasound, it is not possible to exclude sepsis. This requires diagnostic aspiration of fluid and should be explained in the report.

Rectus Femoris/Quadriceps Injury

Rectus femoris (RF) is the most injured anterior thigh muscle because it is the longest and extends across two joints. Injury usually results from kicking in football and other explosive sports such as sprinting. Dependent on the degree and acute nature of injury, management can range from conservative (rest from sport, followed by strength and stretching exercises) to surgery; therefore, accurate reporting of the site and severity of injury is important.[17,18]

Acute apophyseal injury of RF can occur at the AIIS in skeletally immature athletes. Ultrasound can confirm tendon avulsion and associated displacement of bone and cartilage fragment which may require surgical reattachment.

Other sites of injury in more mature athletes are the distal myotendinous junction (Fig. 7.28), the junction of the conjoined direct and indirect tendons with the muscle belly (known as a peripheral injury), or at the deep myotendinous junction of the indirect head, referred to as a central aponeurosis injury (Fig. 7.29). The central injury is associated with a longer rehabilitation time.

Chronic injury to the distal myotendinous junction can mimic a mass due to retraction of the muscle belly

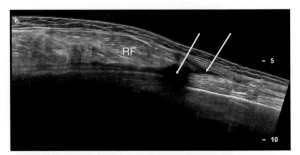

Fig. 7.28 Distal myotendinous rupture of rectus femoris. Longitudinal section showing retraction of the rectus femoris muscle *(RF)* and refraction shadowing and fluid at the site of a complete rupture *(arrows)* of the distal myotendinous junction.

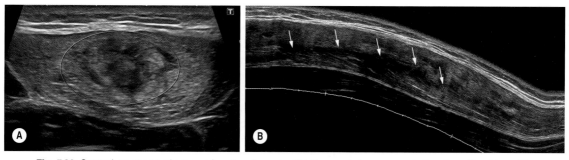

Fig. 7.29 Central aponeurosis tear of rectus femoris. **(A)** The central aponeurosis tear is outlined in red in transverse section. **(B)** Longitudinal section shows the longitudinal extent of the tear and haematoma *(arrows)*.

during extension of the knee and contraction of the quadriceps muscles.

Grading of RF muscle injury is often performed in athletes with MR imaging. This can help with management of injury and predict return to sport.[18] It can be difficult to grade injury using ultrasound; however, when reporting it is important to describe the site of injury and dimensions of the injured muscle. When muscle injury is acute, a large amount of haematoma may be present (Fig. 7.30); this should be mentioned in the report. Haematoma may take several weeks to be reabsorbed and it may be useful to rescan the patient to monitor healing progression and the formation of fibrotic scar tissue – particularly in elite sport as this may alter prognosis. Ultrasound can also look for complications of tissue healing for example myositis ossifcans. The increased pressure caused by extensive intramuscular haematoma can cause compartment syndrome due to restriction to the blood flow to the muscles and nerves. If the patient experiences severe pain and numbness in the affected limb this should be treated as a medical emergency as they may require fasciotomy to release the pressure and prevent permanent damage to the muscles.

> **REPORT—RECTUS FEMORIS CENTRAL APONEUROSIS INJURY (A&E REFERRAL) (FIG. 7.29)**
> Clinical History: 22-year-old, pain in the anterior thigh, slight swelling/bruising following a football injury.
> Ultrasound Report: There is a tear along the length of the central aponeurosis of the rectus femoris muscle with a small amount of haematoma which measures 80 mm × 40 mm × 40 mm.
> The rest of the quadriceps muscles appear normal.
> Conclusion: Tear of the central aponeurosis rectus femoris.

The direct tendon of RF is a potential site of tendinosis and calcium hydroxyapatite crystal deposition. Ultrasound-guided lavage and aspiration have been successfully used for percutaneous treatment.

A crush (blunt force trauma) to the anterior thigh may result in contusion/haematoma within the (deep quadriceps muscles) vastus intermedius as it is forced against the femur.

(Injury to the distal conjoint quadriceps tendon will be covered more extensively in Chapter 8.)

Iliopsoas Bursitis/Tendinopathy

Iliopsoas pathology results in pain during flexion in the anterior hip and is more common in athletes and in patients with chronic hip conditions. Patients with total hip replacement may also develop iliopsoas pathology due to scar tissue or loosening of the prosthesis causing granulation tissue and impingement.[19,20]

When inflamed, the distended iliopsoas bursa is identified medial and deep to the iliopsoas complex. It may also extend along the psoas musculature in the abdomen to simulate a psoas abscess. The fluid-filled

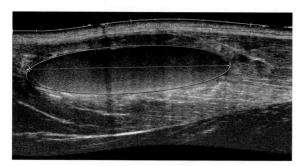

Fig. 7.30 Muscle injury of rectus femoris with extensive haematoma. Longitudinal section of the anterior thigh showing an acute haematoma in the rectus femoris muscle *(red outline)*.

bursa may be seen to communicate with the hip joint (Fig. 7.31) especially in patients with chronic hip joint disease. Iliopsoas tendinopathy results in a hypoechoic thickened tendon with loss of the normal fibrillar pattern.

Adductor Tendinopathy/Tear

Fig. 7.32 is an example of tendinopathy of the adductor origin in a 50-year-old male with pain in the right pubic region. There is marked thickening of the right adductor origin compared with the normal asymptomatic left side.

It can be difficult to determine whether adductor tendinopathy/enthesopathy, is the cause of symptoms as it is commonly also seen in the asymptomatic side. Pain from pressure as the transducer is pressed over the region is

clinically suggestive. Hyperaemia may be detected using colour Doppler but does not occur consistently. Cortical irregularity and calcification are often present, especially in athletes, but these usually represent chronic changes and are often asymptomatic. Calcification at the enthesis can be due to incomplete fusion of secondary ossification centres (observed up to age 26) and may therefore be normal.

The most specific ultrasound feature as a cause of pain is an intrasubstance tear, seen as an anechoic cleft on the deep side of the tendon adjacent to the periosteum. Such tears usually develop upwards through the common rectus abdominis and adductor longus aponeurosis and can result in tendon rupture. In acute situations, usually in athletes, rupture of the tendon results in significant retraction of the adductor longus muscle from its bony attachment

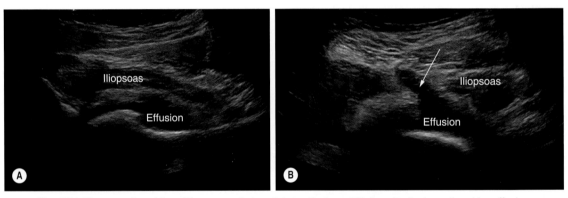

Fig. 7.31 Iliopsoas bursitis with a co-existing joint effusion. (A) Longitudinal section hip effusion. **(B)** Transverse section showing communication with the iliopsoas bursa *(arrow)*.

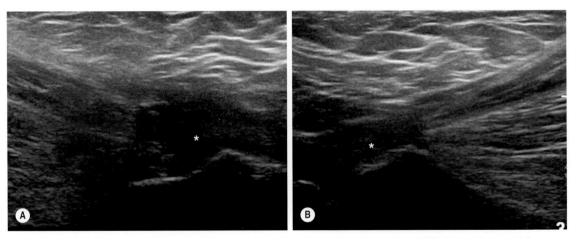

Fig. 7.32 Adductor tendinopathy. Shows marked thickening and tendinopathy of **(A)** right adductor origin *(*)*, compared with the normal **(B)** left side *(*)*.

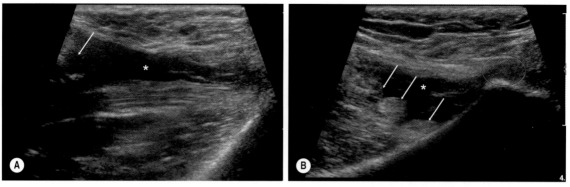

Fig. 7.33 Adductor tear. (A and B) Longitudinal section right medial thigh showing fluid/haematoma *(*)* at the site of an adductor injury. Muscle retraction *(arrows)* is noted and the fibrocartilage is also absent *(red outline)* as it has avulsed from the pubis.

with haematoma at the site of the tear (Fig. 7.33). The extent of the rupture depends on the involvement of the muscular insertion, which should be carefully assessed. Tendon rupture can be associated with an avulsion fracture, particularly in adolescents. It is important to try and assess the degree of rupture as surgery may be offered, especially if the fibrocartilaginous/bony enthesis is avulsed.[21]

Other causes of pubalgia include a Sportsman's hernia (an injury of the common aponeurosis), osteitis pubis, and bone marrow oedema of the pubic tubercle. These cannot be assessed with ultrasound and therefore patients with pain in this region may have primary imaging with MRI rather than ultrasound. Inguinal regional hernias should also be considered as a cause of pain in this region.

REPORT—ADDUCTOR AVULSION (FIG. 7.33) (GP REFERRAL)

Clinical History: 40-year-old male recreational cricketer with pain in the medial thigh and groin. Previous history of injury whilst bowling several weeks ago? palpable defect medial thigh, ? adductor injury,? inguinal hernia.

Ultrasound Report: There is an avulsion injury to the adductor origin with retraction of the tendon and fibrocartilage to a distance of 46 mm from the pubis. Haematoma is seen at the site of injury. Surgical opinion is advised.

Greater Trochanteric Pain Syndrome

Previously it was thought that pain in the lateral hip was due to bursitis; however, it has been shown to be due to a variety of conditions and it is now termed greater trochanteric pain syndrome.[22] Pain may radiate down the lateral thigh and can be difficult to differentiate clinically from hip joint and lumbar pain. More common in females than males, weakness of the gluteal muscles causes instability of the hip and may result in a Trendelenburg (waddling) gait.

The most common cause of lateral hip pain is tendinopathy of the gluteus minimus/medius tendons (Fig. 7.34). This includes deposition of entheseal and hydroxyapatite calcification as in the shoulder (Fig. 7.35).

Fluid in the peritrochanteric bursae (bursitis) is seen less often and may be associated with tendon tears. Gluteus medius/minimus tendon tears are more common in patients who have osteoarthritis, fracture, in 20% of patients who have had total hip arthroplasty with failure of abductor repair, and in runners and athletes involved in high-impact sports.

In Fig. 7.36, fluid is seen in the trochanteric bursa between the iliotibial band and gluteus medius tendon in a 67-year-old patient with lateral hip and Fig 7.37 is an example of bursal fluid associated with tendon rupture.

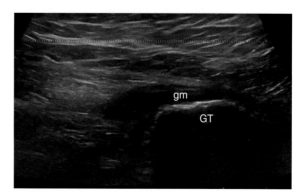

Fig. 7.34 Gluteus medius tendinopathy. Gluteus medius tendon *(gm)*, greater trochanter *(GT)*.

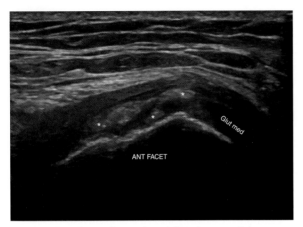

Fig. 7.35 Calcific tendinopathy of the gluteus minimus tendon. Transverse section greater trochanter showing deposits of hydroxyapatite calcification *(*)* in the gluteus minimus tendon.

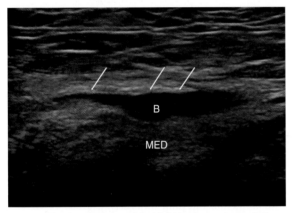

Fig. 7.36 Trochanteric bursitis. Fluid in the trochanteric bursa *(B)* between the iliotibial band *(arrows)* and gluteus medius tendon *(MED)*.

REPORT—TROCHANTERIC BURSITIS (COMMUNITY MUSCULOSKELETAL SERVICES REFERRAL) (FIG. 7.36)

Clinical History: Pain in the lateral hip? trochanteric bursitis.

Ultrasound Report: There is a small amount of fluid within the trochanteric bursa between the iliotibial tract and gluteus medius tendon indicating bursitis. The gluteal tendons appear intact.

REPORT—GLUTEUS MEDIUS TENDON RUPTURE (FIG. 7.37) (GP REFERRAL)

Clinical History: 74-year-old with pain in the lateral hip and difficulty walking. Previous history of THR, is having physiotherapy.

Ultrasound Report: There is a complete rupture of the gluteus medius tendon. The ruptured tendon end is retracted to a distance of 19 mm from the greater trochanter. Fluid is seen within the subgluteus medius bursa in keeping with either bursitis or secondary to the tendon rupture.

The gluteus minimus tendon is intact.

Thickening and tendinopathy of the iliotibial tract/band can occur at the level of GT but also at the iliac origin causing pain. This condition is more common in runners and cyclists performing repetitive movements.

Treatment of greater trochanteric pain syndrome varies. Tendinopathy and bursitis may respond well to nonoperative measures including rest, core and hip strengthening, stretching, and local steroid/platelet rich plasma injection.[23] Surgery is reserved for refractory

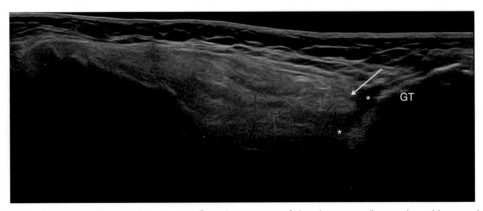

Fig. 7.37 Gluteus medius tendon rupture. Complete rupture of the gluteus medius tendon with retraction of the tendon *(arrow)* from the greater trochanter *(GT)* and fluid in the bursa *(*)*.

cases that have failed with conservative measures including bursectomy, iliotibial band lengthening, and repair of gluteal tears.

Often the ultrasound appearances of the lateral hip structures are normal; in these cases diagnostic steroid/local anaesthetic injection may be offered.

A note of caution: prior to administering therapeutic injection and when reporting the ultrasound examination, it is important to correlate the ultrasound findings with the patient's symptoms. The pathology described may be present when there is no pain and may also be seen in the contralateral asymptomatic side.

Hamstring Pathology

The hamstring common tendon origin can be difficult to assess with ultrasound, especially if the patient is large, as it is a deep structure. Attenuation and anisotropy artefacts may give the tendon features of chronic tendinopathy when the patient is asymptomatic; consequently, contralateral comparison may not help. It is therefore necessary to correlate the patient's symptoms with the ultrasound appearances.

Bursitis of the ischial bursa can be a cause of pain typically when sitting and although the patient may be symptomatic on scanning, effusion/hyperemia of the bursa may be difficult to see on ultrasound. Ultrasound guided steroid injection may be requested to manage this condition.

The site of injury to the HMC and the grading used to assess the degree of injury are akin to RF. Avulsion injury occurs more commonly in young athletes. MR imaging is often superior to ultrasound for accurate assessment of the degree of tendon retraction and morphological features for the surgeon contemplating repair.

Partial tearing/strain of the HMC mostly occurs in the region of the myotendinous junction of BF for reasons already described in the anatomy section. As well as sporting activity, risk factors for HMC injury include increasing age, previous history of posterior thigh pain (hamstring strain and back-related referred pain), knee injury, and osteitis pubis. Management is dependent on the grade of injury, therefore attempts should be made to accurately describe the site and size of injury, presence of haematoma, and scar tissue.[3,18]

Fig. 7.38 shows images of a chronic tear of the ST muscle in a 45-year-old weightlifter. The injury occurred 3 months prior to the scan and the patient felt repeated symptoms (pain and pulling in the hamstrings) during deadlifts. The tear is situated in the superficial aspect of the muscle affecting only a small portion of the muscle bulk. The patient was referred by the musculoskeletal interface clinic. He had been advised to refrain from sport whilst undertaking specific physiotherapy exercises.

REPORT—CHRONIC MUSCLE TEAR SEMIMEMBRANOSUS (MUSCULOSKELETAL INTERFACE CLINIC REFERRAL) (FIG. 7.38)

Clinical History: 45-year-old weightlifter felt pain and pulling 3 months ago after deadlifting.

Ultrasound Report: There is a small chronic tear affecting the superficial fibres of the semitendinosus muscle. The size of the tear measures 36 mm × 32 mm × 31 mm and is at the site of the previous injury in the proximal thigh. The rest of the hamstring muscles and common tendon origin appear normal.

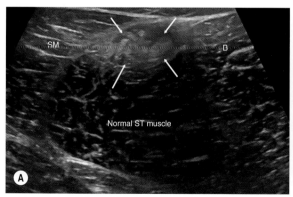 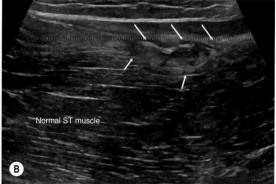

Fig. 7.38 Semitendinosus muscle tear. **(A)** Transverse section and **(B)** longitudinal section posterior thigh. Tear in the superficial aspect of semitendinosus *(ST) (arrows)*. B, Biceps femoris; *SM*, semimembranosus.

TIP

When reporting acute muscle injury in the thigh, it is important to identify and report the type of injury (e.g., avulsion, myotendinous, intramuscular), size (dimensions or proportion of muscle bulk affected), and presence of haematoma.

Snapping Syndromes

Some patients experience pain and snapping sensations in the anterior and lateral hips related to iliopsoas instability and tightness of the iliotibial tract. Snapping occurs when normal translocation of the tendons is replaced by abrupt sudden movements. More common in athletes involved in dance, gymnastics, martial arts, and running, these patients can be assessed on ultrasound using dynamic manouvers.[24,25]

It is important to remember, however, that labral tears, loose bodies, and osteophytes in the hip joint can also cause clicking and therefore other imaging should also be considered to exclude these.

REPORTING TERMINOLOGY FOR NORMAL FINDINGS[26]
- No evidence of a joint effusion or synovitis in the anterior hip joint. If intra-articular pathology is suspected, different imaging may be required.
- Normal appearances of the iliopsoas tendon with no evidence of tendinopathy or iliopsoas bursitis.
- Normal appearances of the hamstring origin at the ischial tuberosity, no evidence of ischial bursitis.
- The gluteal tendons are intact with no evidence of tear or tendinopathy. Normal appearances of the iliotibial tract. No features of peritrochanteric bursitis.

MULTIPLE CHOICE QUESTIONS

1. What is the correct term for pain in the lateral hip?
   a) Greater trochanter syndrome
   b) Trochanteric bursitis
   c) Greater trochanteric pain syndrome
2. Which muscles constitute the adductor group?
   a) Pectineus, adductor brevis, adductor longus, adductor magnus, gracilis
   b) Pectineus, adductor brevis, adductor longus, adductor magnus, sartorius
   c) Adductor brevis, adductor longus, adductor magnus
3. Where is the recommended starting point for ultrasound of the anterior hip joint?
   a) Femoral neck
   b) Femoral head and acetabulum
   c) Iliopsoas complex

4. Which bursa is associated with the insertion of the hamstrings?
   a) Iliopsoas
   b) Semimembranosus
   c) Ischial
5. What are the actions of the rectus femoris muscle?
   a) Extensor of the knee and hip
   b) Flexor of the hip and an extensor of the knee
   c) Flexor of the hip

REFERENCES

1. Collin D, Geijer M, Göthlin JH. Computed tomography compared to magnetic resonance imaging in occult or suspect hip fractures. A retrospective study in 44 patients. Eur Radiol. 2016;26:3932–3938.
2. Saied AM, Redant C, El-Batouty M, et al. Accuracy of magnetic resonance studies in the detection of chondral and labral lesions in femoroacetabular impingement: systematic review and meta-analysis. BMC Musculoskelet Disord. 2017;18:83.
3. Robinson P. Essential Radiology for Sports Medicine. New York: Springer-Verlag; 2010.
4. Thompson J. Netter's Concise Atlas of Orthopaedic Anatomy. Philadelphia: Saunders/Elsevier; 2002.
5. Molini L, Precerutti M, Gervasio A, Draghi F, Bianchi S. Hip: anatomy and US technique. J Ultrasound. 2011;14(2):99-108.
6. Davis JA, Stringer MD, Woodley SJ. New insights into the proximal tendons of adductor longus, brevis and gracilis. BR J Sports Med. 2012;46:871–876.

7. Pfirrmann CWA, Chung CB, Theumann NH, Trudell DJ, Resnick D. Musculoskeletal imaging: greater trochanter of the hip: attachment of the abductor mechanism and a complex of three bursae—MR imaging and MR bursography in cadavers and MR imaging in asymptomatic volunteer's radiology. Radiology. 2001;221(2). https://doi.org/10.1148/radiol.2211001634.

8. Bianchi S, Martinoli C. Ultrasound of the Musculoskeletal System. Berlin Heidelberg: Springer-Verlag; 2007.

9. Beggs I, Bianchi S, Bueno A, et al. European Society of Musculoskeletal Radiology: Musculoskeletal technical guidelines IV. Hip. 2016. Available at: https://essr.org/content-essr/uploads/2016/10/hip.pdf

10. Nestorova R, Vlad V, Petranova T, et al. Ultrasonography of the hip. Med Ultrason. 2012;14:217–224.

11. Jacobson JA, Khoury V, Brandon CJ. Ultrasound of the groin: techniques, pathology, and pitfalls. Am J Roentgenol. 2015;205:513–523.

12. Rudin D, Manestar M, Ullrich O, Erhardt J, Grob K. The anatomical course of the lateral femoral cutaneous nerve with special attention to the anterior approach to the hip joint. J Bone Joint Surg Am. 2016;98(7):561–567.

13. Zhu J, Zhao Y, Liu F, Huang Y, Shao J, Hu B. Ultrasound of the lateral femoral cutaneous nerve in asymptomatic adults. BMC Musculoskelet Disord. 2012;13:227.

14. Balius R, Pedret C, Iriarte I, Sáiz R, Cerezal L. Sonographic landmarks in hamstring muscles. Skeletal Radiol. 2019;48(11):1675–1683.

15. Bierma-Zeinstra SMA, Bohnen AM, Verhaar JAN, Prins A, Ginai-Karamat AZ, Lamériset JS. Sonography for hip joint effusion in adults with hip pain. Ann Rheum Dis. 2000;59:178–182.

16. Rowbotham EL, Grainger AJ. Ultrasound-guided intervention around the hip joint. AJR Am J Roentgenol. 2011;197:W122–W127.

17. Robinson P. Sonography of common tendon injuries. AJR Am J Roentgenol. 2009;193:607–618.

18. Grassi A, Quaglia A, Canata GL, Zaffagnini S. An update on the grading of muscle injuries: a narrative review from clinical to comprehensive systems. Joints. 2016;4(1):39–46.

19. Adler RS, Buly R, Ambrose R, Sculco T. Diagnostic and therapeutic use of sonography-guided iliopsoas peritendinous injections. AJR Am J Roentgenol. 2005;185:940–943.

20. Cheung YM, Beverly M. Iliopsoas bursitis following total hip replacement. Arch Orthop Trauma Surg. 2005;124(10):720–723.

21. Pesquera L, Reboul G, Silvestre A, Poussange N, Meyer P, Dallaudière B. Imaging of adductor-related groin pain. Diagn Interv Imaging. 2015;96:861–869.

22. Long SS, Surrey DE, Nazarian LN. Sonography of greater trochanteric pain syndrome and the rarity of primary bursitis. AJR Am J Roentgenol. 2013;201(5):1083–1086.

23. Jacobson JA, Yablon CM, Henning PT, et al. Greater trochanteric pain syndrome: percutaneous tendon fenestration versus platelet-rich plasma injection for treatment of gluteal tendinosis. J Ultrasound Med. 2016;35:2413–2420.

24. Deslandes M, Guillin R, Cardinal E, Hobden R, Bureau NJ. The snapping iliopsoas tendon: new mechanisms using dynamic sonography. AJR Am J Roentgenol. 2008;190:576–581.

25. Yen YM, Lewis CL, Kim YJ. Understanding and treating the snapping hip. Sports Med Arthrosc Rev. 2015;23(4):194–199.

26. Guidelines for Professional Practice SCOR, BMUS, December 2020 https://www.bmus.org/static/uploads/resources/Guidelines_for_Professional_Ultrasound_Practice_v3_OHoz76r.pdf

Ultrasound of the Knee and Calf

Sara Riley

CHAPTER OUTLINE

LEARNING OBJECTIVES

After reading this chapter you should have gained an understanding of:

- The relevant anatomical structures of the knee/calf
- Ultrasound technique and normal appearances of the knee/calf, including tips and pitfalls
- Common pathologies of the knee/calf, including clinical presentation, management of the conditions, and report writing
- The place of other imaging modalities

INTRODUCTION

Ultrasound provides excellent resolution for the superficial structures of the knee and calf but should not be the imaging modality of choice for generalised knee pain, assessment of intra-articular structures, or disorders of the patellofemoral articulation. For these reasons primary imaging may be with plain radiograph/magnetic resonance (MR).

Ultrasound of the knee/calf is performed with a high-frequency transducer, although a lower frequency may be better suited to the deep posterior structures.

ANATOMY OF THE KNEE AND CALF

The knee is a condyloid joint with three compartments (tricompartmental). The three hyaline cartilage articulations are between the medial and lateral femoral condyles and the tibia, and the femur and patella (patellofemoral joint). The function of the patella (a sesamoid bone) is to act as a fulcrum, to increase the leverage that the quadriceps tendon can exert on the femur in knee extension.

Joint Capsule

The joint capsule is a dual-layered structure with a fibrous connective tissue outer layer to stabilise the joint and an inner synovial layer for lubrication, thinner in the anterior and posterior aspects to enable flexion and extension and thicker on the medial and lateral sides to allow for small rotational movements but prevent dislocation.

The outer fibrous layer of the joint capsule is complex. It is attached to the bony femoral and tibial condyles and the head of fibula. On the lateral side there is a space for the popliteus tendon. On the medial and lateral sides, the collateral ligaments are strong stabilising structures. The medial collateral ligament (MCL) extends from the medial femoral condyle to the tibia in the coronal plane and is composed of deep and superficial fibres; the deep fibres extend to the medial meniscus. The distal MCL inserts on to the tibia deep to the pes anserine (PA) common tendon (Fig. 8.1). The lateral or fibular collateral ligament (LCL) originates from the lateral femur and extends over the popliteus tendon to insert on the lateral aspect of the fibula head along with the biceps femoris tendon (see Fig. 8.1).

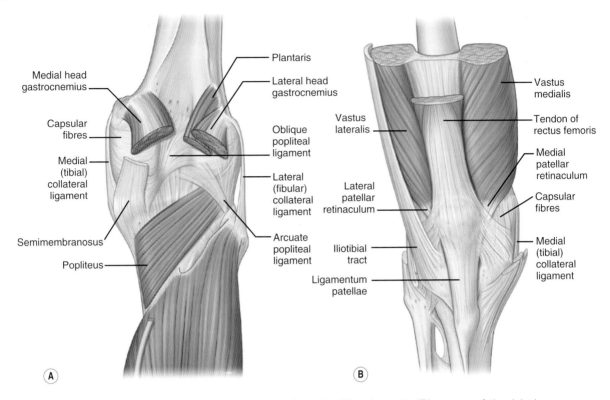

Fig. 8.1 Posterior and anterior knee anatomy. Posterior **(A)** and anterior **(B)** aspects of the right knee showing the joint capsule and the contributions from the various muscles and ligaments crossing the joint. (From Soames R, Pastanga N. Anatomy of Human Movement, Structure and Function. 7th ed. London: Elsevier; 2019; 290).

Along with the patellar tendon/ligament, ligamentous bands of the medial and lateral patella retinaculum contribute to the anterior joint capsule. The retinacula have deep and superficial fibres and blend with the adjacent musculoskeletal structures, vastus medialis, vastus lateralis, iliotibial tract, sartorius, and collateral ligaments to prevent dislocation of the patella (see Fig. 8.1).

There is no outer joint capsule superior to the patella, only an inner synovial layer.

The anterior and posterior cruciate ligaments are intra-articular stabilising ligaments. They extend from the femur to the proximal tibia as intracapsular but extrasynovial structures. The fibrocartilage menisci are intra-articular C-shaped cushioning structures between the femur and the tibia on both the medial and lateral aspects of the joint. These structures are not seen in their entirety on ultrasound and therefore MR is normally the imaging of choice when injury is suspected.

The inner synovial layer of the joint capsule is extensive; it has a prominent suprapatellar recess, also known as the suprapatellar bursa/pouch, which extends superiorly from the knee joint between the patella and the femur. This communicates with the medial and lateral joint recesses, which extend over the medial and lateral aspects of the femoral condyles beneath the patellar retinaculum. In the sagittal plane, the quadriceps/suprapatellar fat pad is located anteriorly between the suprapatellar recess and quadriceps tendon, and the pre-femoral fat pad is located between the suprapatellar recess and the femur (Fig. 8.2). The infrapatellar (Hoffa's) fat pad is an intracapsular but extrasynovial fat pad between the anterior knee joint and the patellar tendon (see Fig. 8.2). This plays an important mechanical role in the knee by altering its shape, absorbing some of the compressive stress exerted on the patella and patellar tendon, and allowing for expansion of the synovial membrane.[1]

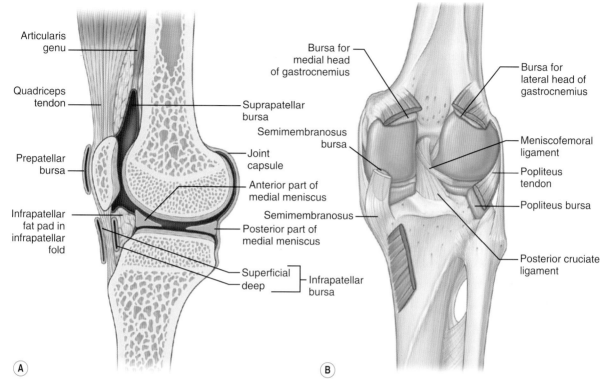

Fig. 8.2 Articular structures of the knee. Paramedian section **(A)** and posterior aspect **(B)** of the left knee showing the reflections of the synovial membrane and bursae of the knee. (From Soames R, Pastanga N. Anatomy of Human Movement, Structure and Function. 7th ed. London: Elsevier; 2019; 293).

Bursae

There are many bursae around the knee joint; a few are shown in Fig. 8.2.

Anteriorly:

- Suprapatellar bursa, as mentioned previously, which communicates with the joint
- Subcutaneous prepatellar bursa between the skin and patella/patellar tendon
- Subcutaneous/superficial infrapatellar bursa between the skin and tibial tuberosity (anterior to the distal patellar tendon)
- Deep infrapatellar bursa between the patellar tendon and proximal tibia

Medially:

- Pes anserine bursa deep to the pes anserine tendons
- Semimembranosus-tibial collateral ligament bursa, which has an inverted U shape located at the joint line between the MCL and the semimembranosus tendon

- MCL bursa which lies between the deep and superficial fibres of the ligament

Laterally:

- Between the joint capsule and lateral head of gastrocnemius
- Between the popliteus tendon and posterior tibia and fibula

Posterior:

A more commonly recognised bursa lies in the medial popliteal fossa between the semimembranosus tendon and medial head of gastrocnemius (SMG bursa). This is shown in Fig. 8.2 as two separate structures but is one continuous bursa. When distended with excess fluid, this is called a Baker's cyst. This bursa communicates to the knee joint in 50% of adults and becomes a common recess for joint fluid and intraarticular loose bodies.

Proximal Tibiofibular Joint

The proximal tibiofibular joint (TFJ) should not be forgotten in the lateral aspect of the knee. It is a plane synovial articulation between the head of the fibula and the lateral condyle of the tibia. Communication with the knee joint has been reported on MR arthrography in up to 64% of adults and it is often termed the "fourth compartment" of the knee. A fibrous capsule surrounds the joint articulation which is also strengthened by ligaments.[2]

The common peroneal/fibular nerve is closely related to the TFJ as it descends along the lateral aspect of the popliteal fossa and curves around the anterolateral aspects of the fibular head and neck.

Tendons

Anteriorly the "extensor mechanism" is formed by the quadriceps (QT) and patellar (PT) tendons. QT inserts on the superior patellar pole, superficial fibres extend over the patella to merge with the fibres of the PT, which inserts on the tibial tuberosity (see Fig. 8.1). The tendons do not have a synovial sheath but paratenon (see Chapter 2).

Medially and anteriorly, the sartorius, gracilis, and semitendinosus tendons insert on the tibia with the distal fibres of the MCL as the conjoint pes anserine tendon. In Latin this means "goose foot" due to the similarity of its shape. A helpful mnemonic to remember the individual tendon components is "**S**ay **G**race before **T**ea." Posterior and proximal to pes anserine, the semimembranosus tendon primarily inserts on the tibia just beyond the tibia articular surface (Fig. 8.3). Posteriorly, the medial and lateral heads of the gastrocnemius originate from the posterior aspect of the femoral condyles.

Laterally, the long head of the biceps femoris tendon has two arms which insert on the lateral aspect of the fibula with the LCL and more anteriorly on the fibula.

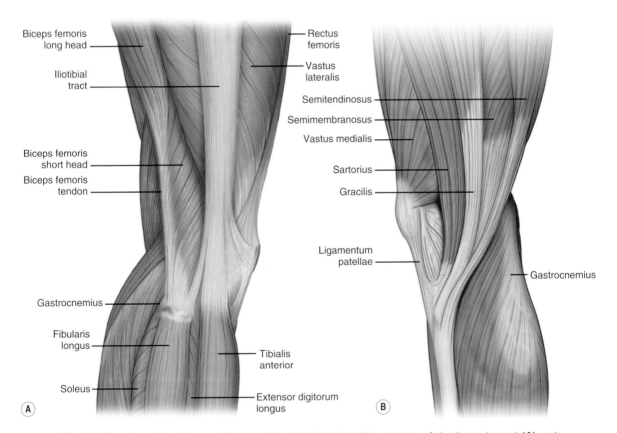

Fig. 8.3 Muscle and tendon anatomy on the lateral and medial aspects of the knee. Lateral **(A)** and medial **(B)** aspects of the right knee showing the muscles crossing the joint. (From Soames R, Pastanga N. Anatomy of Human Movement, Structure and Function. 7th ed. London: Elsevier; 2019; 302).

The short head of the biceps femoris also has two insertions: on the proximal fibula and on the proximal tibia. The popliteus tendon originates at the lateral aspect of the femur, lies within a groove or sulcus of the femur, and courses obliquely with its muscle belly located between the posterior aspect of the tibia and the tibial artery and vein. Anterolaterally, the iliotibial tract/band inserts on to Gerdy's tubercle of the proximal tibia (see Fig. 8.3). Chapter 7 describes the thigh musculature related to the tendons described above.

Popliteal Neurovascular Bundle

Posteriorly in the popliteal fossa, the neurovascular bundle includes the tibial nerve, a branch of the sciatic nerve, and the popliteal artery and vein (Fig. 8.4). Fig. 8.4 also illustrates the position of the common fibular/peroneal nerve.

Calf

The structures of the calf lie in four osseofascial compartments divided by the interosseous membrane of the leg, transverse intermuscular septum, and the anterior intermuscular (crural) septum (Fig. 8.5).

Anteriorly, from medial to lateral, are the tibialis anterior, extensor hallucis longus, and extensor digitorum longus muscles. The neurovascular structures are the anterior tibial vessels and the deep peroneal nerve.

Laterally, there are peroneus brevis and peroneus longus muscles. The deep branch of the peroneal nerve emerges from between the peroneus longus and extensor digitorum muscles, piercing the superficial crural fascia to become subcutaneous in location.

Superficial posterior: The medial and lateral heads of the gastrocnemius muscle converge with the soleus muscle

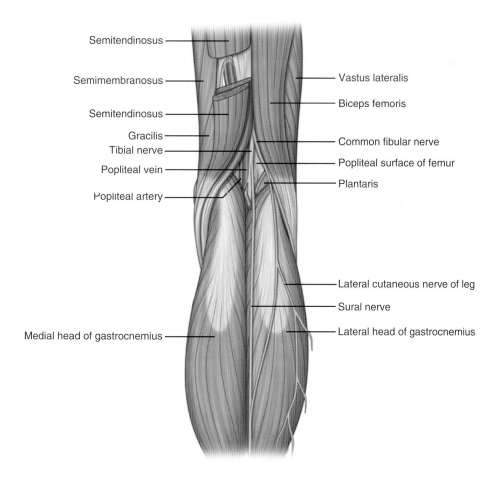

Fig. 8.4 Posterior knee anatomy. (From Soames R, Pastanga N. Anatomy of Human Movement, Structure and Function. 7th ed. London: Elsevier; 2019; 303).

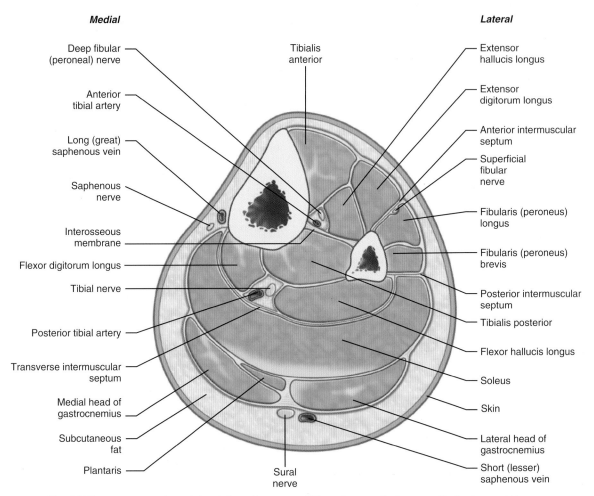

Fig. 8.5 Transverse section of the right calf anatomy. (From Soames R, Pastanga N. Anatomy of Human Movement, Structure and Function. 7th ed. London: Elsevier; 2019; 337).

to form the Achilles tendon. The plantaris muscle origi-nates from the lateral femur. Its tendon is thin and lies between the muscle bellies of the medial head of the gastrocnemius and soleus muscles in the proximal calf, and on the medial aspect of the Achilles tendon in the distal calf, before inserting onto the calcaneus or less commonly, onto the Achilles tendon. Collectively, the medial and lat-eral gastrocnemius and soleus are referred to as the triceps surae. The sural nerve lies in this compartment.

Deep posterior/medially: From anterior to posterior are the tibialis posterior, flexor digitorum longus, and flexor hallucis longus muscles. The neurovascular bun-dle includes the posterior tibial vessels and nerve.[1]

The distal tendons are described in Chapter 9.

ULTRASOUND TECHNIQUE AND NORMAL APPEARANCES

Anterior Knee

The patient lies supine with the knee slightly flexed, allowing assessment of the extensor mechanism under tension to prevent misleading secondary features of tendon rupture.[3–5] This position may be difficult for pa-tients with tendon injury and a rolled-up towel or tissue roll can be positioned under the knee for patient comfort. The transducer is placed in longitudinal section (LS) proximal to the superior pole of the patella along the long axis of QT (Fig. 8.6A). This is a broad tendon, and complete evaluation requires a medial to lateral sweep in

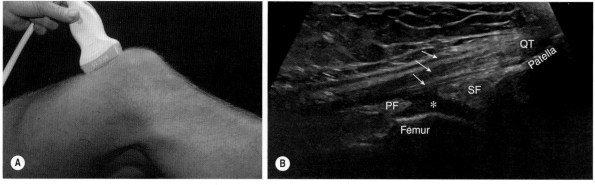

Fig. 8.6 Longitudinal section suprapatellar region. **(A)** Knee flexed and transducer placed superior to the patella. **(B)** Quadriceps tendon *(QT)*. Arrows show the trilaminar tendon slips, suprapatellar joint recess *(*)*, pre-femoral *(PF)* and suprapatellar *(SF)* fat pads.

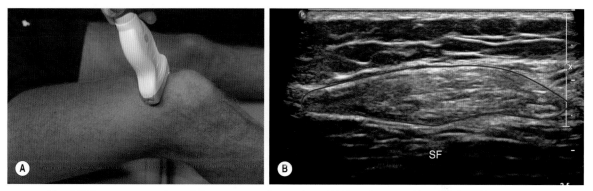

Fig. 8.7 Transverse section of the suprapatellar region. **(A)** Transducer position. **(B)** Quadriceps tendon *(red outline)* superficial to the suprapatellar fat pad *(SF)*.

LS and transverse sections (TS). QT is composed of slips from the quadriceps muscles, rectus femoris anteriorly, vastus intermedius posteriorly, and vastus medialis and lateralis forming the middle layers. A trilaminar appearance is formed by thin layers of fat interposed between the tendon bundles (Fig. 8.6B).[6–8] In TS (Fig. 8.7), care should be taken to avoid anisotropy by small angulations of the transducer.[7,8] Deep to the QT, the suprapatellar joint recess/bursa, and pre-femoral and suprapatellar fat pads are visualised. A small sliver of fluid noted in the suprapatellar recess is normal (Fig. 8.6B).

In comparison to the adult knee, Fig. 8.8 shows un-ossified cartilage in a child's knee; this can be mistaken for an effusion by the inexperienced operator.[9]

If the transducer is moved inferiorly, across the patella from the suprapatellar region in LS, an almost imperceptible continuous fascia exists overlying the patella connecting the quadriceps and patellar tendons (Fig. 8.9).

Keeping the knee in flexion, moving the transducer inferior to the lower pole of the patella (Fig. 8.10A), the full length of the PT is seen from its origin to its insertion on the tibial tuberosity (Figs. 8.9 and 8.10B).[6] It is also a broad tendon requiring careful evaluation of its full extent in LS and TS (Fig. 8.11). When checking for neovascularity in tendinopathy, the knee must be extended to relax the tendon and prevent compression of small blood vessels. Superficial to the PT, in the subcutaneous layers are the prepatellar and superficial infrapatellar bursae, which are not visible unless pathological. Adjacent to the tibial tuberosity it may be normal for the deep infrapatellar bursa to contain a small amount of fluid and comparison with the contralateral side is helpful.

The medial and lateral joint recesses can be assessed for effusion and synovitis by moving the transducer in TS from the medial and lateral edges of the patella towards the femoral condyles. The patella retinaculum is superficial to

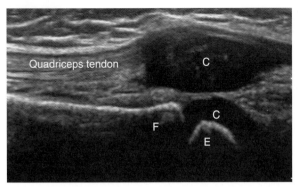

Fig. 8.8 Longitudinal section 2-year old anterior knee. Femoral metaphysis *(F)*, epiphysis *(E)*, and unossified cartilage *(C)*.

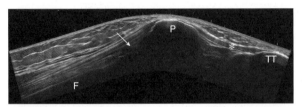

Fig. 8.9 Longitudinal section of the extensor mechanism. *Arrow,* Quadriceps tendon; **,* patellar tendon; *F,* femur; *P,* patella; *TT,* tibial tuberosity.

the joint recesses (Fig. 8.12). Injury to the retinaculum is normally a consequence of patella dislocation. Dislocation injuries are often complex and involve many structures, including the collateral and patellofemoral ligaments and insertional fibres of the quadriceps tendon, and are associated with osteochondral lesions. MR is the imaging of choice for this type of injury.[10]

Part of the femoral trochlear cartilage can be seen in the TS with the knee flexed to 90 degrees, placing the transducer superior to the patella and angling inferiorly towards the femoral condyles (Fig. 8.13). Normal cartilage should appear uniform in thickness (2 to 3 mm); focal thinning and crystal deposition may be evident in osteoarthritis and crystal arthropathies such as gout or pseudogout (see Chapter 10).[11]

◎ TIPS

Evaluate the extensor mechanism in slight flexion for rupture, and in extension for neovascularity in tendinopathy

Do not mistake cartilage in a paediatric knee for an effusion.

Medial Knee

The patient remains supine with the knee flexed but externally rotates the hip.[3–6]

The MCL is seen along the medial joint line (Fig. 8.14); a long fibrillar structure, it should be scanned in both LS and TS sections along its length. The proximal MCL is thicker than the distal ligament. The deep and superficial fibres are separated by an imperceivably thin strip of echogenic fat and a bursa which is not visible unless inflamed. Deep to the MCL, the medial meniscus is seen as a triangular and hyperechoic structure.

To identify the conjoint pes anserine tendon the transducer is moved slightly anterior to the distal MCL (Fig. 8.15A). Here the tendon insertion merges with the MCL. At this point, small blood vessels lie deep to the tendon and should not be mistaken for neovascularity in

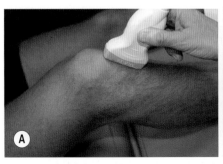

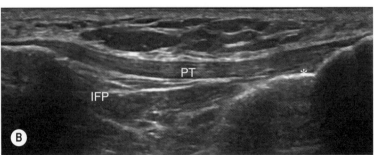

Fig. 8.10 Longitudinal section infrapatellar region. **(A)** Knee flexed, transducer placed inferior to the patella. **(B)** Patellar tendon *(PT)* Hoffa's fat pad *(IFP)*, and deep infrapatellar bursa *(*)*.

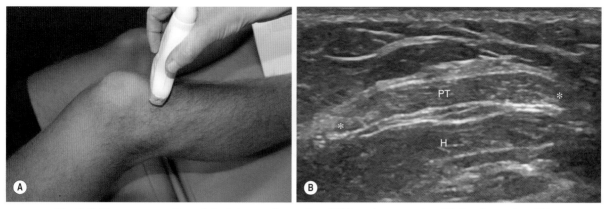

Fig. 8.11 Transverse section of the infrapatellar region. (A) Transducer position. **(B)** Patellar tendon *(PT)*, medial and lateral edges of the tendon *(*)*, Hoffa's fat pad *(H)*.

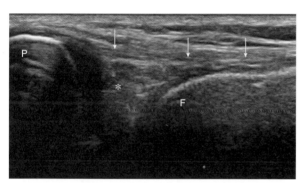

Fig. 8.12 Transverse section medial joint recess *(*)*, patellar retinaculum *(arrows)*, medial femoral condyle *(F)*, patella *(P)*.

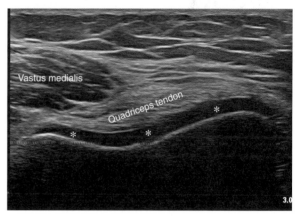

Fig. 8.13 Transverse section flexed knee. Femoral trochlear cartilage *(*)* deep to the quadriceps tendon.

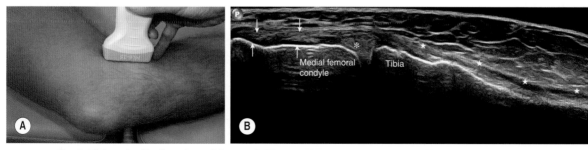

Fig. 8.14 Longitudinal section of the medial knee. (A) Transducer placement. **(B)** Proximal medial collateral ligament (MCL) *(between the arrows)*, distal MCL *(stars)*, medial meniscus *(*)*.

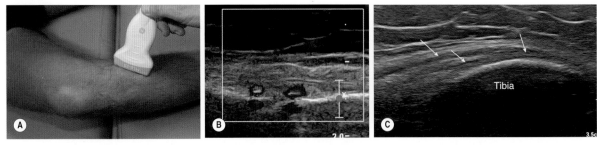

Fig. 8.15 Longitudinal section of the anteromedial knee. **(A)** Distal aspect of the transducer is rotated anteriorly. **(B)** Normal vessels deep to the pes anserine (PA) tendon/medial collateral ligament. **(C)** Elongated PA tendon fibres *(arrows)*.

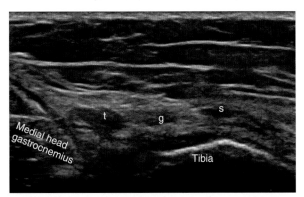

Fig. 8.16 Individual pes anserine tendons in transverse section. *t*, semitendinosus; *g*, Gracilis; *s*, sartorius.

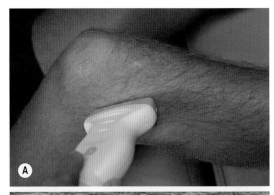

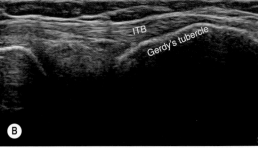

Fig. 8.17 (A) Longitudinal section anterolateral knee. **(B)** Iliotibial band *(ITB)* insertion.

tendinopathy (Fig. 8.15B). To lengthen out the PA tendon fibres as in Fig. 8.15C, the transducer is moved obliquely and more anteriorly. Proximal to the PA tibial insertion, the individual tendons can be seen separately in TS; sartorius is the most anterior, semitendinosus posterior, with gracilis in between (Fig. 8.16).

Lateral Knee

In the supine position the patient internally rotates the hip and slightly flexes the knee. The patient can turn slightly onto their side if they are unable to rotate the hip sufficiently.[3–6]

Starting at the lateral edge of the patella in LS, the iliotibial tract is the first structure seen as the transducer is moved posteriorly. It should be a thin flat fibrillar structure with slight expansion at its insertion onto Gerdy's (tibial) tubercle (Fig. 8.17).

Moving posteriorly in LS, to the position shown in Fig. 8.18, the popliteus tendon is seen in its transverse plane

in the groove on the lateral femoral condyle. Popliteus is fully evaluated by moving the transducer through 90 degrees, orientated posteriorly; a toggling movement helps to avoid anisotropy. The groove for popliteus is a useful landmark in LS for visualising the LCL as its proximal attachment is seen superficial to the groove. By stabilising the proximal end of the transducer on the femur and rotating, the distal end of LCL is elongated to its insertion onto the fibula (Fig. 8.19). Valgus (outward) angulation

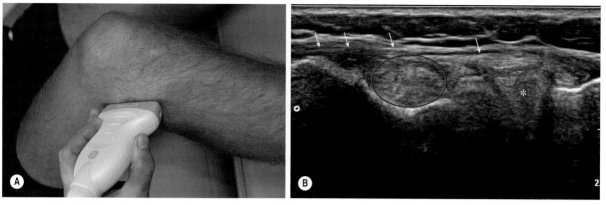

Fig. 8.18 Longitudinal section lateral knee. **(A)** Transducer positioned to show, **(B)** the lateral collateral ligament *(arrows)*, popliteus *(red outline)*, and lateral meniscus *(*)*.

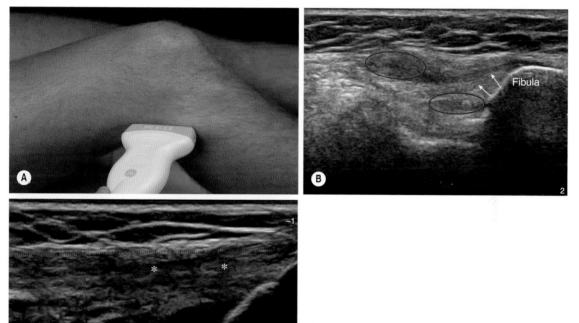

Fig. 8.19 Longitudinal section lateral knee. **(A)** Transducer is rotated to demonstrate **(B)** the distal insertion of lateral collateral ligament *(arrows)*, and anisotropy of biceps femoris *(red outlines)*. **(C)** Biceps femoris tendon.

of the knee can create a wavy appearance to the LCL as the ligament is not under tension, mimicking rupture.[7] The biceps femoris tendon insertions (see Fig. 8.19C) are then identified in longitudinal section by anchoring the probe over the distal LCL and by rotating the proximal end of the probe slightly posteriorly. The normal tendon may appear tendinopathic due to anisotropy of

the complex insertion as the fibres bifurcate to travel superficially and deep to the LCL.

The anterior body of the lateral meniscus is seen at the lateral joint line as an echogenic structure deep to the LCL in longitudinal section (see Fig. 8.18B).

The hypoechoic nerve fascicles of the common peroneal nerve should be visible by scanning in a transverse section at the level of the fibular head[7] (Fig. 8.20). By moving the transducer slightly anterior from this position, the TFJ can be identified (Fig. 8.21).

Posterior Knee

For evaluation of the posterior knee/popliteal fossa, often performed to exclude a "Baker's cyst," the patient is placed prone with the knee extended.[6] This may be difficult for elderly patients and scanning with the patient in a decubitus position with a pillow between their knees may achieve a similar result.

There are different ways of finding the correct anatomical site of the SMG bursa. One technique is to start in the proximal calf with the transducer in TS and identify the two heads of the gastrocnemius muscle (Fig. 8.22). Following the medial head of gastrocnemius (MHG) superiorly into the popliteal fossa, the tendon of semimembranosus will be on the medial aspect of the MHG, with the SMG bursa found in-between (Fig. 8.23). Alternatively, start in the distal thigh where the semitendinosus tendon lies superficial to the semimembranosus muscle ("cherry on the cake sign," see Chapter 7). From here, the semimembranosus muscle can be tracked distally into the popliteal fossa until its tendon is seen on the medial side of the MHG. A pitfall can occur by misinterpreting anisotropy of the semimembranosus and semitendinosus tendons as a small Baker's cyst.[7,8]

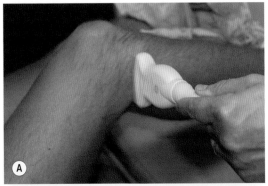
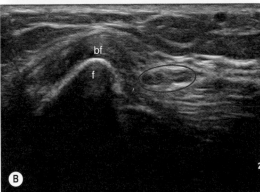

Fig. 8.20 Common peroneal nerve in tranverse section. (A) Transducer position. **(B)** Head of fibula *(f)*, common peroneal nerve *(red outline)*, biceps femoris insertion *(bf)*.

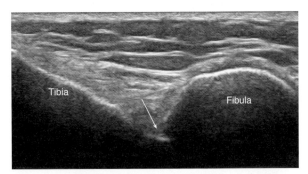

Fig. 8.21 Proximal tibiofibular joint. *Arrow* points to the joint.

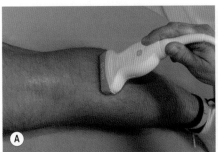
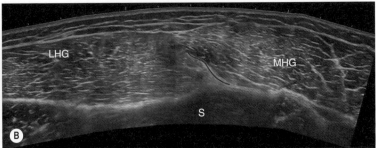

Fig. 8.22 Posterior left calf in transverse section. (A) Transducer positioned in the proximal calf. **(B)** Medial *(MHG)* and lateral *(LHG)* heads of gastrocnemius, soleus *(S)*, and myotendinous junction of the Achilles tendon *(red line)*.

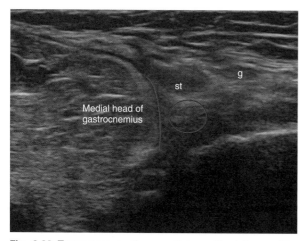

Fig. 8.23 Transverse section medial popliteal fossa. *Blue line* shows the position of the semimembranosus-gastrocnemius bursa. *red circle*, semimembranosus tendon; *st*, semitendinosus; *g*, gracilis tendon.

The popliteal vessels are seen in TS and LS sections in the popliteal fossa along with the tibial nerve (Fig. 8.24). Slight flexion of the knee will enable better visualisation of the popliteal vein as it can be compressed in extension. Deep vein thrombosis in rare circumstances can be a complication of a large or ruptured Baker's cyst and a popliteal aneurysm should be considered as a differential diagnosis for a popliteal mass.[7]

> **TIP**
>
> Ensure that the correct anatomical landmarks of the semimembranosus tendon and medial head of gastrocnemius are visualised before attempting a diagnosis of a Baker's cyst.

Calf

The individual calf muscles are more easily recognised by starting at the level of the ankle and finding the tendons in transverse section. By moving the transducer proximally, the myotendinous junctions are visualised. The muscles can then be examined in both TS and LS. It is important to recognise the normal anatomy of the myotendinous junction of the muscles (see Chapter 2) as in adults, this is where injury is commonly found.

PATHOLOGY

Joint Effusion

A knee joint effusion is seen as excessive fluid distension of the suprapatellar, medial, and lateral joint recesses.[12] In the suprapatellar recess, fluid separates the prefemoral and suprapatellar fat pads (Fig. 8.25). Flexion and extension and changes in patient position may move fluid from one part of the joint to another.

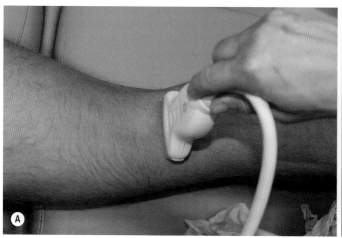

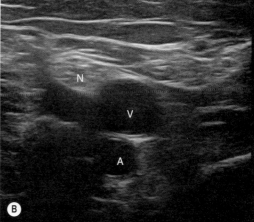

Fig. 8.24 Transverse section of the neurovascular bundle in the popliteal fossa. **(A)** Transducer placed centrally in the popliteal fossa. **(B)** Popliteal vein *(V)*, artery *(A)*, and tibial nerve *(N)*.

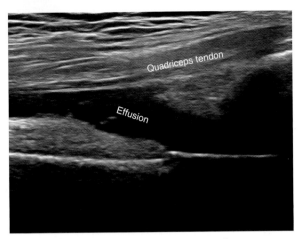

Fig. 8.25 Joint effusion in the suprapatellar recess.

REPORT—JOINT EFFUSION (A&E REFERRAL) FIG. 8.25

Clinical History: 13-year-old female, right knee pain, swelling and raised CRP. No history of injury. ? synovitis.

Ultrasound Report: There is a moderate amount of fluid in the right suprapatellar bursa. No evidence of synovial hypertrophy or neovascularity seen on Power Doppler. The contralateral left knee appears normal.

Conclusion: Right knee effusion. Infection is not excluded on ultrasound; if sepsis is a clinical concern, diagnostic aspiration is advised.

As in other joints, care should be taken to distinguish synovial hypertrophy from joint sepsis with the use of Power Doppler and compressibility of the fluid. Ultrasound can be used to guide knee joint aspiration in patients with uncertain diagnosis.

Joint effusion is likely to be due to some form of intra-articular insult, though this may be transitory, and it does not necessarily indicate the presence of an identifiable cause. The effusion can be symptomatic and limit a return to normal function and so aspiration in some cases can be therapeutic.

In trauma, ultrasound appearances of an effusion can raise the suspicion of intra-articular injury. For instance, blood within the effusion (haemarthrosis) shows as diffuse low-level echoes, stranding, and clot retraction. Blood and fat within a suprapatellar effusion (lipo-haemarthrosis) presents as a fat-fluid level and suggests intra-articular knee fracture; ultrasound is more sensitive than radiography.[7]

Quadriceps/Patellar Tendinopathy and Rupture

Pathology of the extensor mechanism ranges from tendinopathy to partial or complete rupture.

Requests for ultrasound of tendinopathy are more frequent for the patellar than quadriceps tendon. Manifesting as anterior knee pain, proximal patellar tendinopathy is more common than distal tendinopathy. Proximal patellar tendinopathy, also referred to as jumper's knee or Sinding-Larson-Johansson disease in children, often affects athletes in sports that involve jumping, such as basketball. The patellar tendon (PT) is broad and proximal tendinopathy is usually focal, present in the deep fibres of the mid-tendon as in Fig. 8.26. In more advanced cases interstitial clefts or tears may develop in the tendon.

This condition can be difficult to treat. Based on current literature, conservative management includes rest, addressing biomechanical issues, and progressive loading of the tendon. In recalcitrant tendinopathy, other options include taping, transverse friction massage, injecting platelet rich plasma, extracorporeal shock wave therapy, and ultimately surgical excision of the diseased portion of tendon.[13,14]

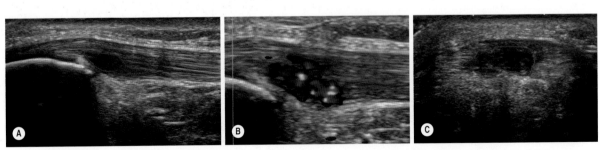

Fig. 8.26 Proximal patellar tendinopathy. (A/B) longitudinal sections and **(C)** transverse section of the proximal patellar tendon, showing tendinopathy *(red outlines)* and neovascularity of the deep fibres.

Tendinopathy of the distal PT is less common and usually affects young males involved in kicking and jumping sports. In the developing skeleton, it is termed Osgood-Schlatter disease (OSD). On ultrasound there may be swelling of the unossified cartilage and overlying soft tissues, fragmentation and irregularity of the ossification centre, as well as tendinopathy. It is important not to equate isolated "fragmentation" of the apophysis with OSD, as there may be secondary ossification centres; therefore OSD should not be considered unless the patient is symptomatic.

It is worth mentioning that the PT is often thickened following total knee replacement (TKR). This may not be symptomatic and therefore care should be taken not to over report its significance.

REPORT—PROXIMAL PATELLAR TENDINOPATHY (GP REFERRAL) FIG. 8.26

Clinical History: 20-year-old male basketball player, right anterior knee pain.

Ultrasound Report: There is focal tendinopathy of the deep middle fibres of the right proximal patellar tendon with neovascularity at the site of tendinopathy but no tear.

Rupture of the extensor mechanism often results from a forced eccentric contraction (contracting while lengthening) against an outside force.[10] This can happen during high-energy accidents such as motor vehicle crashes and during sporting activities, or during low-energy injuries such as falls from a standing position onto a bent knee. The other risk factors of rupture are increasing age, repetitive microtrauma, genetics, systemic disease, and long-term medication. Patients will report acute onset of pain and inability to perform a straight leg raise (SLR). A palpable defect in either the QT or PT tendon may be apparent, although this can be difficult to feel when the knee is swollen, and haematoma is present.

Initially the patient should have a plain radiograph to rule out a fracture. X-ray of a patient with rupture may show a high (Alta) or low patella (Baja) in PT and QT rupture, respectively; there may also be avulsion of a bone fragment.

In young patients, an avulsion sleeve injury may occur where there is a chondral or osteochondral avulsion of the tendon as seen on both X-ray and ultrasound in Fig. 8.27.

Distinguishing between a partial and complete rupture of the extensor mechanism and/or tears of the quadriceps musculotendinous junctions are important to help with management of the patient.

Partial tears can be treated nonoperatively with immobilisation of the leg in full extension followed by a progressive mobility and strengthening program, the patient resuming normal activity anywhere from 3 to 6 months after the injury.

High grade partial tears (where a large percentage of tendon fibres are torn) and complete rupture require surgical repair/reattachment of the tendon. This is normally performed within 1 to 2 weeks of injury for the best results. If left untreated, the outcome is poor with muscle atrophy of the quadriceps. On ultrasound, complete rupture shows

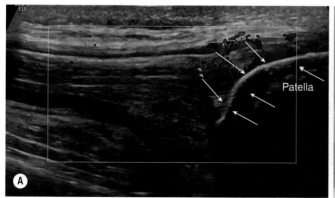
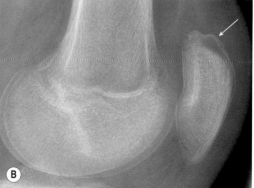

Fig. 8.27 Avulsion sleeve injury of the quadriceps tendon (QT). Arrows show the osteochondral fragment on ultrasound **(A)** and **(B)** Lateral X-ray.

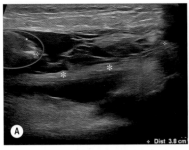
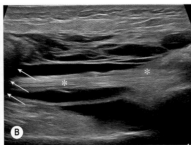
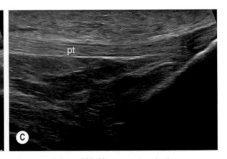

Fig. 8.28 Longitudinal section of a high-grade partial quadriceps tendon rupture. **(A)** Knee extended and **(B)** knee flexed. Rupture tendon end of quadriceps *(red outline)* with refractory shadow *(arrows)*, intact vastus intermedius fibres *(*)*. **(C)** Intact taut patellar tendon *(pt)*.

as full thickness and full width disruption of the QT or PT tendon with separated tendon ends or avulsion of the tendon from the patella. A measurement of the distance in LS between tendons ends or from the retracted tendon end to patella should be reported.

Ultrasound assessment can be difficult as there is often extensive haematoma present. The following features may aid diagnosis:

- the presence of refraction shadowing at the retracted tendon end
- a wavy appearance to the patella tendon, which is a secondary sign of complete QT rupture, due to inferior translation of the patella. This sign can help confirm findings; however, care should be taken to assess with the knee in slight flexion as this wavy appearance can be seen in a non-ruptured quadriceps tendon when the knee is completely extended.

Fig. 8.28 shows the images of a 75-year-old male with a high-grade QT rupture. The vastus intermedius tendon (VI) fibres are still intact and are demonstrated under tension when the patient has his knee flexed. The rest of the quadriceps tendon has ruptured, and the conjoint tendon end is retracted to a distance greater than 3 cm from the patella. Interestingly, the patella tendon is still taut as the patella has not moved inferiorly because of the maintained VI fibres.

Fig. 8.29 is an example of complete PT rupture in a 70-year-old male who fell with his knee bent beneath him.

REPORT—COMPLETE PT RUPTURE (A&E REFERRAL) (FIG. 8.29)

Clinical History: 70-year-old male. Anterior knee swelling following fall, knee bent beneath him. No palpable defect in the PT but unable to SLR, ? PT rupture.

Ultrasound Report: There is a complete rupture of the patellar tendon in the mid-portion, 1 cm from the inferior pole of the patella. The gap between the tendon ends with the knee in extension, is 10 mm with intact distal tendon fibres at the tibial tuberosity. There is organising haematoma superficial to the ruptured tendon.

The quadriceps tendon is intact.

A potential pitfall in the evaluation of chronic rupture is interposed scar tissue; this can give a complete tear the appearance of a partial tear.[7,8]

In trauma patients, during examination of the extensor mechanism, fractures of the patella may be identified on ultrasound as cortical defect, or step-off deformity. A bipartite patella should not be mistaken for a fracture. This is found when the superolateral ossification centre is unfused.

REPORT—HIGH-GRADE PARTIAL QT RUPTURE (A&E REFERRAL) (FIG. 8.28)

Clinical History: 75-year-old male. ? palpable defect in the QT following fall. Unable to SLR. History of chronic kidney disease.

Ultrasound Report: There is a high-grade partial rupture of the quadriceps tendon. The vastus intermedius tendon fibres are intact but the rest of the quadriceps tendon has ruptured. The tendon end is retracted to 3.8 cm from the patella when the knee is extended. The patella tendon is still intact. There is haematoma at the site of the tear and a suprapatellar effusion.

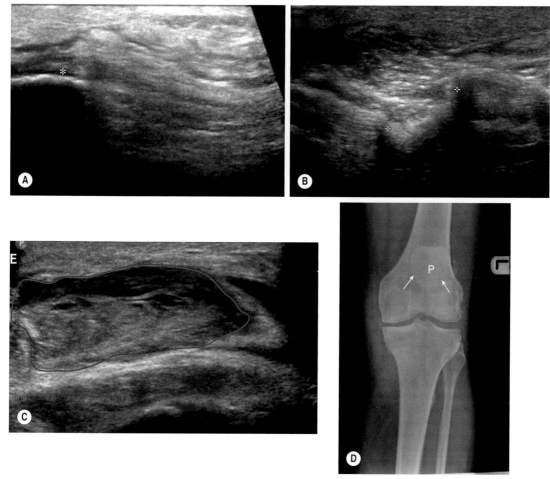

Fig. 8.29 Ruptured patella tendon. (A) Small stump of intact tendon attached to the inferior pole of patella *(*)*. **(B)** Ruptured tendon ends (with refractory shadowing) *(calipers)*. **(C)** Haematoma seen superficial to the distal tendon end in transverse section *(red outline)*. **(D)** X-ray shows superior and lateral migration of the patella (*P* and *arrows*).

> **TIP**
>
> Secondary signs of complete rupture of the quadriceps tendon are a low positioned patella and a wavy contour of the patella tendon.

Fat Pad Injury/Inflammation/Impingement

Pathology of the fat pads in the anterior knee should be considered as another cause of anterior knee pain and swelling. Repeated mechanical stress during flexion, extension, and rotation movements causes tissue alteration due to inflammatory, oedematous, and haemorrhagic reactions which result in swelling and loss of plasticity of the infrapatellar/Hoffa's fat pad (IFP). Oedema and haemorrhage of the IFP can be seen on ultrasound; however, MR imaging gives a more comprehensive assessment of the condition and can evaluate associated bone oedema and nodule formation. Treatment is rest, anti-inflammatory medication, and strengthening exercises of vastus medialis to prevent patellar maltracking which can contribute to the problem. The images in Fig 8.30 show fat pad impingement and proximal PT tendinopathy in a 25-year-old postman.

It is important to take imaging findings in clinical context, as "abnormal" appearances are common in asymptomatic patients.

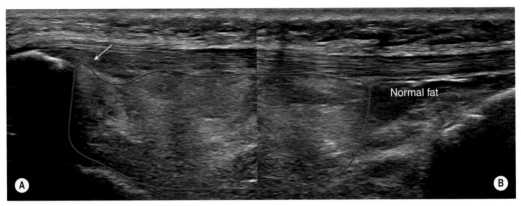

Fig. 8.30 Panoramic view of the infrapatellar region. **(A and B)** Oedema *(red outline)* of the fat pad and tendinopathy of the proximal patellar tendon *(arrow).*

> **REPORT—IFP INFLAMMATION/PROXIMAL PATELLAR TENDINOPATHY (A&E REFERRAL) (FIG. 8.30)**
>
> Clinical History: 25-year-old postman. Anterior knee swelling, struggling to SLR, ? patellar tendon rupture/tendinopathy.
>
> Ultrasound Report: There is focal tendinopathy of the deep proximal fibres of the patellar tendon which is intact. Marked oedema of the infrapatellar fat pad is also seen proximally.
>
> An MR scan is advised for a more comprehensive assessment of the adjacent bony structures for oedema, stress fracture.

The subcutaneous prepatellar fat pad contains multiple fibrous septa which reinforce its adherence to the skin, distributing mechanical stress. Injury to the fat pad occurs acutely as the result of a direct blow or fall as a Morel-Lavallée closed degloving injury. On ultrasound, serous fluid fills a space between the sheared tissues and may become encapsulated.

Bursitis

There are many potential sites of bursitis/inflammation of the bursae around the knee, some of which are already mentioned in relation to other pathologies, sites of tendinopathy, and trauma. Bursitis may also occur secondary to inflammatory arthritis/gout.[15–17]

One of the most common indications for ultrasound of the knee is to look for a Baker's cyst which as mentioned in the anatomy section is fluid within the

SMG bursa. When distended this causes a lump at the back of the knee which may be concerning and painful for the patient. Location is important and care must be taken to ensure that a popliteal cystic mass is in the correct position (Fig. 8.31A) before reporting it as a Baker's cyst.[7,8] There are other bursae in this region which may become inflamed and a cystic sarcoma in the popliteal fossa should also be considered. If associated with osteo or inflammatory arthritis, the bursa may have a complex appearance on ultrasound and may contain synovial hypertrophy +/− hyperaemia on Doppler. Calcified 'loose bodies' may be visible, usually floating within the bursal effusion. (see Rheumatology chapter). The bursa may rupture and cause swelling which can mimic symptoms of a deep vein thrombus. In these patients, fluid may be seen tracking inferiorly in the calf, superficial to the MHG muscle.

Baker's cysts are usually managed conservatively but may be aspirated or injected with steroid under ultrasound guidance, although there is a significant rate of recurrence.[18]

> **REPORT—BAKER'S CYST (GP REFERRAL) (FIG. 8.31A/B)**
>
> Clinical History: 60-year-old with a mass in the popliteal fossa, ? Baker's cyst.
>
> Ultrasound Report: There is a large cystic lesion which measures 53 mm × 39 mm × 33 mm arising from between the medial head of gastrocnemius and semimembranosus tendon.
>
> Conclusion: Baker's cyst.

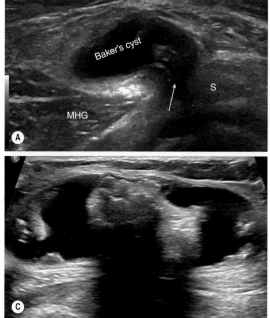

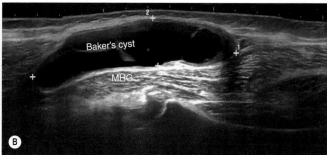

Fig. 8.31 Baker's cyst. **(A)** Transverse section Baker's cyst. The arrow shows the neck of the distended bursa as it extends towards the joint. **(B)** Longitudinal section of the bursa superficial to the MHG. **(C)** Transverse section shows a different Baker's cyst containing calcific loose bodies. *MHG,* Medial head of gastrocnemius ; *S,* Semimembranosus tendon.

Chronic injury to the prepatellar bursa occurs with repetitive microtrauma from kneeling (e.g., tradesmen, carpet fitters, plumbers). In initial stages this shows as thickening of the prepatellar fat on ultrasound. In moderate cases, fluid is seen between the fat lobules and in severe cases, fluid collections are seen in the region of the prepatellar and superficial infrapatellar bursae. These cases are normally reported as mild, moderate, or marked prepatellar bursitis.

In Fig. 8.32 the image shows marked acute-on-chronic prepatellar bursitis in a 40-year-old paramedic who had to repeatedly kneel at work. He had ignored the swelling in the anterior knee for months until the symptoms had become severe.

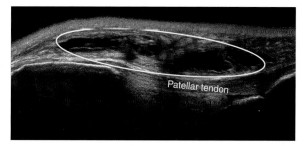

Fig. 8.32 Prepatellar bursitis. Fluid superficial to the patellar tendon *(white outline)* in a case of marked prepatellar bursitis.

REPORT—PREPATELLAR BURSITIS (FIG. 8.32) (A&E REFERRAL)

Clinical History: 40-year-old paramedic, swelling prepatellar region for months, ? bursitis.

Ultrasound Report: There is a large loculated cystic lesion which measures 53 mm × 15 mm × 38 mm superficial to the patellar tendon and patella.

Conclusion: Marked prepatellar bursitis.

Meniscal Tear/Cyst

Ultrasound would not be the imaging of choice for suspected meniscal disease as it cannot visualise the whole of the meniscus; in fact, the deeper meniscal tears not seen on ultrasound are more likely to be clinically significant. However, a cyst arising from a degenerate meniscus may be the cause of a soft tissue swelling (Fig. 8.33) and it may be possible to see a tear in the superficial portion of the meniscus on ultrasound.

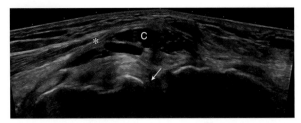

Fig. 8.33 Lateral meniscal cyst. Large loculated cyst (*C*) displacing the lateral collateral ligament (***). Hypoechoic cleft in the lateral meniscus (*arrow*) suggesting a tear.

REPORT—LATERAL PARAMENISCAL CYST (FIG. 8.33)(GP REFERRAL)

Clinical History: 40-year-old with a mass in the lateral knee ? nature.

Ultrasound Report: There is a large cystic lesion which measures 44 mm × 16 mm × 22 mm deep to the LCL, with no neovascularity. There is disruption of the superficial aspect of the lateral meniscus.

Impression: parameniscal cyst with degenerative changes in the lateral meniscus. An MR scan is advised for a more comprehensive assessment of the meniscus and lateral joint structures.

◎ TIP

When assessing structures with an intra-articular component (e.g., menisci and cruciate ligaments) remember that ultrasound is unable to assess the full extent of injury and MRI should be considered.

Collateral Ligament Injury

Laterally, the LCL and conjoint biceps tendon are seldom injured in isolation; therefore, imaging is often with MR.

MCL injuries are the most common ligamentous injuries of the knee. They are usually the result of sports injury resulting from valgus stress to the knee from force to the outside of the knee or sudden change in direction. The patient presents with swelling and pain in the medial knee. A good history and physical examination to assess widening of the medial joint whilst applying valgus force may provide the diagnosis; however,

imaging may be required when injury is chronic or when multiple ligamentous injuries are suspected. MR would be the imaging of choice especially in complex injury as the cruciate ligaments and menisci may also be involved.

Ultrasound may be helpful at point-of-care in an acute setting to help with initial assessment. Typical ultrasound features of MCL injury are thickening and reduced echogenicity of the ligament, loss of the normal taut fibrillar structure of the ligament, and surrounding fluid.[19,20] Dynamic ultrasound imaging of the medial joint space in valgus stress may be useful, as the degree of joint space widening is related to injury grade. Scanning the contralateral MCL is vital as age related changes are common.

Management of MCL injury is usually conservative with knee bracing followed by active rehabilitation, even in high-grade injury. In some patients, a chronic painful condition can develop where an ossified (Pelligrini-Steida) lesion forms adjacent to the femoral condyle in the injured proximal MCL. Initially thought to be the result of an avulsion fracture, it is now thought to be due to calcified haematoma as it can take weeks after injury for the calcification to form. The case in Fig. 8.34 is a good example of this condition. This patient was referred for steroid injection to the MCL region because of pain related to a chronic MCL tear and Pelligrini-Steida lesion. This had been diagnosed on X-ray and MRI 6 weeks after the patient had a fall. It was not responding well to rehabilitation 8 months after the original injury.

Other Sites of Tendinopathy in the Knee

Pes anserine tendinopathy causes similar symptoms to a sprain of the MCL, including pain over the inside of the knee below the joint line. The patient may experience pain when climbing stairs or when contracting the hamstring muscles against resistance. Stretching the hamstring muscles may also cause pain. Repetitive sporting activities such as running, cycling, and breaststroke swimming can result in tendinopathy and bursitis; other risk factors include valgus knee deformity, flat feet, and instability, as well as diabetes, osteoarthritis, and obesity. Patients with TKR may also develop this condition. As well as features of tendinopathy, bursitis is often seen deep to the PA tendons. Comparison with the asymptomatic side can be helpful as fluid is present in the bursa in 5% of asymptomatic knees. Care should be

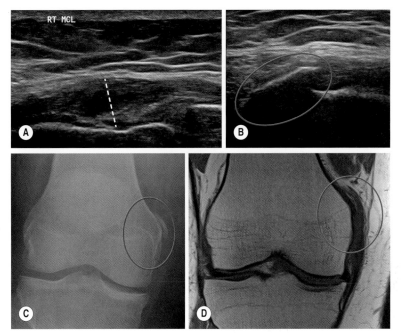

Fig. 8.34 Medial collateral ligament injury. **(A)** Chronic tear of MCL showing thickened proximal fibres *(dashed line)*. Pelligrini-Steida lesion *(red outline)* on **(B)** ultrasound, **(C)** X-ray, and **(D)** MRI. *MCL,* Medial collateral ligament.

made to ensure that the fluid-filled PA bursa is in the correct location as medial meniscal cysts, large Baker's cysts, and MCL bursitis are other causes of cystic medial knee lesions. Treatment is with physiotherapy, and steroid injection into the bursa may also help.[16,17]

Iliotibial band syndrome is a nontraumatic overuse injury common in runners and cyclists, with a bias towards female athletes. It is thought to be due to repetitive knee flexion and extension with an underlying weakness of the hip abductors. Patients present with pain directly over the iliotibial band insertion. They often have pain along the length of the iliotibial tract and into the lateral hip. Ultrasound evidence of iliotibial band syndrome includes hypoechoic thickening of the iliotibial band and adjacent oedema.[3]

Proximal Tibiofibular Joint/Common Peroneal Nerve Pathology

Due to its superficial position, disorders of the TFJ may present as a palpable mass. Degenerative arthritis of the TFJ may accompany osteoarthritis of the knee or occur in isolation. A ganglion may arise from the joint (Fig. 8.35) which may compress or extend into the common peroneal nerve.

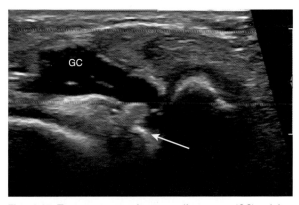

Fig. 8.35 Transverse section ganglion cyst *(GC)* arising from the proximal tibiofibular joint *(arrow).*

The common peroneal nerve branches close to the neck of the fibula where it is prone to injury during fracture of the fibula and it can be a site of neuromas in the stump in below knee amputees.

The TFJ and popliteus tendon are often involved in injuries to the posterolateral corner of the knee from road traffic accidents or falls where the knee is overextended. The TFJ may also be injured through impacts which force the knee out to the side. This type of injury will usually require MR imaging as multiple structures, including the posterior cruciate ligaments, may be involved.

Interesting Knee Case

A 54-year-old female presented from her GP with swelling and pain for several months in the infrapatellar region.

Ultrasound shows a large cystic mass in the infrapatellar region, deep to the patellar tendon within Hoffa's fat pad (Fig. 8.36). There were no suspicious features, and the ultrasound diagnosis was infrapatellar fat pad ganglion. MR was performed to assess for any extension deep to the patella or connection with any other structures and confirm the benign features. A surgical referral was advised.

In the literature, these lesions are quite rare and usually require open rather than arthroscopic surgical excision as they are extrasynovial in the infrapatellar fat pad.[21]

Tennis Leg

A tear of the myotendinous junction of the MHG (Fig. 8.37B) is a common injury classically seen in middle-aged athletes who play tennis but can be induced by playing squash, skiing, and athletics. The injury can also occur with nonsporting activity, such as running to catch a bus. Extension of the knee and forced dorsiflexion of the ankle seem to be the most frequent biomechanical causes of the injury. The patient feels a sudden sharp pain in the posterior aspect of the calf,

with a sensation of something "snapping." There is usually focal tenderness and swelling. Treatment is rest followed by a progressive exercise programme.[22]

Rupture of the plantaris tendon can also present with similar symptoms and should be considered when investigating this injury. It is also prudent to assess for involvement of the distal Achilles tendon in these cases.

REPORT—TENNIS LEG (GP REFERRAL) (FIG. 8.37B).
Clinical History: 40-year-old. Pain playing football with his son 5 weeks ago. Suspected muscle tear which is still causing problems, referred for physiotherapy.
Ultrasound Report: There is a chronic tear with scarring at the myotendinous junction of the medial head of gastrocnemius muscle over a distance of 55 mm. The Achilles tendon is intact distally.

REPORTING TERMINOLOGY FOR NORMAL FINDINGS
No evidence of a joint effusion or synovitis.
No evidence of a solid or cystic lesion seen in the popliteal fossa. No Baker's cyst. The popliteal artery is of normal calibre.
Normal appearances of the quadriceps and patellar tendons. Normal fibrillar pattern. No evidence of tendon tears, calcification, or enthesitis.[23]

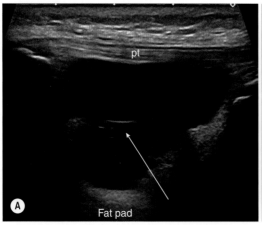
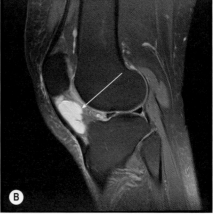

Fig. 8.36 Infrapatellar ganglion. (A) Large cystic infrapatellar ganglion (arrow) deep to the patellar tendon *(pt).* **(B)** Magnetic resonance images of the lesion.

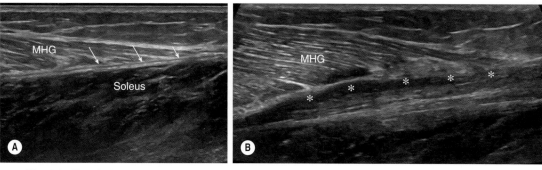

Fig. 8.37 Tennis leg. (A) Longitudinal section normal myotendinous junction of MHG *(arrows)* and soleus. **(B)** Longitudinal section chronic tear showing scar tissue *(*)* at the myotendinous junction of the MHG. *MHG,* Medial head of gastrocnemius.

MULTIPLE CHOICE QUESTIONS

1. What makes up the trilaminar structure of the quadriceps tendon from anterior to posterior?
   a) Vastus medialis, vastus intermedius, vastus lateralis
   b) Rectus femoris, vastus medialis, vastus lateralis, vastus intermedius
   c) Rectus femoris, vastus medialis, vastus intermedius, vastus lateralis
2. Where is a Baker's cyst situated?
   a) Between the lateral head of gastrocnemius and semimembranosus
   b) Between the medial head of gastrocnemius and semitendinosus
   c) Between the medial head of gastrocnemius and semimembranosus
3. In a complete rupture of the quadriceps tendon, what type of patella position would occur?
   a) Patella alta
   b) Patella baja
   c) Medial position

4. Which structures are referred to as the Triceps Surae
   a) Medial and lateral gastrocnemius, soleus
   b) Achilles, plantaris, tibialis posterior
   c) Gastrocnemius, Achilles, tibialis posterior
5. Proximal patellar tendinopathy in children is also referred to as:
   a) Osgood-Schlatter's disease.
   b) Pelligrini-Steida disease.
   c) Sinding-Larson-Johansson disease.

REFERENCES

1. Sinnatamby CS. Last's Anatomy: Regional and Applied. 12th ed. Edinburgh/New York: Churchill Livingstone/Elsevier; 2011.
2. Forster BB, Lee JS, Kelly S, et al. Proximal tibiofibular joint: an often-forgotten cause of lateral knee pain. AJR Am J Roentgenol. 2017;188:W359–366.
3. Bianchi S, Martinoli C. Ultrasound of the Musculoskeletal System. Berlin Heidelberg: Springer-Verlag; 2007.
4. McNally E. Practical Musculoskeletal Ultrasound. Oxford: Churchill Livingstone; 2014.
5. Jacobson JA. Fundamentals of Musculoskeletal Ultrasound. Philadelphia: Elsevier; 2018.
6. Beggs I, Bianchi S, Bueno A, et al. ESSR musculoskeletal technical guidelines V. Knee. ESSR: 2016. Available at: https://essr.org/content-essr/uploads/2016/10/knee.pdf
7. Alves TI, Girish G, Brigido MK, Jon A, Jacobson JA. US of the knee: scanning techniques, pitfalls and pathologic conditions. Radiographics. 2016;36:1759–1775.

8. Jamander DA, Robertson BL, Jacobson JA, et al. Musculoskeletal sonography: important imaging pitfalls. AJR Am J Roentgenol. 2010;194:216–225. Available at: https://www.ajronline.org/doi/full/10.2214/AJR.09.2712.

9. Windschall D, Trauzeddel R, Haller M, et al. Pediatric musculoskeletal ultrasound: age- and sex-related normal B-mode findings of the knee. Rheumatol Int. 2016;36(11):1569–1577.

10. Tintinalli JE, Stapczynski J, Ma J, Yealy D, Meckler G, Cline D. Tintinelli's Emergency Medicine: a Comprehensive Study Guide. 8th ed. New York: McGraw-Hill, Medical Pub. Division; 2015.

11. Roberts HM, Moore JP, Thom JM. The reliability of suprapatellar transverse sonographic assessment of femoral trochlear cartilage thickness in healthy adults. J Ultrasound Med. 2019;38(4):935–946.

12. Johnson MW. Acute knee effusions: a systematic approach to diagnosis. Am Fam Physician. 2000;61(8):2391–2400.

13. Reinking MF. Current concepts in the treatment of patellar tendinopathy. Int J Sports Phys Ther. 2016;11(6):854–866.

14. Rutland M, O'Connell D, Brismée JM, Sizer P, Apte G, O'Connell J. Evidence-supported rehabilitation of patellar tendinopathy. N Am J Sports Phys Ther. 2010;5(3)166–178.

15. Ward EE, Jacobson JA, Fessell DA, Hayes CW, van Holsbeeck M. Sonographic detection of Baker's cysts comparison with MR Imaging. AJR Am J Roentgenol. 2001;176:373–380. https://www.ajronline.org/doi/full/10.2214/ajr.176.2.1760373.

16. Rennie WJ, Saifuddin A. Pes anserine bursitis: incidence in symptomatic knees and clinical presentation. Skeletal Radiol. 2005;33(7):395–398.

17. Sarifakioglu B, Afsar SI, Yalbuzdag SA, Ustaömer K, Bayramofülü M. Comparison of the efficacy of physical therapy and corticosteroid injection in the treatment of pes anserine tendino-bursitis. J Phys Ther Sci. 2016;28(7):1993–1997.

18. Smith MK, Lesniak B, Baraga MG, Kaplan L, Jose J. Treatment of popliteal (baker) cysts with ultrasound-guided aspiration, fenestration, and injection: long-term follow-up. Sports Health. 2015;7(5):409–414. doi:10.1177/1941738115585520.

19. Andrew K, Lu A, Mckean L. Review: medial collateral ligament injuries. J Orthop. 2012;14(4):550–554.

20. Lee JI, Song IS, Jung YB, et al. Medial collateral ligament injuries of the knee: ultrasonographic findings. J Ultrasound Med. 1996;15(9):621–625.

21. Nikolopoulus I, Krinas G, Kipriadis D, et al. Large infrapatellar ganglionic cyst of the knee fat pad: a case report and review of the literature. J Med Case Rep. 2011;5:351.

22. Jamadar D, Jacobson JA, Theisen SE, et al. Sonography of the painful calf: differential considerations. AJR Am J Roentgenol. 2002;179:709-716. Available at: https://www.ajronline.org/doi/10.2214/ajr.179.3.1790709.

23. Guidelines for Professional Practice SCOR, BMUS, December 2020. https://www.bmus.org/static/uploads/resources/Guidelines_for_Professional_Ultrasound_Practice_v3_OHoz76r.pdf.

Ultrasound of the Ankle and Foot

Andrew Longmead and Alison Hall

CHAPTER OUTLINE

LEARNING OBJECTIVES

After reading this chapter you should have gained an understanding of
- Relevant anatomical structures of the foot and ankle
- Ultrasound technique and normal appearances of these structures
- Common pathologies and their ultrasound appearances

INTRODUCTION

Ultrasound can be used to examine many superficial structures around the foot and ankle and is helpful in the diagnosis of soft tissue pathologies. Whilst cortical bone can be demonstrated, it is important to remember that intraarticular pathology cannot be excluded and some associated ligaments cannot be fully assessed with ultrasound. This chapter outlines anatomy and ultrasound technique of many accessible structures around the foot and ankle and gives examples of common pathologies.

PATIENT POSITIONING, EQUIPMENT, AND PHYSICAL EXAMINATION

As with all diagnostic ultrasound examinations, both patient and operator comfort are paramount and in foot and ankle scanning, the patient should be seated on an examination couch and the limb gently moved into the appropriate position for scanning. Both high and medium frequency probes should be available (6–15 MHz) as the skin on the sole of the foot will attenuate sound and necessitate a lower frequency than other superficial structures.

Referrals for ankle/foot scanning should be specific and appropriate to symptoms; however, it is often necessary to scan the opposite aspect—for example, scanning both medial and lateral ankle tendons—as one may cause issues in the other and degenerative changes may be asymptomatic, but may guide future prognosis and treatment. A guide to common sites and causes of symptoms are outlined below. This is not an exhaustive list and not all pathologies can be reliably detected using ultrasound. Those that are, will be explored in more detail in this chapter.

Anterior ankle:
- Degenerative/inflammatory joint disease, anterior impingement, tenosynovitis

Posterior ankle
- Achilles tendinopathy, bursitis, enthesitis, posterior impingement, Os trigonum

Medial ankle
- Tendinopathy/tenosynovitis, tarsal tunnel syndrome, deltoid injury

Lateral ankle
- Tendinopathy/tenosynovitis, sinus tarsi syndrome, subtalar joint disease, ATFL injury, fibular stress fracture

Plantar heel pain
- Plantar fasciopathy, bursitis, fat pad atrophy, calcaneal stress fracture

Midfoot pain
- Degenerative/inflammatory joint disease, ganglia,

Forefoot pain
- 1st MTPj – Hallux valgus/rigidus, gout, Degenerative joint disease, sesamoiditis

- 2nd -4th MTPj – Morton's neuroma, plantar plate disruption/hammer toe, stress fracture
- 5th MTPj – bursitis, inflammatory joint disease

ANTERIOR ANKLE AND DORSAL MIDFOOT

Anterior Ankle Joint—Anatomy

The ankle includes three main joints—the tibiotalar (talocrural joint), subtalar, and inferior tibiofibular joints (Fig. 9.1). The tibiotalar joint forms a hinged sy-

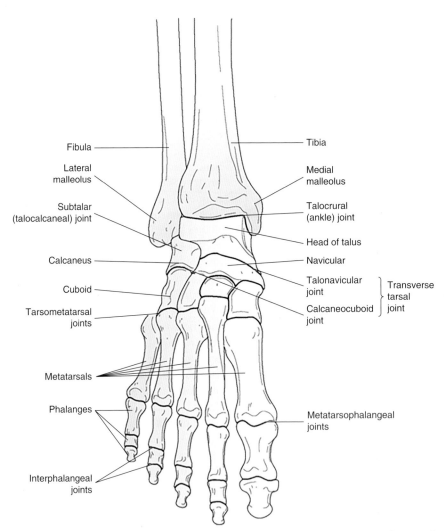

Fig. 9.1 Anterior Ankle and Foot. (From https://musculoskeletalkey.com/measurement-of-range-of-motion-of-the-ankle-and-foot/)

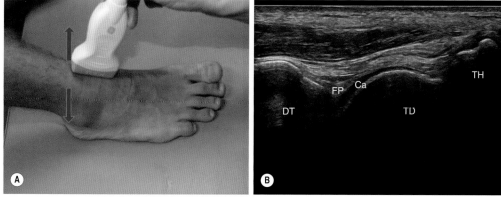

Fig. 9.2 (A) Ankle joint ultrasound technique. Red arrows denote probe movement across the joint. **(B)** Ankle joint ultrasound image. Distal tibia *(DT)*, fat pad *(FP)*, cartilage *(Ca)*, talar dome *(TD)*, talar head *(TH)*.

novial articulation between the distal tibia and fibula and the talus allowing dorsiflexion and plantarflexion of the foot. The joint capsule extends distally over the talar neck and the anterior joint recess which contains a fat pad and deep to this, cartilage, which can be seen over the articular surface of the talus.

Anterior Ankle Joint—Ultrasound Technique

The anterior ankle is best assessed with the knee flexed and the foot flat on the examination table. There is limited acoustic access of the tibiotalar joint due to overlying bony structures; however, clear views of the anterior ankle recess can be obtained with a longitudinal view between the medial and lateral malleoli. When assessing the joint, it is important to slide the probe across the entire width of the joint from medial to lateral to exclude any focal pathology (Fig. 9.2A).

The fat pad is seen as a hyperechoic triangle of soft tissue deep to the extensor tendons/muscles, overlying the articular cartilage of the talus (Fig. 9.2B).

Extensor Tendons and Retinacula— Anatomy

Three extensor tendon groups run on the anterior aspect of the ankle joint region (Fig. 9.3):
- Tibialis anterior (TA)
- Extensor hallucis longus (EHL)
- Extensor digitorum longus (EDL)

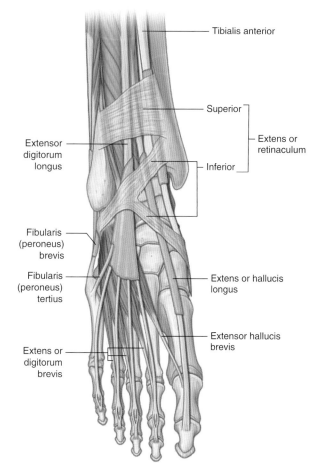

Fig. 9.3 Anterior Ankle Anatomy Showing Tendons and Retinacula.

These tendons are held in position by two retinacula, fibrous bands which extend horizontally across the anterior aspect of the ankle.

TA is the most medial tendon in the anterior ankle with its muscle originating from the lateral tibial condyle. It inserts into the plantar aspect of the medial cuneiform and base of the first metatarsal to provide dorsiflexion and inversion of the foot.

Lateral to this is the smaller EHL whose muscle originates from the anterior surface of the fibular. EHL tendon passes below the superior and inferior extensor retinacula and inserts into the base of the distal phalanx of the great toe.

The most lateral of the extensor tendons is the conjoined EDL whose muscle originates from the lateral condyle of the tibia and the interosseous membrane. The tendon continues beneath the inferior extensor retinaculum, after which it splays into four slips that extend distally and insert into the distal and middle phalanges of the second to fifth toes.

In over 90% of the population, an accessory tendon—peroneus tertius—may be present,[1] located lateral to EDL, although its location is variable making visualisation with imaging unpredictable. This tendon originates from the mid face of the fibular and extends underneath the retinaculum to insert onto the base of the fifth metatarsal.

Deep to the anterior ankle tendons lies the peroneal neurovascular bundle which continues along the dorsum of the foot, branching out towards the tarsal and metatarsal joints (Fig. 9.4).

This bundle comprises the anterior tibial artery and deep peroneal nerve. As it courses distally, the nerve passes from the lateral to the medial side of the dorsalis pedis artery. The deep peroneal nerve is primarily responsible for activation of the muscles to allow dorsiflexion of the foot, extension of the toes, and assisting the dominating tibialis anterior with inversion of the foot.

Extensor Tendons and Retinacula—Ultrasound Technique

Keeping the patient in the position described previously, the anterior tendon compartments, neurovascular bundle, and retinacula are best identified with the transducer held in transverse section (TS) at a level just distal to the medial malleolus (Fig. 9.5A).

Both retinacula are approximately 1 mm thick and appear as echogenic bands overlying the tendons (Fig. 9.5B)

The tendons are seen in TS and traced by sliding the transducer distally towards their insertions. The

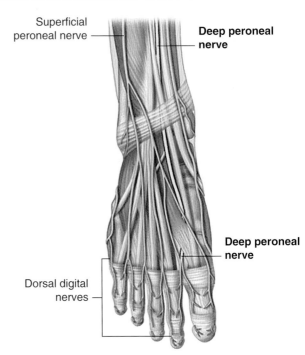

Fig. 9.4 Anterior Ankle Nerve Anatomy. (From https://link.springer.com/chapter/10.1007/978-3-319-27482-9_69)

transducer can then be rotated through 90 degrees, allowing longitudinal assessment (Fig. 9.5C)

> **TOP TIP**
>
> When scanning the tendons around the foot and ankle, identify the tendon in transverse and scan from the myotendinous junction to the distal insertion to ensure you are scanning the correct tendon. By scanning up to the myotendinous junction, you will appreciate the position of the corresponding muscle.

Dorsal Midfoot—Anatomy

On assessing the dorsal midfoot, below the skin and subcutaneous soft tissue layers there are two superficial muscle groups, the extrinsic and intrinsic muscles. The extrinsic muscles originate from the lower leg and are mainly responsible for movements such as inversion, eversion, plantar, and dorsiflexion of the foot, and their tendon components are easily visualised as the superficially located extensor tendons as previously mentioned in this chapter.

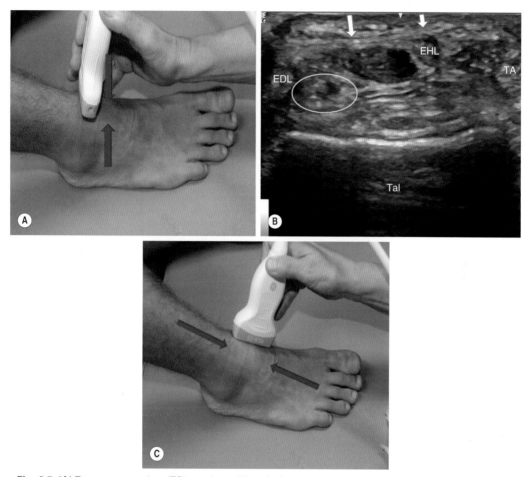

Fig. 9.5 (A) Transverse section *(TS)* anterior ankle soft tissues—ultrasound technique. Red arrows denote probe movement across the tendons. **(B)** TS anterior ankle soft tissues—ultrasound image. Tibialis anterior *(TA)*, extensor hallucis longus *(EHL)*, extensor digitorum longus *(EDL)*, talus *(Tal)*, retinaculum *(white arrows)*, peroneal neurovascular bundle *(yellow circle)*. **(C)** Anterior ankle soft tissues—ultrasound technique longitudinal. Red arrows denote probe movement along the tendons.

The main intrinsic muscles, extensor digitorum and extensor hallucis brevis muscles, originate from within the foot and are responsible for fine motor movements such as flexion and extension of individual toes.

Deep to the muscle layers there is complex bony anatomy which constitutes five tarsal bones—navicular, cuboid and medial, intermediate, and lateral cuneiforms—and five metatarsals (Fig. 9.6). Articulations are complex and many are not visible with ultrasound but the dorsal surfaces can be appreciated whilst scanning the midfoot.

Dorsal Midfoot—Ultrasound Technique

The dorsal surfaces of the tarsal and metatarsal joints are those most readily assessed with ultrasound and given the talus, navicular, intermediate cuneiform, and second metatarsals are aligned longitudinally, they can be used to navigate and identify the adjacent joints.

As the bi-lobed surface of the talus is easily recognised, it is a recommended place to begin the scan (Fig. 9.7) Alternatively, the operator may choose to start the scan distally over a particular toe, scanning proximally to work out which joint is symptomatic/pathological.

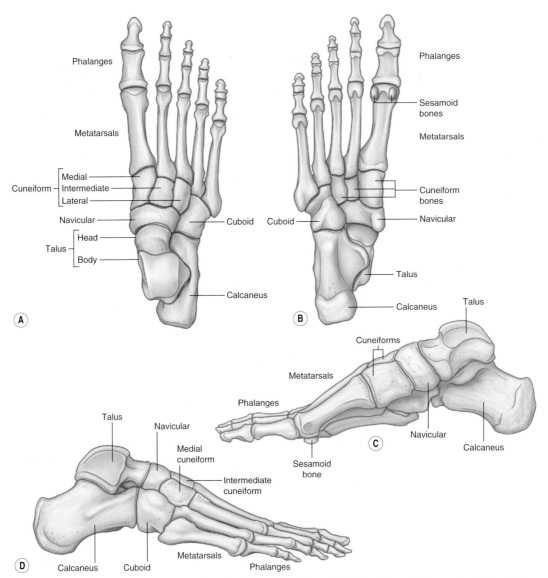

Fig. 9.6 Bone Anatomy of the Foot. Superior **(A)**, inferior **(B)**, medial **(C)** and lateral **(D)** aspects of the right foot. (From Soames R, Palastange N. Anatomy and Human Movement Structure and Function. 7th ed. London: Elsevier; 2019.)

◎ TOP TIP

It is important to be accurate when identifying specific symptomatic tarsal joints as future treatments may include injection or surgery. The midfoot is complex, so start either proximally over the talus or distally over the appropriate metatarsal so that you can work out exactly which joint is the cause of pain.

Anterior Ankle and Dorsal Midfoot—Common Pathology and Clinical Management
Tendon Pathology

Degenerative pathology of the anterior extensor tendons is uncommon, with TA the most likely to be affected due to friction against the inferior extensor retinaculum or underlying osteophytes, leading to tendinopathy,

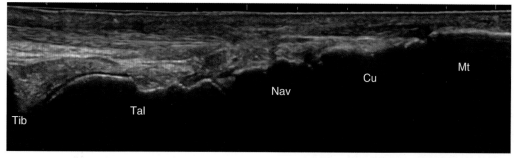

Fig. 9.7 Ultrasound panoramic image dorsal view of central bones of the midfoot: tibia *(Tib)*, talus *(Tal)*, navicular *(Na)*, cuneiform *(Cu)*, metatarsal *(Mt)*.

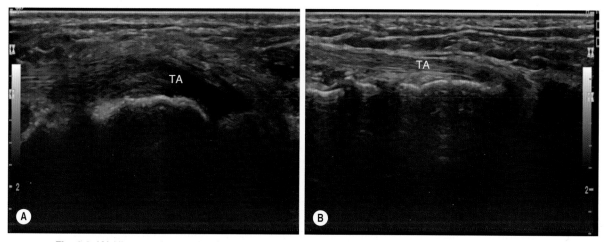

Fig. 9.8 (A) Ultrasound example of insertional tendinopathy of tibialis anterior *(TA)*—thickened tendon with loss of the normal fibrillar pattern. **(B)** Ultrasound normal TA tendon insertion.

enthesopathy, (Fig. 9.8) and eventually, rupture. Other causes include trauma, inflammatory arthropathy, or systemic conditions such as diabetes mellitus.

Ultrasound appearances of tendinopathy have been discussed in previous chapters and include hypoechogenicity, thickening, and loss of the normal fibrillar pattern. Later stages may include hypoechoic tendon splits and eventually the structural discontinuity and retraction of a complete tear.[2]

Initial treatment of symptoms may include PRICE (protection, rest, ice, compression, and elevation), nonsteroidal antiinflammatories, physical therapy, and orthotics, but if these are ineffective and there is significant pathology on imaging, surgery may be considered.[3]

Joint Effusion, Synovial Hypertrophy, and Synovitis

It is well recognised that ultrasound evaluation of larger joints is limited due to restricted access provided by bony interfaces and that intraarticular pathology cannot be excluded. As this can lead to a high rate of false negative ultrasound scans, if there is clinical concern for pathology within a large joint, further imaging should be suggested.[4]

In the tibiotalar joint, joint fluid or synovitis can be seen displacing the fat pad in the anterior joint recess (Fig. 9.9).

Causes include trauma, inflammation, infection, or degeneration and although clinical history can assist in differentiating between them, ultrasound alone may not exclude or confirm a particular pathology but may

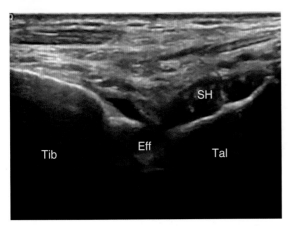

Fig. 9.9 Ultrasound example of synovial hypertrophy *(SH)* and effusion *(Eff)* at the tibio *(Tib)* talar *(Tal)* joint.

be used to aid aspiration for analysis. It is common to see a small amount of fluid within this joint deep to the fat pad[5] and comparison with the contralateral joint can highlight physiologically normal from abnormal amounts of fluid.

Joint Disease of the Midfoot

Using the technique to navigate the complex midfoot bony anatomy as described previously in this chapter, the dorsal surface of the relevant joint may be identified and the degree of osteophytes, synovial thickening, and/or enthesopathy assessed and correlated with symptoms (Fig. 9.10). Active synovitis seen on Doppler within symptomatic joints affected by osteoarthritis

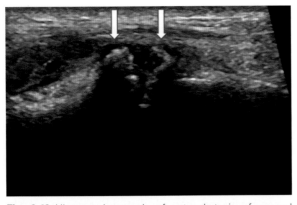

Fig. 9.10 Ultrasound example of osteophytosis of second tarsometatarsal joint *(white arrows)*.

(OA) is not uncommon[6] and should not be mistaken for an inflammatory arthritis such as rheumatoid disease. The overlying tendons and the deep peroneal nerve can be irritated by osteophytes and ganglia are commonly seen arising from the dorsal joints or tendon sheaths (see Chapter 11). Ultrasound guided injections of steroid and local anesthetic may be effective in treating the symptoms of joint disease and ganglia can be aspirated with surgical interventions being employed if symptoms are considerable and persistent.[7]

MEDIAL ANKLE

Flexor Tendons, Retinacula and Tarsal Tunnel—Anatomy

Three flexor tendons are located over the medial aspect of the ankle joint (Fig. 9.11)
- Tibialis posterior (TP)
- Flexor digitorum longus (FDL)
- Flexor hallucis longus (FHL)

These tendons are covered by synovial sheaths which range in length, a few centimeters above and below the medial malleolus. In 20% of the population, FHL tendon sheath communicates with the tibiotalar joint cavity and effusion may communicate between them.[8]

TP is the largest and most anterior of the tendons, originating as a muscle from the posterolateral tibia, posteromedial fibula, and interosseous membrane. The tendon forms just above the medial malleolus and passes posterior to it, extending distally to insert on to the navicular, with additional slips to the plantar portions of the second, third, and fourth metatarsals, second and third cuneiforms, and cuboid. The muscle is primarily responsible for plantar flexion and inversion.

Located immediately adjacent and posterior to TP is FDL which is smaller in caliber. The FDL muscle originates from the posterior tibia and the tendon runs beneath the medial malleolus, along the inner aspect of the talar shelf. This courses along and around the plantar lateral aspect of the foot, where the tendon splits into four branches that insert on the plantar surface at the base of the distal phalanges of the second, third, fourth and fifth toes.

The deepest and most posterior of the three tendons is FHL whose muscle arises from the inferior two-thirds of the posterior surface of the body of the fibula and

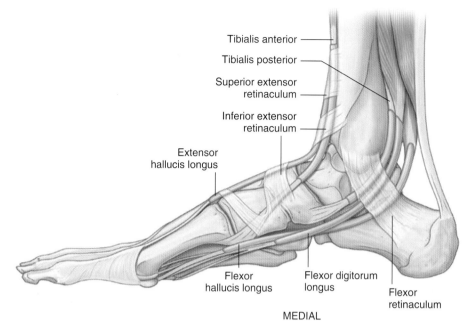

Tibialis anterior

Tibialis posterior

Superior extensor retinaculum

Inferior extensor retinaculum

Extensor hallucis longus

Flexor hallucis longus

Flexor digitorum longus

Flexor retinaculum

MEDIAL

Fig. 9.11 Medial Ankle—Flexor Tendons, Sheaths, and Retinacula. (From Soames R, Palastange N. Anatomy and Human Movement Structure and Function. 7th ed. London: Elsevier; 2019.)

extends distally as a tendon along the posterior aspect of the talus, the plantar aspect of the foot, and inserts into the distal phalanx of the great toe (Fig. 9.12).

Around the medial malleolus, the flexor tendons, along with the posterior tibial neurovascular bundle, are contained within a fibro-osseous tunnel known as the tarsal tunnel where the flexor retinaculum forms the roof. This retinaculum extends from the medial malleolus to the medial calcaneal process. The FHL tendon is contained within its own separate retinaculum.

Flexor Tendons, Retinacula and Tarsal Tunnel—Ultrasound Technique

The medial aspect of the ankle is best examined with the knee slightly flexed and the foot externally rotated so that the lateral malleolus rests on the examination table (Fig. 9.13A).

The medial tendons are identified in TS by placing one edge of the transducer on the medial malleolus and the other edge pointing to the most posterior aspect of

the plantar heel (see Fig. 9.13A). TP is situated adjacent to the medial malleolus, FDL, and the neurovascular bundle, and FHL found deeper and posterior to the neurovascular bundle (Fig. 9.13B)—it can be challenging to visualise but can be identified dynamically by flexing and extending the great toe.

Each tendon should be tracked from their musculotendinous junctions to their distal insertion in both TS and longitudinal section (LS). A small amount of fluid is commonly seen in asymptomatic patients around TP distally and a useful rule of thumb is that the cross-section area of the fluid should not exceed that of the adjacent tendon.[9]

On assessing TP, an accessory navicular bone (os navicularum) may be seen at the distal insertion which is a normal variant, present in approximately 10% of the population[10] (Fig. 9.14).

Medial Ligaments—Anatomy

Overlying the medial aspect of the ankle joint and seated deep to the medial tendons is a strong, broad, triangular

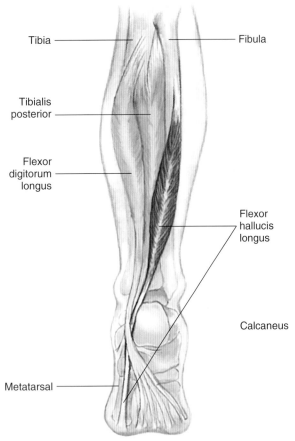

Fig. 9.12 Posterior View of Medial Ankle Muscles/Tendons. (From https://www.sportsinjurybulletin.com/the-flexor-hallucis-longus/)

ligament complex—the deltoid. The deltoid ligament is a multifascicular group of ligaments which functions as a strong restraint, limiting abnormal talar abduction and pronation. It can be divided into a superficial and deep group of fibres originating from the medial malleolus, fanning out to insert in the talus, calcaneus, and navicular bones. The specific, smaller ligaments are shown in Fig. 9.15 but are difficult to discern from each other on ultrasound.

Medial Ligaments—Ultrasound Technique

As described earlier, the deltoid ligament complex is often difficult to assess, not least because their ultrasound imaging is prone to anisotropy due to the variation in the trajectory of each portion, and subtle pathology may be missed. In view of this, and with the likelihood of concomitant intraarticular pathology following ankle injury, many centres do not routinely use ultrasound but would rather refer for magnetic resonance imaging (MRI) assessment in this area.

To allow evaluation of the deltoid ligament if ultrasound is used, the patient is asked to maintain the position described for the medial ankle tendons (see Fig. 9.13A) with the foot slightly dorsiflexed. An advised starting point is to place the proximal edge of the transducer over the medial malleolus and rotate the distal end anteriorly and posteriorly to cover the base of the triangle (Fig. 9.16).

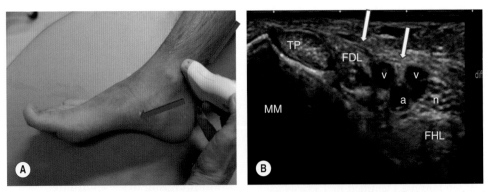

Fig. 9.13 (A) Transverse ultrasound technique medial tendons/neurovascular bundle. Red arrows denote probe movement along the tendons. **(B)** Transverse ultrasound image medial tendons/neurovascular bundle. *a,* Artery; *FDL,* flexor digitorum longus; *FHL,* flexor hallucis longus; *MM,* medial malleolus; *n,* nerve; *TP,* tibialis posterior; *v,* vein; *white arrows,* flexor retinaculum.

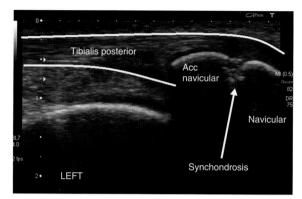

Fig. 9.14 Ultrasound Example of Accessory Navicular/Os Navicularum. (From https://ankleandfootcentre.com.au/ultrasound-imaging-accessory-navicular-bone/)

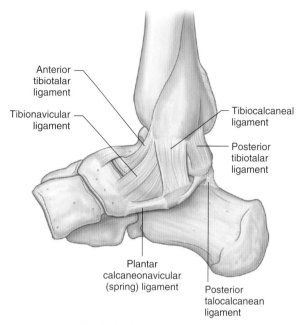

Fig. 9.15 Deltoid Ligaments.

> ### ◎ TOP TIP
>
> Identifying and interpreting ultrasound appearances of individual ligaments around the ankle is possible but can be challenging. If the patient has significant symptoms and there is obvious damage to some ligaments, or if no specific injury can be detected with ultrasound, there may well be damage to intraarticular structures and alternative imaging may be more worthwhile

Medial Ankle—Common Pathology and Clinical Management

Tendon Pathology

The medial ankle tendons are prone to pathological change due to the compressive element of loading as they bend around the malleolus. TP tendon is the most affected of the flexor tendons in terms of degenerative changes. This is multifactorial and may be due to extrinsic factors such as poor biomechanics, overuse, or adjacent bony arthritic changes irritating the tendon, or intrinsic factors such as diabetes, rheumatoid arthritis, or vascular disease. These factors may cause the tendon to become weak and tendinopathic with oedema and loss of the normal fibrillar pattern. Tenosynovitis may also be evident as a thickened synovial sheath showing hyperemia on Doppler with or without effusion (Fig. 9.17).

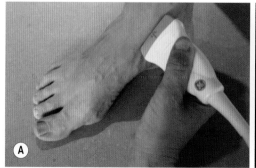

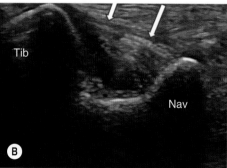

Fig. 9.16 (A) Ultrasound technique deltoid ligament—tibionavicular portion. **(B)** Ultrasound image deltoid ligament—tibionavicular portion. Tibia *(Tib)*, navicular *(Nav)*, ligament *(white arrows)*.

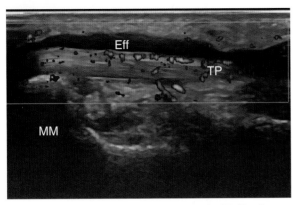

Fig. 9.17 Longitudinal Ultrasound Example TP Tendinopathy/Tenosynovitis. Medial malleolus *(MM)*, tibialis posterior tendon *(TP)*, effusion *(Eff)*.

As TP tendon is heavily involved with support of the arch, its failure, known as tibialis posterior dysfunction,[11] can lead to flat footedness deformity (pes planus) which ultimately leads to failure of some of the medial ligaments. If dysfunction continues without intervention, the tendon may stretch, become thin and atrophic, then tear (Fig. 9.18).

Depending on the stage of the disease process and symptoms, initial treatment of TP dysfunction may include PRICE, orthoses, stabilizing tape, eccentric exercise, pain medication, and patient education.[12] Chronic tendinopathy requires activity modification and tendon loading which is gold standard, first-line tendon treatment (see Chapter 2). If there is active tenosynovitis, steroid injections may be considered, but with the pos-

sibility of weakening an already pathological tendon, they should be given with extreme caution. Conservative treatments, including orthotics, should be exhausted before interventional treatment. With moderate to severe TP dysfunction or rupture, surgical options may be considered, including soft tissue reconstruction and tendon transfers.[11]

Insertional tendinopathy in the presence of an accessory navicular bone. Type 2 os navicular, where there is a connection between the navicular and accessory bone, essentially forming a pseudoarthrosis, may be symptomatic. The cause of pain is thought to be repetitive tension and shear stress across the synchondrosis as a result of the pull of the TP tendon.[10] On ultrasound, the accessory bone can be identified with evidence of adjacent tendinopathy, often showing neovascularity on Doppler when compared with the asymptomatic side. Initial treatment may include a guided steroid injection before any surgical fixation is considered.

Tarsal tunnel syndrome. Tarsal tunnel syndrome is an entrapment neuropathy of the tibial nerve or one of its branches either inside, or just distal to the tarsal tunnel.[13] It may be caused by compression from the retinaculum, a space occupying lesion such as a ganglion (Fig. 9.19), neuroma, varicosity of the adjacent vessels, or by tenosynovitis of an adjacent tendon. This can cause symptoms as far distal as the first, second, or fourth toes due to nerve distribution.

Treatment will depend on the cause of compression but may include the correction of foot biomechanics, aspiration of ganglia, or surgery.[13]

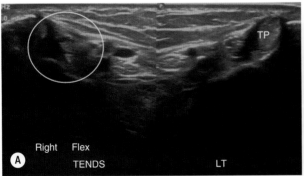
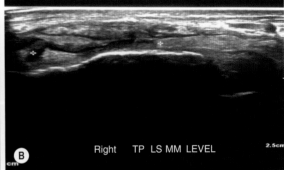

Fig. 9.18 (A) Ultrasound example of absent tibialis posterior tendon *(yellow circle)*—split screen comparison of the asymptomatic side showing normal tendon on the left *(TP)*. **(B)** Longitudinal ultrasound example ruptured tibialis posterior tendon—calipers across a full thickness tear.

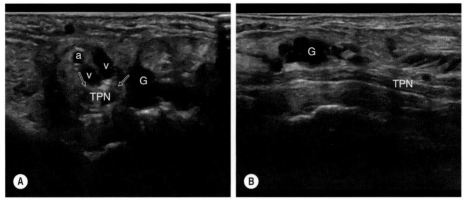

Fig. 9.19 Ultrasound example of tarsal tunnel ganglion abutting the nerve in **(A)** transverse and **(B)** longitudinal section. *a,* Tibialis posterior artery; *G,* ganglion; *TPN,* tibialis posterior nerve; *v,* posterior tibial vein.

Medial Ligament Pathology

Medial ankle ligaments are infrequently injured in isolation and as stated previously, other cross-sectional imaging is often used for completeness. Injuries range from eversion stress causing ligament sprains to partial, full, or avulsion tears (Fig. 9.20).[14,15] Depending on the severity of the injury, ultrasound appearances will vary from a thickened, hypoechoic, oedematous ligament to less common full thickness defect with retraction. Because of the fanning out of ligament fibres in multiple directions, anisotropy can occur making it extremely difficult to exclude subtle pathology, and comparison with the asymptomatic side is essential.

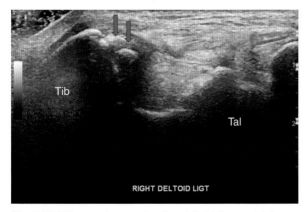

Fig. 9.20 Ultrasound example of a deltoid ligament injury – bony avulsion of the ligament from the tibia *Tib, (blue arrows).*

LATERAL ANKLE

Peroneal Tendons and Retinacula—Anatomy

Two tendons are located on the lateral aspect of the ankle (Fig. 9.21). They are the:
- Peroneal brevis (PB)
- Peroneal longus (PL)

PB muscle arises from the distal two-thirds of the fibula, forming as a tendon 2 to 3 cm proximal to the tip of the fibula, continuing distally posterior and inferior to the lateral malleolus and running anteriorly over the surface of the lateral calcaneus before inserting into the base of the fifth metatarsal. The muscle assists in weak plantar flexion and eversion of the foot.

PL muscle arises from the head and upper two-thirds of the fibula running superficial to PB and forming a tendon more proximally which runs around the malleolus before diverging from PB at the peroneal tubercle and running under the foot to insert into the plantar aspect of the medial cuneiforms and base of the first metatarsal. The main action of PL is plantar flexion of the foot in conjunction with some eversion.

Both PB and PL tendons are contained within a common synovial sheath that extends from approximately 4 cm proximal to the tip of the lateral malleolus, to 1 cm distal to it, where it then splits at the peroneal tubercle into two separate sheaths. It is considered normal to see a trace of fluid within the distal sheaths.[16]

The sheath and tendons are covered by the superior and inferior peroneal retinacula which play an important role in stabilizing the tendons in place (see Fig. 9.21.).

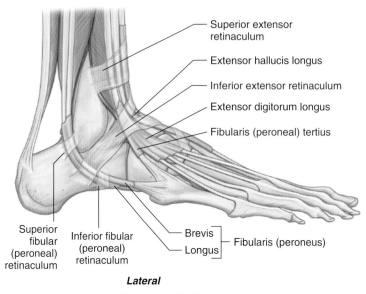

Fig. 9.21 Peroneal Tendons, Tendon Sheath, and Retinacula. (From Soames R, Palastange N. Anatomy and Human Movement Structure and Function. 7th ed. London: Elsevier; 2019.)

In an estimated 10% to 13% of the population an accessory muscle, the peroneal quartus muscle, is present, which arises from the lower third of the fibula, peroneus brevis muscle, and/or peroneus longus muscle. Its distal insertion varies greatly, with the most common insertion seen to be onto the lateral surface of the calcaneus.[17]

Peroneal Tendons and Retinacula— Ultrasound Technique

For optimum assessment, the patient is positioned supine or seated semi-recumbent with the affected leg internally rotated.

The peroneal tendons will be identified in TS by placing the most anterior aspect of the transducer on the lateral malleolus at a 45-degree angle to the heel (Fig. 9.22A). Both tendons can be evaluated in TS along their length around the lateral malleolus to the peroneal tubercle distally (Fig. 9.22B). PB sits on the medial aspect of the malleolus with PL slightly lateral.

Both tendons should be assessed in TS from the musculotendinous junctions to their distal insertion and then the probe should be rotated through 90 degrees to image the tendons in LS (Fig. 9.23A). The distal PL tendon is difficult to visualise but rarely injured. The distal PB

tendon is more commonly injured and can be seen inserting into the base of the fifth metatarsal (Fig. 9.23B).

Lateral Ligaments—Anatomy

On the lateral aspect of the ankle, acting as an important stabilizing mechanism, are four ligaments (Fig. 9.24):
- Anterior inferior tibiofibular ligament AiTFL— extends between the distal ends of the adjacent margins of the tibia and fibula.
- Anterior talofibular ligament (ATFL)—extends between the lateral/anterior malleolus of the fibular, running anteromedially to the surface of the talus.
- Calcaneofibular ligament (CFL)—extends between the tip of the lateral/posterior malleolus running inferiorly to the calcaneus.
- Posterior inferior talofibular ligament (PTFL)—less visible than ATFL and rarely involved in ankle sprains. This ligament is not usually assessed as part of routine US of the lateral ankle.[18,19]

Lateral Ligaments—Ultrasound Technique

The patient should be positioned on the bed ideally in a supine position with their knee flexed and the plantar surface of the foot placed flat on the bed.

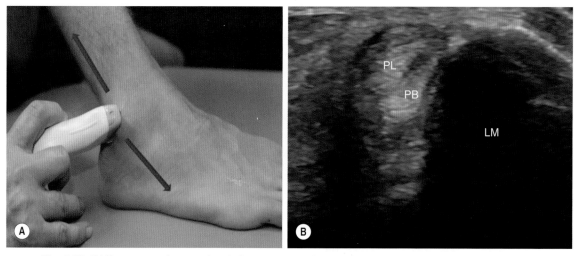

Fig. 9.22 (A) Transverse ultrasound technique peroneus longus and brevis tendons. *Red arrows* denote probe movement along the tendons. **(B)** Transverse ultrasound image. *LM,* Lateral malleolus; *PB,* peroneal brevis; *PL;* peroneal longus.

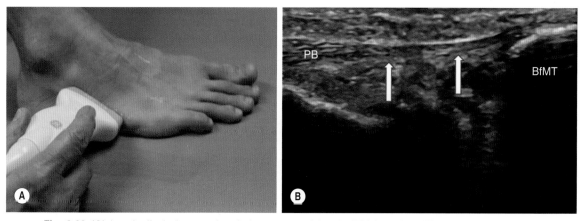

Fig. 9.23 (A) Longitudinal ultrasound technique peroneal brevis (PB) insertion. **(B)** Ultrasound image PB insertion. Peroneal brevis (*PB* and *white arrows*), base of fifth metatarsal *(BfMT).*

The ATFL is best assessed with the ultrasound probe placed on the anterior aspect of the lateral malleolus with the probe face parallel to the sole of the foot (Fig. 9.25A). The ligament is seen as a regular, linear structure traversing the gap between talus and fibula (Fig. 9.25B). To check the integrity of the ligament, placing the ankle in slight inversion is advised.

To image the AiTFL, from this position, maintain the posterior edge of the transducer on the lateral malleolus and rotate the anterior edge anticlockwise until the tibia is located with the thin AiTFL ligament running between the two bones (Fig. 9.26).

For assessment of the CFL, the patient should be asked to internally rotate the ankle slightly. The transducer should be placed distal to the posterior edge of the lateral malleolus showing the transverse section of the peroneal tendons (Fig. 9.27A). The transducer should then be slid distally along the tendons until the CFL becomes visible running almost horizontally, deep to the tendons, along the surface of the calcaneus (Fig. 9.27B). Anisotropy can be

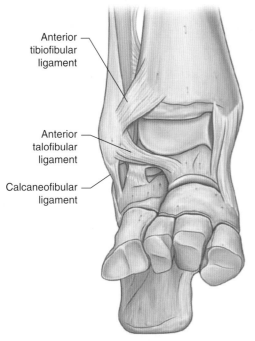

Fig. 9.24 Lateral Ligamentous Complex Anatomy. (From Soames R, Palastange N. Anatomy and Human Movement Structure and Function. 7th ed. London: Elsevier; 2019.)

reduced by dorsiflexing the ankle to enable optimal visualisation of the fibula end of the ligament[20] (Fig. 9.27C).

> ◎ **TOP TIP**
>
> Moving the foot during scanning will stress/stretch ligaments and tendons which may reduce anisotropy and make them easier to see.

Lateral Ankle—Common Pathology and Clinical Management

Tendon Pathology

As with the medial tendons, there are a number of causes which may lead to pathology of the lateral tendons but of particular importance laterally is impingement of PL on PB, usually due to poor biomechanics. In the early to mild stages of tendinopathy, PB becomes enlarged, oedematous, and increasingly U-shaped on TS scanning, engulfing PL which often remains normal in appearance. This is commonly known as the "sun and moon" appearance on ultrasound (Fig. 9.28). If left untreated, longitudinal splitting of PB may occur which gives the appearances of three tendons within the sheath and eventually one or both portions of PB may rupture completely.[21]

Insertional tendinopathy and bony avulsion may also occur at PB insertion onto the base of the fifth metatarsal, most commonly as a result of trauma. Alternative pathologies here include fractures to the base of the fifth metatarsal, peroneus tertius tendinopathy/enthesopathy (if present), and, on the plantar aspect, enthesopathy of the lateral band of the plantar fascia.

Inflammation of the peroneal tendons and sheath may occur in a similar way as the medial tendons. Causes include poor biomechanics, trauma, overuse, or an inflammatory arthropathy. Depending on the degree of the disease process, ultrasound assessment may show thickened tendons and/or sheath, with or without effusion and hyperemia on Doppler assessment (Fig. 9.29).

Potential treatment of tendinopathy and tenosynovitis consists of PRICE, nonsteroidal anti-inflammatory medication, rest, activity modification, and orthoses

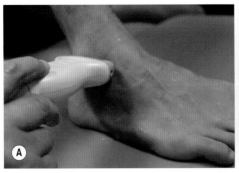

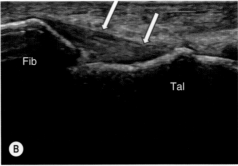

Fig. 9.25 **(A)** Ultrasound technique anterior talofibular ligament. **(B)** Ultrasound image anterior talofibular ligament *(white arrows)*. *Fib,* Fibula; *Tal,* talus.

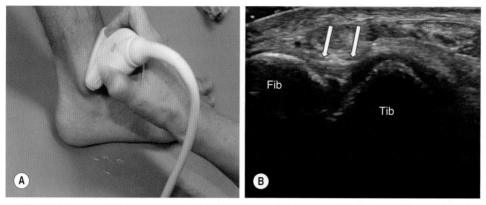

Fig. 9.26 (A) Ultrasound technique anterior inferior tibia fibular ligament. **(B)** Ultrasound image. Anterior inferior tibia fibular ligament *(white arrows)*. *Fib,* Fibula; *Tib,* tibia.

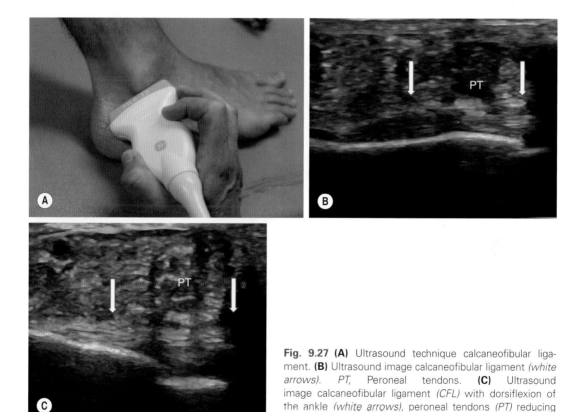

Fig. 9.27 (A) Ultrasound technique calcaneofibular ligament. **(B)** Ultrasound image calcaneofibular ligament *(white arrows)*. *PT,* Peroneal tendons. **(C)** Ultrasound image calcaneofibular ligament *(CFL)* with dorsiflexion of the ankle *(white arrows)*, peroneal tendons *(PT)* reducing anisotropy and lifting the peroneal tendons.

with lateral forefoot posting in mild cases. In refractory cases, immobilisation devices of the ankle may be utilised. Surgical options are available including synovectomy or procedures to deal with the adjacent causes such as peroneal tubercle resection.[22]

Lateral Ligament Pathology

Lateral ligament sprains as a result of hyperinversion are among the commonest of all ankle injuries, with ATFL the most likely to be affected.[20] When other ligaments are affected, it is usually CFL, with injuries to AiTFL

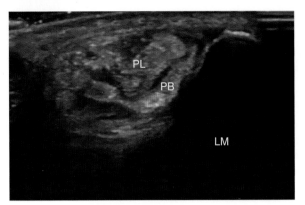

Fig. 9.28 Transverse Ultrasound Example of Peroneus Brevis Tendinopathy: "Sun and Moon Appearances." *PB,* Peroneal brevis; *PL,* peroneal longus; *MM,* medial malleolus.

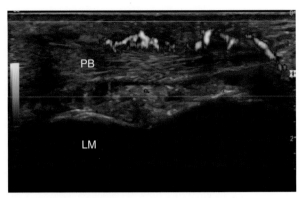

Fig. 9.29 Longitudinal Ultrasound Example of Peroneal Tenosynovitis. *PB,* Peroneus brevis; *LM,* lateral malleolus.

being rare and often indicating significant intraarticular pathology/instability.[20] Again, in the case of multiple ligament damage, appropriate alternative cross-sectional imaging is often requested.

Depending on the degree of injury, the ligament may show a number of ultrasound features ranging from mild oedema and thickening to small defects or complete tears/avulsion. A full thickness tear will be seen as a hypoechoic area of discontinuity within the ligament or a complete avulsion of the bone surface at an insertion (Fig. 9.30).

Assessing the ligament dynamically by placing the tendon under stress may assist in demonstrating the degree of tear.

It is generally regarded that successful treatment of acute ankle sprain can be achieved with individualised, aggressive, and nonoperative measures. Indications for the surgery are usually associated with unstable ankle fractures, OCD (osteochondral defects), loose bodies, or peroneal tendon tears and are indicated on an individual patient basis.

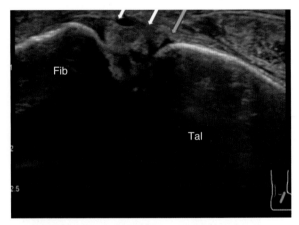

Fig. 9.30 Ultrasound example anterior talofibular ligament (ATFL) tear: Fibula *(Fib)*, talus *(Tal)*, ATFL *(white arrows)*, site of tear *(blue arrow)*.

POSTERIOR ANKLE

Posterior Ankle—Anatomy

The Achilles tendon is situated adjacent to the posterior aspect of the distal tibia and is the strongest and thickest tendon in the human body capable of sustaining loads up to 17 times body weight. It is approximately 12 to 15 cm long and varies in width from 1.2 to 2.5 cm.

Males have a larger cross-sectional area than females. It is formed by the gastrocnemius and soleus muscles and is a flat broad tendon proximally, becoming more rounded distally before flattening in the last 4 cm before it inserts into the posterior aspect of the calcaneus (Fig. 9.31).

As the tendon descends, it rotates through 90 degrees and the medial fibres are posterior by the time the tendon inserts. This rotation is thought to impart elastic properties upon the tendon allowing it to re-coil after stretch. The Achilles tendon is encased medially, laterally, and posteriorly by a highly vascular, membranous covering—the paratenon—which extends proximally from the musculotendinous fascia to the distal calcaneal periosteum.

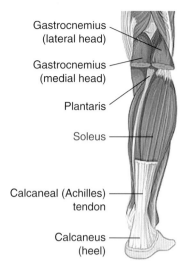

Gastrocnemius
(lateral head)

Gastrocnemius
(medial head)

Plantaris

Soleus

Calcaneal (Achilles)
tendon

Calcaneus
(heel)

Fig. 9.31 Achilles Tendon.

Studies have shown a relatively avascular portion of the tendon approximately 2 to 6 cm proximal to the tendon insertion which corresponds to the maximum area of rotational stress.[23] Under normal circumstances blood vessels do not permeate from the paratenon into the tendon substance. Deep to the distal Achilles tendon is a fat pad sitting between the tendon and FHL muscle, historically called Kager's fat pad.

The plantaris is a vestigial muscle, absent in 7% to 20% of people.[24] It consists of a small muscle belly developing into a long thin tendon that forms part of the posterosuperficial compartment of the calf. The muscle originates from the lateral supracondylar line of the femur and courses in an inferior and medial direction, forming a long thin tendon which runs along the medial aspect of the Achilles tendon to its insertion on the calcaneus. Anatomical studies have shown that the calcaneal insertion may occur independently of the Achilles tendon[24] which is of interest as the plantaris tendon may remain intact when the Achilles tendon ruptures. Although less common, the plantaris tendon may rupture in isolation.

Two bursae are seen in the distal Achilles region (Fig. 9.32).

The retrocalcaneal bursa is located between the anteroinferior aspect of the Achilles tendon and the posterosuperior surface of the calcaneum and Kager's fat pad. In its normal state it contains a trace of fluid and reduces friction caused by movement of the Achilles tendon against the bone. The subcutaneous calcaneal bursa is an acquired bursa and located posteriorly and superficially, between the tendon and the underlying skin.

Posterior Ankle—Ultrasound Technique

Ultrasound examination of the Achilles tendon (and plantaris if present) is usually performed with the

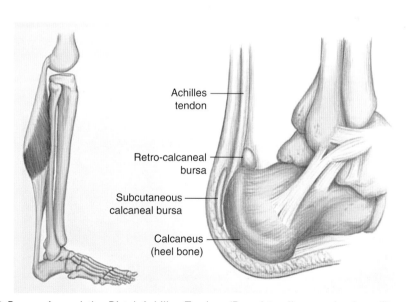

Achilles
tendon

Retro-calcaneal
bursa

Subcutaneous
calcaneal bursa

Calcaneus
(heel bone)

Fig. 9.32 Bursae Around the Distal Achilles Tendon. (From https://www.webmd.com/fitness-exercise/picture-of-the-achilles-tendon#1)

patient prone with their foot relaxed and hanging over the end of the couch. This allows full visualization of the calf and heel, enabling movement of the foot for dynamic scanning.

The transducer should be placed on the posterior aspect of the calf in TS, just above the heel (Fig. 9.33A) where the Achilles tendon is easily visualised (Fig. 9.33B). The tendon can then be scanned proximally up to the myotendinous junction and distally to its insertion.

The transducer should then be rotated through 90 degrees and moved proximally and distally to show the tendon in its longitudinal plane (Fig. 9.34).

The Achilles tendon is seen in LS as an echogenic, linear, fibrillar structure which increases in depth from the myotendinous portion to the mid portion, then remains similar in depth through to the insertion. The maximum AP diameter should not reach over 6 mm[25] and comparison with the contra lateral side is essential, although bilateral abnormalities are not uncommon. Colour/power Doppler should be used to detect any neovascularity within the tendon which would be abnormal. Note it is important to keep the tendon in a relaxed state when using Doppler as tension may obliterate any tiny new vessels.

The retrocalcaneal bursa is seen lying deep to the distal tendon, adjacent to the upper border of the calcaneus, and often containing a trace of fluid. The superficial Achilles bursa may not be seen in normal circumstances

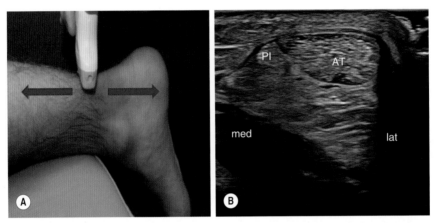

Fig. 9.33 (A) Transverse ultrasound technique Achilles and plantaris tendons. *Red arrows* denote probe movement along the tendons. **(B)** Transverse ultrasound image Achilles and plantaris tendons. *AT,* Achilles tendon; *Pl,* plantaris tendon.

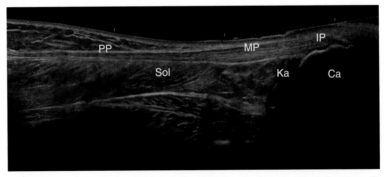

Fig. 9.34 Extended/Panoramic View of the Achilles Tendon in Longitudinal Section. *Ca,* Calcaneum; *IP,* insertional portion; *Ka,* Kager's fat pad; *MP,* mid portion; *PP,* proximal portion of the Achilles tendon, *Sol,* soleus muscle.

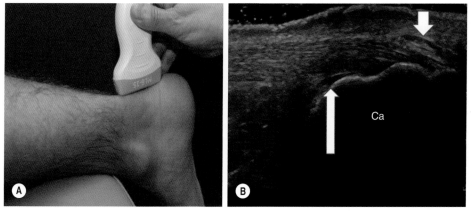

Fig. 9.35 (A) Ultrasound technique retrocalcaneal and superficial Achilles bursae. **(B)** Ultrasound image distal Achilles insertion–retrocalcaneal bursa *(long arrow)*, superficial Achilles bursa *(short arrow)*, calcaneus *(Ca)*.

but lies between the skin and the distal insertion of the tendon. Very light pressure of the transducer and a generous amount of gel is required as the bursa can very easily be compressed (Fig. 9.35).

Posterior Ankle—Common Pathology and Clinical Management

Achilles Tendinopathy

Common ultrasound appearances of diseased tendons were discussed in Chapter 2 and may be acute or chronic and due to intrinsic or extrinsic causes. The Achilles tendon is particularly prone to tendinopathy which may be associated with overuse, poor biomechanics, some systemic diseases, and

drug use such as Quinolones and long-term glucocorticoids.[26]

Clinically, the main symptom of Achilles tendinopathy is pain with either global or focal thickening. "Noninsertional tendinopathy" is the term used for degenerative change affecting the middle third of the tendon, whereas "insertional tendinopathy" is the term used for changes affecting the distal third.[27] Distal disease may also be due to an inflammatory arthropathy affecting the distal insertion/enthesis whilst other systemic diseases, such as gout or hyperlipidemia, may accumulate deposits throughout the tendon.[28] On ultrasound, appearances of tendinopathy are seen as thickening, loss of the normal fibrillar pattern, and relative hypoechogenicity due to oedema (Fig. 9.36).

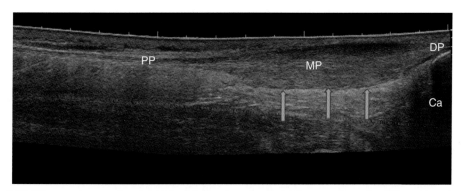

Fig. 9.36 Ultrasound example of middle third/noninsertional Achilles tendinopathy (AT), evident by the fusiform thickening of the tendon with relatively normal depth proximally, and at the distal insertion proximal to the calcaneum. *Blue arrows*, Thickened AT; *Ca*, calcaneus; *DP*, distal portion AP; *MP*, midportion AT; *PP*, proximal portion AT.

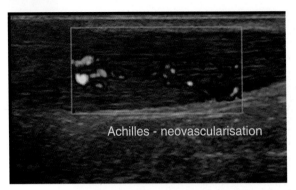

Fig. 9.37 Ultrasound example of neovascularity (new blood flow) on power doppler within the achilles tendon.

Neovascularity within the affected portion of tendon is usually seen as a result of increased blood supply intended to assist tendon matrix regeneration and correlates well with pain[29] (Fig. 9.37).

Depending on the area of tendinopathy and severity, there is evidence for a range of nonsurgical interventions. Conservative options, including initial PRICE, physiotherapy and orthotics,[30] should always be the first line of treatment, followed by tendon loading (see Chapter 2) and may take several months to achieve desired outcomes.

More recent treatments, such as extra corporeal shockwave therapy, plasma rich protein, cryotherapy, and prolotherapy injection, are designed to induce a healing response[31] but have varying success rates according to the evidence. High-volume saline injections are sometimes used to strip the invading vessels and adjacent nerves from the tendon in an attempt to reduce pain[32] but it has been recognised that these therapies carry some risk of tendon rupture and so are usually carried out following specialist referral. Steroid injections are thought to carry the greatest risk of rupture and are now rarely given. Surgical procedures can be used in insertional Achilles tendinopathy to remove degenerative tissue and associated calcification and in some cases tendon grafting is used; however, there is no gold standard treatment due to varying clinical results between studies.[31]

Achilles Tendon Tears

As stated previously, the Achilles tendon is particularly prone to injury in the mid-distal portion, 2 to 6 cm proximal to the calcaneal insertion. There are several theories to this, one of which is thought to be due to relatively poor vascularity to that area.[33] Another common site of injury and tear is the myotendinous junction, in particular the medial head of gastrocnemius (see Chapter 8), and this area should always be included in an Achilles assessment.

Partial thickness tears often appear as an area of fibre disruption/cystic degeneration within the tendon (Fig. 9.38) and can continue to develop into defects that extend across the full depth of tendon tissue, often as a result of relatively low impact trauma.

Identifying the edges of a full thickness tear can be challenging if there is late presentation of the injury and significant haematoma is present; however, the torn edges commonly demonstrate refraction artefact which may help the examiner to identify the extent of the damaged segment (Fig. 9.39).

Dynamic imaging may also help as passive movement of the foot or gentle squeezing of the calf muscles (Thompson test) during scanning may help to identify any gap between the torn tendon ends as one tendon end moves without translation of movement to the other tendon end.

The clinical importance of an intact plantaris tendon becomes most relevant when there is an Achilles tendon tear. If present, the plantaris tendon often supports a weakened Achilles, making clinical tests for possible rupture difficult and there are cases where a ruptured Achilles has been undiagnosed clinically, due to the actions of the intact plantaris, and ultrasound is useful to confirm or exclude this. The plantaris tendon may also be harvested to replace ruptured tendons in the hand or foot—in these cases, the sonographer may simply be asked to determine the presence or absence of a plantaris tendon for harvesting.[34]

Treatments of complete tendon tears would include conservative treatment or surgery and the decisions may be based on imaging appearances as well as clinical features such as patients age, comorbidities, etc.

Conservative treatments would include stabilizing the foot in a boot with the foot in equinus/plantar flexion in an attempt to oppose the tendon ends and allow healing.

Surgery would involve debridement and suturing of the tendon or tendon transplantation and success would depend on the size of tear, amount of tendon affected, and the degree of tendon disease.

Accurate assessment of tendon tears is vital to assist surgeons in these clinical decisions.[35] In addition to an

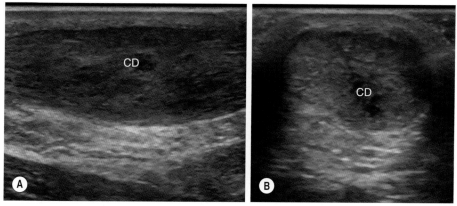

Fig. 9.38 Ultrasound example of cystic degeneration *(CD)* within a tendinopathic Achilles tendon in longitudinal **(A)** and transverse section **(B)**.

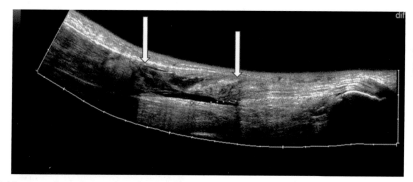

Fig. 9.39 Ultrasound panoramic image of a full thickness tear demonstrating refraction artefact at the edges of the damaged segment *(white arrows)*. Calipers show measurement from the upper border of the calcaneus to the distal edge of the tear.

opinion as to the degree of tendinopathy, the position of the tear in relation to the calcaneus should be calculated and documented—with the patient prone and the foot relaxed, the distance between the distal edge of the torn tendon and the posterior aspect of the upper border of the calcaneus should be measured (see Fig. 9.39).

In order to give the size of the gap between the tendon ends, the foot should remain in neutral and a measurement between the proximal and distal tendon stumps should be given (Fig. 9.40).

Then, the foot should be placed in equinus (plantar flexion) (Fig. 9.41) to see if the tendon ends oppose (Fig. 9.42), or if there is herniation of Kager's fat pad into the gap as this would prevent healing if conservative treatments are being considered (Fig. 9.43).

> ◎ **TOP TIP**
>
> In many centres, orthopedic surgaeons welcome objective information from an ultrasound scan of a ruptured Achilles tendon in order to aid treatment options. This includes the site and size of the tear and information on the state of the remaining tendon.

Ultrasound assessment of postoperative/surgically treated Achilles tendon is sometimes requested to evaluate if the tendon is grossly intact. The postoperative tendon will always appear abnormal, even if asymptomatic, and suture material is often seen within it but the most helpful assessment on ultrasound is dynamic scanning during

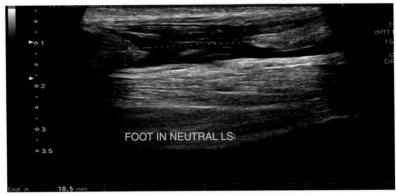

Fig. 9.40 Longitudinal Ultrasound Example of Full Thickness Achilles Tear. Calipers measure the gap between the tendon ends with the foot in a neutral position.

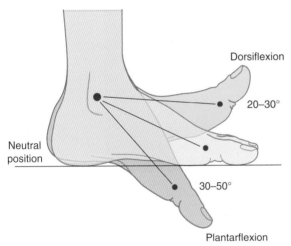

Fig. 9.41 Movement of Foot During Dorsiflexion and Plantarflexion. (From Soames R, Palastange N. Anatomy and Human Movement Structure and Function. 7th ed. London: Elsevier; 2019.)

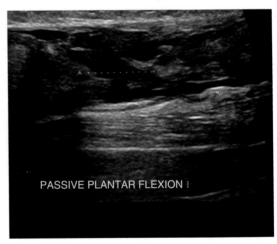

Fig. 9.42 The same patient as 9.40 showing a reduction in the gap between the tendon ends when the foot is put into plantar flexion.

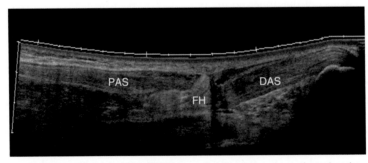

Fig. 9.43 Ultrasound panoramic image of full thickness Achilles tear where there has been herniation of Kager's fat pad into the "gap." *DAS,* Distal Achilles stump; *FH,* fat herniation; *PAS,* proximal Achilles stump.

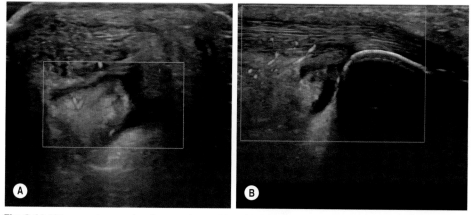

Fig. 9.44 Ultrasound example of retrocalcaneal bursitis in transverse **(A)** and longitudinal section **(B)**.

flexion and extension of the ankle to exclude any major disruption to the repaired tendon.[35]

Paratenonitis, Retrocalcaneal, and Subcutaneous Calcaneal Bursitis

Paratenonitis is an inflammatory condition which may have a biomechanical or systemic cause. It can occur in repetitive/overuse injuries, caused by friction between the Achilles tendon and the paratenon but also may also be a feature of a seronegative inflammatory arthritis.[36] Ultrasound appearances include hypoechoic thickening and hyperemia of the paratenon on the superficial surface of the tendon—signs can sometimes be very subtle and therefore comparison with the nonsymptomatic contralateral side is advised.

Retrocalcaneal and superficial Achilles bursitis can be associated with an overuse injury and can coexist with tendinopathy or inflammatory conditions.[37,38] Ultrasound appearances would include effusion and/or hyperemia of the bursae often with vessels invading the adjacent tendon (Figs. 9.44 and 9.45).

Ultrasound guided aspiration and/or steroid injection may be utilised as a form of treatment for the symptoms of pain and swelling, but the underlying cause must be simultaneously addressed to avoid recurrence.

Achilles Enthesopathy and Haglund's Disease

Achilles enthesopathy refers to any disorder at the point of insertion of the tendon fibres onto the calcaneum, and ultrasound appearances may include irregularity of the fibrocartilage and bony calcaneal surfaces along

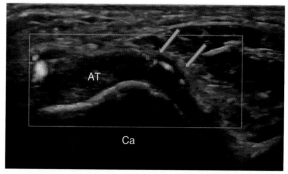

Fig. 9.45 Transverse Ultrasound Example of Doppler Flow in the Superficial Achilles Bursitis Covering the Distal Achilles Tendon. *AT,* Achilles tendon; *blue arrows,* hyperemic superficial Achilles bursa; *Ca,* Calcaneus.

with tendon swelling and loss of the fibrillar pattern, with or without associated calcification, spurs, and hypervascularity on Doppler.

These appearances may occur in isolation but there is a specific noninflammatory condition, "Haglund's" syndrome, which involves a triad of conditions[38]:
- Hypertrophied prominence of the posterosuperior calcaneal tuberosity proximal to the insertion point of the Achilles tendon-Haglund's deformity
- Retrocalcaneal bursitis
- Tendinopathy of the anterior distal portion of the Achilles tendon (Figs. 9.46 and 9.47)

Calcaneal spurs alone are not a sign of Haglund's syndrome and are commonly seen in the asymptomatic patients.

Rest and other conservative measures such as antiinflammatory medication and orthotics may be used to

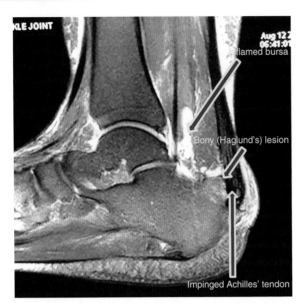

Fig. 9.46 MRI Showing Appearances of Haglund's Syndrome. (From Vaishya R, Agarwal AK, Azizi AT, Vijay V. Haglund's syndrome: a commonly seen mysterious condition. Cureus. 2016;8(10):e820. doi:10.7759/cureus.820)

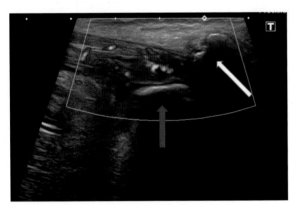

Fig. 9.47 Ultrasound Example of Haglund's Deformity with Neovascularity in the Distal Achilles Tendon. Hypertrophied prominence of posterior calcaneal tuberosity Haglund's deformity *(red arrow)*, calcific calcaneal spur at the Achilles insertion *(white arrow)*.

treat these insertional conditions but if symptoms persist, surgical treatment may be considered.[38]

PLANTAR HEEL

Plantar Heel—Anatomy

The plantar fascia or aponeurosis is a strong fibrous structure linking the plantar aspect of the calcaneus to the toes, maintaining the longitudinal arch of the foot whilst providing a dynamic function in maintaining a normal gait whilst walking.

It originates from the medial tubercle of the calcaneus and is formed of three bands—medial, lateral, and central bands. The central band forms the majority of the fascia.[1]

It extends distally where it divides into five slips that insert into the ligaments, tendons, and plantar plate at the metatarsal heads. The medial band overlies the muscles to the hallux (big toe), while the lateral band inserts on the plantar and lateral aspect of the fifth metatarsal bone, close to the peroneus brevis/peroneus tertius insertions (Fig. 9.48).

In young people, the Achilles tendon communicates with the plantar fascia around the posterior heel, but this communication is lost in older age.

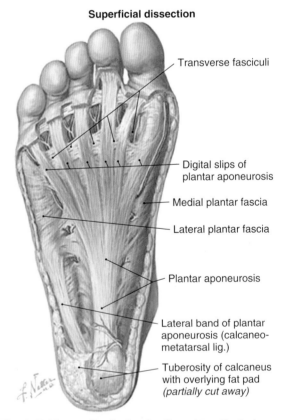

Superficial dissection

Transverse fasciculi

Digital slips of plantar aponeurosis

Medial plantar fascia

Lateral plantar fascia

Plantar aponeurosis

Lateral band of plantar aponeurosis (calcaneo-metatarsal lig.)

Tuberosity of calcaneus with overlying fat pad *(partially cut away)*

Fig. 9.48 Plantar Fascia Bands. (From https://netterimages. com/sole-of-foot-superficial-dissection-labeled-hansen-ca-2e-general-anatomy-frank-h-netter-40194.html)

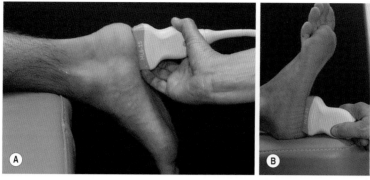

Fig. 9.49 Ultrasound technique plantar fascia with (A) the patient prone and (B) the patient supine.

In addition to the plantar fascia, there are ten intrinsic muscles, arranged in four layers, which are located on the plantar aspect of the foot. Their function is to stabilise the foot and influence movement of the toes.

Plantar Heel—Ultrasound Technique

The plantar fascia can be examined with the patient positioned supine and the heel resting on a pad placed on the examining couch or positioned prone with their feet overhanging the end of the couch (Fig. 9.49).

The skin of the heel may significantly attenuate the ultrasound beam so a lower frequency probe of between 7 and 10 MHz may be required.

The fascia is seen as a smooth, linear, hyperechoic structure which is thickest proximally, thinning as it extends distally and superficially (Fig. 9.50). The recognised maximum depth for a normal plantar fascia is 4 mm, although this can increase slightly with increased height and weight of the patient. Longitudinal "rocking" of the transducer may be necessary in order to bring the fascia perpendicular to the ultrasound beam, thus avoiding anisotropy.

The three bands of the fascia must be visualised by moving the transducer across the width of the plantar heel to identify the maximum thickness of the fascia where it leaves the calcaneal tuberosity. The depth, fibrillar pattern, and echogenicity of the fascia should be evaluated (see Fig. 9.50)

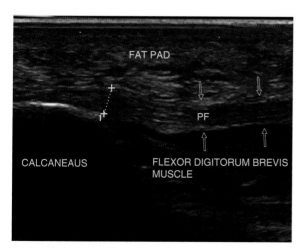

Fig. 9.50 Ultrasound Image of Plantar Fascia (PF) and Associated Structures.

⊚ TOP TIP

Plantar fasciopathy is often a clinical diagnosis following a history of pain at the plantar heel. Ultrasound is often used to confirm the diagnosis with evidence of thickening and oedema of the fascia. Fasciopathy/fasciitis is a self-limiting condition but ultrasound appearances may still be visible even when pain has resolved.

Plantar Heel—Common Pathology and Clinical Management

Plantar Fasciitis/Fasciopathy

Pain and structural change at the proximal insertion of the plantar fascia is a common complaint and is estimated to affect 10% of the population in middle age. On histology and imaging, thickening, oedema, and degenerative structural changes are more common than inflammatory findings and because of this, in recent years, the term plantar fasciopathy has replaced the well-used "plantar fasciitis."[39] Plantar fasciopathy is

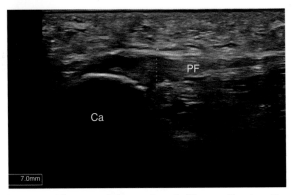

Fig. 9.51 Ultrasound Example of Plantar Fasciopathy. *Ca*, Calcaneus; *PF*, plantar fascia.

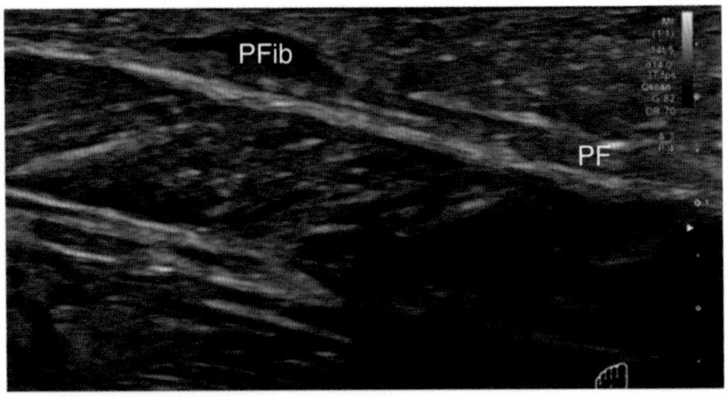

Fig. 9.52 Longitudinal Ultrasound Example of a Plantar Fibroma. *PF*, Plantar fascia; *PFib*, plantar fibroma.

thought to be related to repetitive "trauma" and causes include biomechanical factors, obesity, overuse, and poor footwear. It is a "self-limiting" condition but can take several years to resolve, often having a significant impact on mobility and quality of life.

On ultrasound assessment, a thickness over 4 mm with associated features such as relative hypoechogenicity, loss of fibrillar pattern, and pain, are associated with plantar fasciopathy[39] (Fig. 9.51). In equivocal cases, the affected fascia can be compared with the contralateral side.

The proximal third of the central and medial bands of the fascia are most commonly involved. Spurs on the plantar surface of the calcaneus were thought to be associated with fasciopathy but they are common in asymptomatic individuals and so are not specific. Other conditions associated with plantar fasciopathy include inflammatory arthritides such as psoriatic arthritis (see Chapter 10).

An initial treatment of a simple progressive exercise protocol consisting of high-load strength training may aid in a quicker reduction in pain and improvements in function.[40] Other conservative treatment options such as orthotics, ultrasound-guided steroid or platelet-rich plasma injections can alleviate symptoms, although it can disappear with time. In recalcitrant cases, surgical options may be explored which involves release just distal to the calcaneal insertion.[41]

Plantar Fibroma

Fibrous nodules—plantar fibromas, plantar fibromatosis, or Ledderhose disease—can occur within the plantar fascia, usually in the mid or distal portions, and are often not painful. These nodules can be associated with Dupuytren's contracture in the hand and present as hypoechoic, focal thickenings, continuous with the plantar fascia[39] (Fig. 9.52). Minimal or no internal vascularity is usually seen within these lesions on Doppler assessment so if significant vascularity is detected, alterative etiology and further assessment with MRI may be required in order to further characterise.

If symptomatic, usually due to the site of the nodule, most patients respond to conservative measures including orthotics and/or physical therapy. Surgical options are typically reserved for more aggressive lesions and include local excision, wide local excision, and complete plantar fasciectomy.[39]

FOREFOOT

Forefoot—Anatomy

The forefoot contains five metatarsals (MTs) which articulate with phalanges distally at the synovial metatarsophalangeal joints (MTPjs). The phalanges have proximal and distal joints—proximal interphalangeal (PIPjs) and distal interphalangeal (DIPjs)—except for the first toe, which only has one interphalangeal joint (IPj) (Fig. 9.53). As well as these larger bones, there are a variable number of sesamoid bones that help improve function and are often found as variants, in particular on the plantar surface of the first MT head.

The extensor and flexor tendons are located on the dorsal and plantar aspects of the phalanges and they insert into their respective distal phalanges.

Located on the plantar surface of each MTPj is the plantar plate (PP), a fibrocartilaginous structure similar

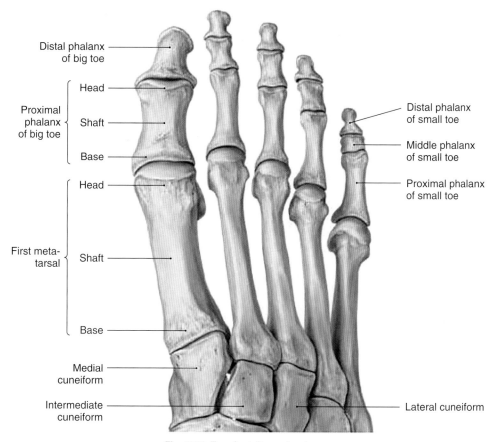

Fig. 9.53 Forefoot Bony Anatomy.

Distal phalanx of big toe

Proximal phalanx of big toe
- Head
- Shaft
- Base

First meta-tarsal
- Head
- Shaft
- Base

Medial cuneiform

Intermediate cuneiform

Distal phalanx of small toe

Middle phalanx of small toe

Proximal phalanx of small toe

Lateral cuneiform

to the volar plate of the hand which blends with the plantar joint capsule and flexor tendons at the metatarsal head. It attaches at the base of the proximal phalanx of the toe and helps to stabilise the joint, being strong and able to withstand considerable pressure whilst allowing dorsi and plantar flexion of the joint (Fig. 9.54).

Located between each toe and passing dorsal to the transverse ligaments at the metatarsal heads, are the interdigital nerves. Adjacent and deep to the nerve at this level are the intermetatarsal bursae (Fig. 9.55).

Forefoot—Ultrasound Technique

To assess dorsal structures of the forefoot, the patient can be scanned supine or sitting with the knee flexed at 90 degrees and the plantar aspect of the foot flat on the couch to give maximum stabilization. The dorsal aspect of the mid- and forefoot can be assessed in longitudinal (Fig. 9.56A) from the midfoot, running distally to the MT shafts, MTP, and IPjs and extensor tendons (Fig. 9.56B). Turning the probe through 90 degrees allows the structures to be imaged in transverse plane.

The intermetatarsal spaces can also be assessed from the dorsal to plantar surfaces using an appropriate narrow-faced transducer with reduced frequency to penetrate the depth of tissue (Fig. 9.57A). This is an alternative approach to visualizing the interdigital neurovascular bundle and interdigital bursa in patients with suspected neuroma (Fig. 9.57B)

The patient can then be asked to extend their knee, with their heel resting on the examination couch, in order to visualise the plantar aspect of the forefoot in transverse and longitudinal planes. From this aspect, the flexor tendons, PP, and surface of the joints (Fig. 9.58) and the intermetatarsal spaces can be seen by sliding the probe medially and laterally (Fig. 9.59).

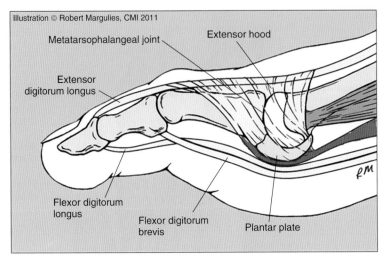

Illustration © Robert Margulies, CMI 2011

Fig. 9.54 Forefoot Metatarsal Joint Anatomy. (From https://regenexx.com/blog/flexor-hallucis-longus-tendon-pain/)

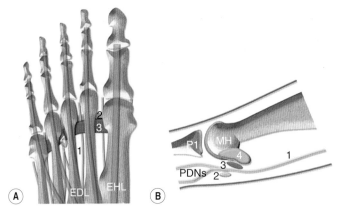

Fig. 9.55 Diagram Showing the Forefoot Anatomy and Location of Morton's Neuroma. *P1,* Phalanx; *2, MH,* Metatarsal head (*1,* interdigital nerve; *2,* Morton's neuroma; *3,* transverse ligament; *4,* intermetatarsal bursa). *EDL,* Extensor digitorum longus; *EHL,* extensor hallucis longus; *PDNs,* proper digital nerves. (From https://www.semanticscholar.org/paper/Practical-US-of-the-forefoot-Bianchi/c4d79376ca7700e831c385c67dcff6e02d4485b7# extracted)

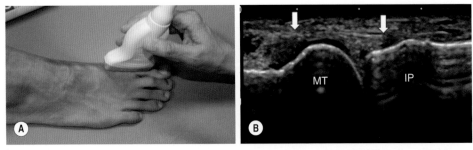

Fig. 9.56 **(A)** Longitudinal ultrasound technique, dorsal metatarsophalangeal joint (MTPj) first toe. **(B)** Ultrasound image first MTPj. *IP,* Phalangeal shaft; *MT,* metatarsal head; *white arrows,* extensor tendon.

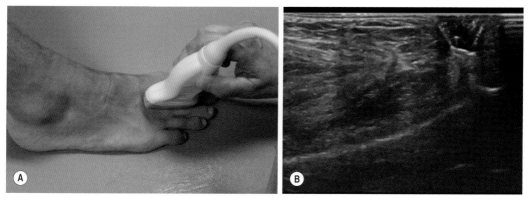

Fig. 9.57 (A) Ultrasound technique dorsal aspect of the second intermetatarsal space. **(B)** Ultrasound image dorsal view, second intermetatarsal space.

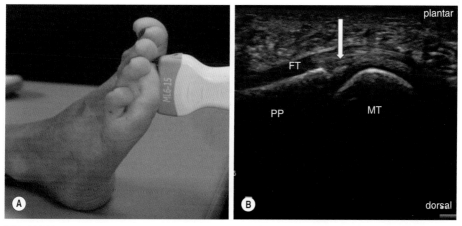

Fig. 9.58 (A) Ultrasound technique plantar aspect, second metatarsophalangeal joint (MTPj). **(B)** Ultrasound image plantar aspect second MTPj. *FT,* Flexor tendon; *MT,* metatarsal head; *PP,* proximal phalanx; *white arrow,* plantar plate.

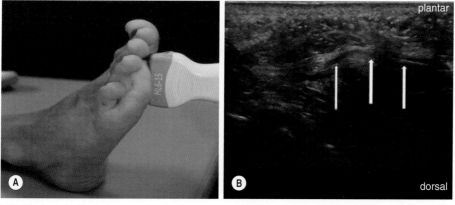

Fig. 9.59 (A) Longitudinal ultrasound technique plantar aspect interdigital space. **(B)** Longitudinal ultrasound image plantar aspect interdigital space. Interdigital nerve *(white arrows).*

Digital pressure can be used by the sonographer by pressing on the dorsal surface of the intermetatarsal space whilst scanning from the plantar surface. This can widen the intermetatarsal space and decrease the depth of soft tissues, optimizing the image. Dynamic examinations of the intermetatarsal spaces can be performed by squeezing the width of the forefoot during scanning in TS (Fig. 9.60).

Forefoot—Common Pathology and Clinical Management

Morton's Neuroma and Intermetatarsal Bursitis

"Morton's" neuroma is a benign thickening of the myelin sheath of the intermetatarsal plantar nerve within the intermetatarsal spaces. It is most commonly seen between the second and third and third and fourth metatarsal heads and is very uncommon in the other spaces.[42]

Symptoms include severe pain, tingling, and numbness of the second, third, or fourth toes and a sensation of "walking on a pebble."

Ultrasound examination for Morton's neuroma can be performed from either the dorsum or the sole of the foot and often both approaches are helpful. The nerve lies closer to the plantar surface of the foot but the sole and plantar soft tissues are more sound-attenuating than those on the dorsal surface which necessitates a lower frequency and a compromise in image resolution.

The appearance of the neuroma is that of a relatively well-defined, hypoechoic, non or partially compressible lesion between the metatarsal heads, deep to the transverse intermetatarsal ligament (Fig. 9.61).

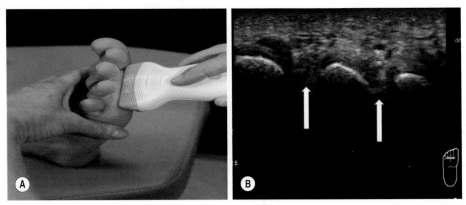

Fig. 9.60 (A) Transverse ultrasound technique plantar aspect metatarsal (MT) heads. **(B)** Transverse ultrasound image plantar aspect MT heads. Interdigital spaces *(white arrows).*

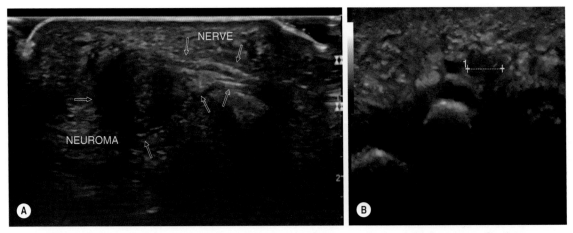

Fig. 9.61 Ultrasound Example Morton's Neuroma in **(A)** Longitudinal and **(B)** Transverse Section.

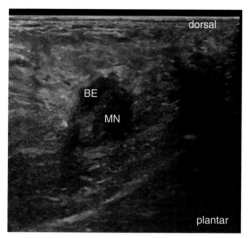

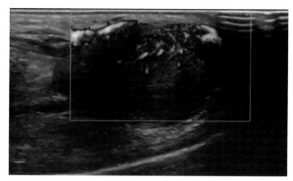

Fig. 9.63 Longitudinal Ultrasound Example Severe Interdigital Bursitis Dorsal Showing Marked Vascularity on Doppler.

Fig. 9.62 Longitudinal Ultrasound Example Neuroma/Bursal Complex Dorsal. *BE,* Bursal effusion; *MN,* Morton's neuroma.

Assessment is advised by starting with a plantar approach, the transducer being in a longitudinal plane, moving to a transverse plane once the lesion has been identified. When in transverse, a metatarsal squeeze test may show the lesion as it bulges from between the metatarsal heads, making the classic "clunk" when this action is performed, known as a Mulder's click. If no lesion is evident from the plantar aspect, it is advised to rescan from the dorsal surface as these lesions can be difficult to identify. If identified, the lesion should be measured in three planes—two measurements in the longitudinal image and one in the transverse image, as with any lesion.

It is not uncommon for Morton's neuroma to coexist with an intermetatarsal bursal effusion (Fig. 9.62) and the two structures may be indistinguishable from each other on ultrasound, which leads to the commonly reported "neuroma/bursal" complex which is probably more accurate than "neuroma" alone. This combination can lead to overestimation of the size of a neuroma on scanning compared to the actual neuroma at surgery.[43] Interdigital pressure of the lesion prior to ultrasound measurement may help overcome this issue.

If the lesion is large and more rounded than the normal fusiform shape of a neuroma, with internal vascularity on Doppler, the practitioner should consider an inflammatory arthritis as a possible underlying cause (Fig. 9.63) (see Chapter 10).

Treatment for Morton's neuroma is initially conservative and includes advice on footwear and orthotics progressing to local injection of steroids or alcohol in some

centres. Surgical treatments consist of neurectomy or neurolysis either via a dorsal or plantar approach.[43] However, postoperatively, if there is failure of nerve retraction, the neural stump can become enlarged and bulbous and may adhere to adjacent bone and soft tissue, causing traction neuritis, often called a "stump" neuroma.[39]

 TOP TIP

The dorsal approach to scanning the intermetatarsal space can be a useful addition to the plantar approach and can help to exclude a neuroma/bursa in the space.

Arthritis

As previously highlighted, ultrasound can demonstrate the presence of degenerative and inflammatory joint pathology in superficial joints such as the MTP/IP joints of the foot because they are relatively easily accessed. Effusions are common in asymptomatic MTPjs and should be differentiated from synovial hypertrophy/synovitis by sonopalpation and correct use of system functions, in particular Doppler (see Chapter 10).

The first MTPj is the joint most affected by OA and OA of the second MTPj may be caused by damage to the joint capsule (see plantar plate section). Ultrasound appearances would include osteophytic change with or without active synovitis in symptomatic joints (Fig. 9.64). Synovitis is unusual in the remainder of the MTPjs or the IPjs and if present, an inflammatory condition should be excluded (see Chapter 10). Ultrasound guided injections can aid symptom relief to assist initial or other conservative management methods.

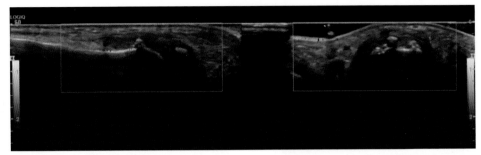

Fig. 9.64 Ultrasound example of osteoarthritis of second metatarsophalangeal joint *(MTPj)* following plantar plate rupture. **(A)** Longitudinal and **(B)** transverse section plantar plate injury.

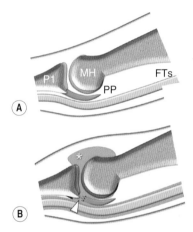

Fig. 9.65 Schematic sagittal drawings showing **(A)** the normal metatarsophalangeal (MTP) joint and **(B)** rupture of the plantar plate. *FTs,* Flexor tendons; *MH,* metatarsal head; *P1,* proximal phalanx; *PP,* joint plantar plate. (From https://www.semantic-scholar.org/paper/Practical-US-of-the-forefoot-Bianchi/c4d7937 6ca7700e831c385c67dcff6e02d4485b7#extracted)

Imaging studies have shown that PP tears are more common than previously thought and occur most commonly at the second MTPj[44] due to increased stresses on a relatively small joint when the larger, more robust first MTPj is arthritic. Small PP tears may cause mild pain with no obvious deformity of the toe but larger defects, with or without bony avulsion of the base of the proximal phalanx, may cause significant localised pain over the plantar surface of the metatarsal head, followed by progressive deformity, eventually resulting in dislocation of the MTPj and visual "hammering" of the toe (Fig. 9.65).

This "hammering" in turn causes abnormal wear of the MTPj and can cause bony changes with active synovitis (see Fig. 9.64). Hammering is possible in other toes though far less common than in the second MTPj.[44]

On ultrasound, careful interrogation of the plantar surface of the metatarsal joint capsule reveals a hypoechoic defect in the PP which can vary in size, with or without a bony avulsion of the base of the distal phalanx (Fig. 9.66).

Conservative treatment of PP injuries may consist of strapping and orthotics to stabilise and remove load from the joint with antiinflammatories where there is synovitis. The PP does not readily repair itself and where conservative treatment has been exhausted, surgery may be required to achieve satisfactory stability and pain reduction.[45]

Stress Fractures

High-resolution sonography has been proven to be highly accurate in the early diagnosis of metatarsal stress fractures before they are radiographically evident, and although X-ray is still the first-line imaging tool, fractures may be picked up incidentally by an experienced practitioner before they become displaced. The clinical history is vital in these cases and reports of a sudden sharp pain with/without bruising that causes significant ongoing symptoms should alert the practitioner to scan over the metatarsal shafts.

Early signs on ultrasound may include periosteal thickening, elevation, or a break in the cortex with prominent neovascularity on Doppler as a result of bone healing. These appearances can be subtle and a cortical break not obvious until there is some movement in the fracture (Fig. 9.67). Adjacent soft tissue changes and oedema may be seen adjacent to the periosteum corresponding to a haematoma. Further imaging and/or urgent referral to orthopaedics should be considered, dependent on the origin of the original referral.

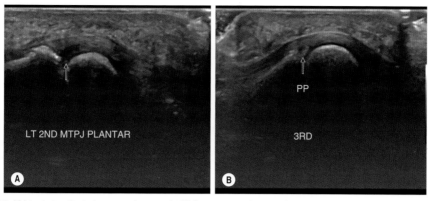

Fig. 9.66 (A) Longitudinal ultrasound example. Yellow arrow shows a hypoechoic tear in the plantar plate *(PP)* of the second metatarsophalangeal joint *(MTPj)*. **(B)** *Yellow arrow* shows an intact PP of the third MTPj.

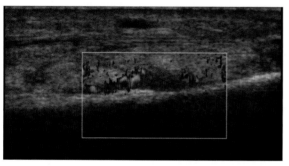

Fig. 9.67 Longitudinal ultrasound example of subtle third metatarsal shaft fracture with periosteal thickening and hyperemia.

> ◎ **TOP TIP**
>
> Stress fractures are often picked up on ultrasound in patients with acute pain of the forefoot. They are difficult to identify on X-ray until there has been some movement of the fracture, whilst ultrasound can detect subtle changes in the periosteum and surrounding soft tissues.

Over time, the production of callus can be detected as thickening or concavity of the bone surface in comparison with an unaffected metatarsal.

MULTIPLE CHOICE QUESTIONS

1. Which tendon lies medial to the extensor hallucis longus tendon on the anterior aspect of the ankle?
   a) Tibialis anterior
   b) Extensor digitorum longus
   c) Peroneus longus
2. Which two metatarsophalangeal joints are most commonly affected by OA?
   a) First MTPj
   b) Second MTPj
   c) Third MTPj
   d) Fourth MTPj
   e) Fifth MTPj
3. What treatment is thought to carry the greatest risk of rupture in patients with Achilles tendinopathy?
   a) High volume saline injection
   b) Physiotherapy

c) Orthotics
   d) Steroid injection
4. What is the most recognised maximum depth on ultrasound for the plantar fascia in an average size person?
   a) 6 mm
   b) 4 mm
   c) 2 mm
5. Which structures insert onto the base of the fifth metatarsal?
   a) Peroneus brevis, peroneus quartus, medial band of the plantar fascia
   b) Peroneus longus, lateral cord of the plantar fascia
   c) Peroneus brevis, lateral cord of the plantar fascia

MCQ Answers
1a, 2a, 3d, 4b, 5c

REFERENCES

1. Kelikian AS, Sarrafian SK. Sarrafian's Anatomy of the Foot and Ankle. Philadelphia, PA, USA: Lippincott Williams & Wilkins; 2011.

2. Khoury V, Guillin R, Dhanju J, Cardinal E. Ultrasound of ankle and foot: overuse and sports injuries. Semin Musculoskelet Radiol. 2007;11:149–161.

3. Mao H, Xu G. Soft tissue repair for tibialis anterior tendon ruptures using plate and screw fixation technique in combination with anterolateral thigh flaps transplantation. J Orthop Surg Res. 2015;10:143.

4. Shalaby MH, Sharara SM, Abdelbary MH. High resolution ultrasonography in ankle joint pain: Where does it stand? Egypt J Radiol Nucl Med. 2017;48(3):645–652.

5. Kumar SA, Deep RP, Bharat A. Ultrasound of ankle and foot in rheumatology. Indian J Rheumatol. 2018;5:43–47.

6. Shu CC, Zaki S, Ravi V, Schiavinato A, Smith MM, Little CB. The relationship between synovial inflammation, structural pathology, and pain in post-traumatic osteoarthritis: differential effect of stem cell and hyaluronan treatment. Arthritis Res Ther. 2020;22:29.

7. Sakamoto A, Okamoto T, Matsuda S. Persistent symptoms of ganglion cysts in the dorsal foot. Open Orthop J. 2017; 11:1308–1313.

8. Schweitzer ME, Van Leersum M, Ehrlich SS, Wapner K. Fluid in normal and abnormal ankle joints: amount and distribution as seen on MRI. AJR Am J Roentgenol. 1994; 162:111–114.

9. Lee S, Oliveira I, Li Y, Welck M, Saifuddin A. Fluid around the distal tibialis posterior tendon on ankle MRI: prevalence and clinical relevance. Br J Radiol. 2019; 92:1104.

10. Abourazzak FE, Shimi M, Azzouzi H, Mansouri S, El Mrini A, Harzy T. An unusual cause of medial foot pain: The cornuate navicular. Eur J Rheumatol. 2015;2(1):33–34.

11. Bubra PS, Keighley G, Rateesh S, Carmody D. Posterior tibial tendon dysfunction: an overlooked cause of foot deformity. J Family Med Prim Care. 2015;4(1):26–29.

12. Kohls-Gatzoulis J, Angel JC, Singh D, Haddad F, Livingstone J, Berry G. Tibialis posterior dysfunction: a common and treatable cause of adult acquired flatfoot. BMJ. 2004;329(7478): 1328–1333.

13. Inthasan C, Pasuk M. Tarsal tunnel syndrome: anatomical facts and clinical implications. J Anat Soc India. 2019;68: 236-241.

14. Alves T, Dong Q, Jacobson J, Yablon C, Gandikota G. Normal and injured ankle ligaments on ultrasonography with magnetic resonance imaging correlation. J Ultrasound Med. 2019;38:513–528.

15. El-Liethy N, Kamal H. High resolution ultrasonography and magnetic resonance imaging in the evaluation of tendino-ligamentous injuries around ankle joint. Egypt J Radiol Nucl Med. 2016;47(2):543–555.

16. Davda K, Malhotra K, O'Donnell P, Singh D, Cullen N. Peroneal tendon disorders. Foot Ankle. 2017;2:281–292.

17. Yousif A, Yousif A, Alasmari W, et al. Peroneus quartus muscle: its incidence and clinical importance. Int J Anat Res. 2017;(543):4691-4694. doi:10.16965/ijar.2017.445.

18. Peetrons P, Creteur V, Bacq C. Sonography of ankle ligaments. J Clin Ultrasound. 2004;32:491–499.

19. Morvan G, Busson J, Wybier M, Mathieu P. Ultrasound of the ankle. Eur J Ultrasound. 2001;14:73–82.

20. Sconfienza LM, Orlandi D, Lacelli F, Serafini G, Silvestri E. Dynamic high-resolution US of ankle and midfoot ligaments: normal anatomic structure and imaging technique. Radiographics. 2015;35:164–178.

21. Taljanovic M, Alcala J, Gimber L, Rieke J, Chilvers M, Latt D. High-resolution US and MR imaging of peroneal tendon injuries. Radiographics. 2015;35:179–199.

22. Al-Nuaimi AHD, Shalan KI. Aging and tenosynovitis of the peroneal tendons: the cause and management MOJ Anat & Physiol. 2019;6(1):25–28.

23. Del Buono A, Chan O, Maffulli N. Achilles tendon: functional anatomy and novel emerging models of imaging classification. Int Orthop. 2013;37(4):715–721.

24. Spina AA. The plantaris muscle: anatomy, injury, imaging, and treatment. J Can Chiropr Assoc. 2007; 51(3):158–165.

25. Pang BS, Ying M. Sonographic measurement of Achilles tendons in asymptomatic subjects: variation with age, body height, and dominance of ankle. J Ultrasound Med. 2006;25(10):1291–1296.

26. Kirchgesner T, Larbi A, Omoumi P, et al. Drug-induced tendinopathy: from physiology to clinical applications. Joint Bone Spine. 2014;81(6):485–492.

27. Courville XF, Coe MP, Hecht PJ. Current concepts review: noninsertional Achilles tendinopathy. Foot Ankle Int. 2009;30(11):1132–1142.

28. Fu Y, Huang QL. Xanthoma combined with gout infiltration of the Achilles tendon: a case report. Clin Med Insights Arthritis Musculoskelet Disord. 2019;12:1179544119865261.

29. Alfredson H, Ohberg L, Forsgren S. Is vasculo-neural ingrowth the cause of pain in chronic Achilles tendinosis? An investigation using ultrasonography and colour Doppler, immunohistochemistry, and diagnostic injections. Knee Surg Sports Traumatol Arthrosc. 2003;11:334–338.

30. Ohberg L, Lorentzon R, Alfredson H. Eccentric training in patients with chronic Achilles tendinosis: normalised tendon structure and decreased thickness at follow up. Br J Sports Med. 2004;38:8–11.

31. Li HY, Hua YH. Achilles tendinopathy: current concepts about the basic science and clinical treatments. Biomed Res Int. 2016;2016:6492597.

32. Boesen AP, Langberg H, Hansen R, Malliaras P, Boesen MI. High-volume injection with and without corticosteroid in chronic midportion Achilles tendinopathy – a randomised double blinded prospective study. Br J Sports Med. 2018;52:A7.

33. Gitto S, Draghi AG, Bortolotto C, Draghi F. Sonography of the Achilles tendon after complete rupture repair: What the radiologist should know. J Ultrasound Med. 2016;35:2529–2536.

34. Ahmed S, Murudkar P, Ahmed K. A study of plantaris tendon and its role in tendon graft. Int J Anat Res. 2017; 5(1):3572–3574.

35. Gitto S, Draghi AG, Bortolotto C, Draghi F. Sonography of the Achilles tendon after complete rupture repair. J Ultrasound Med. 2016;35:2529–2536.

36. Syha R, Springer F, Ketelsen D, et al. Achillodynia - radiological imaging of acute and chronic overuse injuries of the Achilles tendon. RoFo. 2013;185(11): 1041–1055.

37. Balint PV, Sturrock RD. Inflamed retrocalcaneal bursa and Achilles tendonitis in psoriatic arthritis demonstrated by ultrasonography. Ann Rheum Dis. 2000;59(12):931–933.

38. Vaishya R, Agarwal AK, Azizi AT, Vijay V. Haglund's syndrome: a commonly seen mysterious condition. Cureus. 2016;8(10):e820.

39. Draghi F, Gitto S, Bortolotto C, Draghi AG, Ori Belometti G. Imaging of plantar fascia disorders: findings on plain radiography, ultrasound and magnetic resonance imaging. Insights Imaging. 2017;8(1):69–78.

40. Rathleff MS, Mølgaard CM, Fredberg U, et al. High-load strength training improves outcome in patients with plantar fasciitis: a randomized controlled trial with 12-month follow-up. Scand J Med Sci Sports. 2015; 25(3):e292–300.

41. Latt LD, Jaffe DE, Tang Y, Taljanovic MS. Evaluation and treatment of chronic plantar fasciitis. Foot Ankle Orthop. 2020;5(1). https://doi.org/10.1177/2473011419896763.

42. Santiago FR, Muñoz PT, Pryest P, Martínez AM, Olleta NP. Role of imaging methods in diagnosis and treatment of Morton's neuroma. World J Radiol. 2018;10(9):91–99.

43. Valisena S, Petri G, Ferrero A. Treatment of Morton's neuroma: a systematic review. Foot Ankle Surg. 2018; 24(4):271–281.

44. Gregg J, Silberstein M, Schneider T, Marks P. Sonographic and MRI evaluation of the plantar plate: a prospective study. Eur Radiol. 2006;16(12):2661–2669.

45. Baravarian B, Redkar A. Expert insights on treating plantar plate tears. 2016. Available at: http://www.podiatrytoday.com/expert-insights-treating-plantar-plate-tears.

Ultrasound in Rheumatology

Alison Hall and Samantha Hider

CHAPTER OUTLINE

LEARNING OBJECTIVES

- Appreciate the wide variety of inflammatory arthritides, the drugs used for their treatment, and the role of diagnostic ultrasound in inflammatory arthritis.
- Understand the limitations and pitfalls of ultrasound imaging in inflammatory arthritis and how to maximise accuracy using good techniques and system settings.
- Recognise the ultrasound features and clinical presentation of pathologies associated with inflammatory arthritis.
- Have the information required in order to create robust protocols for ultrasound scanning of routine rheumatology patients.

INTRODUCTION

Since the year 2000, rapid developments in ultrasound technology and techniques have enabled visualisation of very small structures and the detection of low velocity blood flow at a microvascular level. The ability of ultrasound to detect pathological changes in soft tissues and bone surface and to assess blood flow using Doppler, coupled with its low cost and accessibility, has led to the widespread use of ultrasound to detect and monitor inflammatory diseases such as inflammatory arthritis (IA).

Diagnostic scans may be carried out by appropriately trained clinicians within a rheumatology department or requested from radiology services on patients with clinical symptoms of a rheumatological disease. In addition to specialised services, the use of ultrasound in the wider musculoskeletal (MSK) field has led to the frequent detection of unexpected pathologies and it is therefore important for all MSK ultrasound practitioners to have the underpinning knowledge and skills to recognise and interpret features of IA, understand how to report them and how to facilitate prompt specialist referral using appropriate patient pathways.

Most ultrasound protocols designed to detect or exclude IA concentrate on joints of the hands and feet as small joint involvement is a key part of diagnostic and classification criteria. Although larger joints such as the shoulder, hip, or knee may be involved, the limitations of ultrasound in detecting intraarticular pathology and the lack of specificity of some ultrasound appearances, has led to the exclusion of large joints from many scanning protocols.

Taking this into account, this chapter aims to cover the small joints of the hands and feet routinely scanned in most protocols, only briefly covering some of the more apposite large joints.

BACKGROUND TO RHEUMATOLOGICAL CONDITIONS

The term "arthritis" is used to describe pain, swelling, and/or stiffness in one or more joint(s). The commonest form of arthritis is osteoarthritis (OA) which affects middle-aged and older adults and most frequently affects the knee, hand, and hip. It is estimated that symptomatic OA affects one in eight men and women in the United States and is a leading cause of disability globally.[1] OA is considered to be a "whole joint" disorder and articular cartilage damage can lead to changes in the sub-chondral bone, ligaments, and joint capsule.[2]

Inflammatory polyarthritis is an umbrella term for a group of diseases including rheumatoid arthritis (RA) and spondyloarthropathies (such as ankylosing spondylitis and psoriatic arthritis [PsA]). In these disorders, immune system dysfunction leads to inflammation within the synovial membrane or joint enthesis (where tendons or ligaments join bone). This leads to joint pain, stiffness, and swelling and untreated may lead to bony damage (erosions) and cartilage loss.

Rheumatoid Arthritis

RA is the commonest IA, with a prevalence of around 0.67%, meaning that approximately 400,000 people in the United Kingdom have RA.[3] RA is twice as common in women as men and the prevalence increases with age.[3] Classically, RA causes a small joint *symmetrical* polyarthritis, which typically affects the metacarpophalangeal (MCP) and proximal interphalangeal joints (PIPj) in the hands.[4]

Spondyloarthropathies

Spondyloarthropathy is the term for a group of disorders which affect both the joints and entheses. This can predominantly affect the back and pelvis, called axial spondyloarthritis (Ax-SpA), or mainly affect peripheral joints (peripheral SpA). Peripheral spondyloarthropathies include PsA, reactive arthritis following infection, and enteropathic arthritis which occurs in association with inflammatory bowel diseases such as Crohn's or ulcerative colitis.[5]

Unlike RA, peripheral SpA is often asymmetric and can present with joint pain and swelling, persistent pain affecting tendon insertions (enthesitis), or swelling of a whole digit (known as dactylitis).

Psoriatic Arthritis

PsA is a peripheral spondyloarthropathy which is often associated with skin psoriasis. Although not all patients with PsA will have active skin psoriasis, many will have a personal or family history of skin or nail psoriasis and conversely, around 30% of all people with skin psoriasis will show clinical signs of PsA. The prevalence of psoriatic arthritis varies according to the definition used but is thought to be around 0.1% to 0.3%, affecting men and women equally, with peak incidence between 30 and 55 years.[6]

Crystal Arthropathies

Crystal arthropathies are a group of conditions caused by intraarticular or soft tissue deposits of crystals. These can be asymptomatic or can cause acute attacks of pain, redness, and swelling around joints or tendons. The two commonest crystal arthropathies are gout, caused by monosodium urate (MSU) crystals, and pseudogout which is caused by calcium pyrophosphate crystal deposition (CPPD).

Gout

Gout is the commonest crystal IA and is more common in men than women and increases with increasing age. Gout is becoming more common as a result of increasing hyperuricemia.[7]

It typically affects the feet (in particular the MTP joints), knees and elbows and may be associated with the development of skin deposits of urate crystals (called tophi). The MSU crystals classically sit on the surface of cartilage and produce a classic "double contour" sign on ultrasound.

Calcium Pyrophosphate Arthritis

Deposits of calcium pyrophosphate crystals can lead to an acute arthritis (acute CPPD arthropathy) where the crystals sit *within* the articular cartilage and may be visible on plain radiographs as calcification within fibrocartilage. CPPD arthritis tends to affect knees, wrists, and ankles, though other joints can be affected. CPPD affects men and women equally and is uncommon under the age of 60.[8]

Aspiration of synovial fluid from an affected joint viewed under polarizing light microscopy can help distinguish between the type of crystal arthropathy.

Investigations for Inflammatory Arthritis

There is no single diagnostic test for IA—making an accurate diagnosis depends on a combination of clinical history and examination supported by relevant investigations.

In terms of blood tests, inflammatory markers such as erythrocyte sedimentation rate (ESR), C-reactive protein (CRP), or plasma viscosity (PV) can be useful in indicating the degree of inflammation and in monitoring response to treatment. Serum uric acid is commonly elevated in gout, although it may be unreliable during an acute flare or be elevated in people with chronic kidney disease (known as hyperuricemia).

Immunological tests may also be helpful, although none are diagnostic. Commonly requested tests include rheumatoid factor (RF), which is an autoantibody, a type of protein made by the immune system that acts against the person's own body tissue. However, a positive RF does not necessarily indicate the presence of RA as it may be positive in people with other inflammatory conditions and in up to 5% of older people. Furthermore, you can be diagnosed with RA and not have the RF factor present in your blood (known as seronegative rheumatoid arthritis). Antibodies to citrullinated proteins, known as ACPA are much more specific (90% to 96% specificity) for RA, although these antibodies may be present for many years before development of the disease. Like RF, they are not diagnostic because only about 60% of patients with RA have these antibodies.[9]

Although plain radiographs of hands and feet are often requested, (and indeed presence of classic erosions on X-ray is a poor prognostic sign), they may be normal in early disease.

Treatment

The management of IA has revolutionised over the last two decades, with the advent of highly targeted biologics treatments and the more aggressive use of conventional disease modifying treatments such as methotrexate either singly or in combination. Guidelines for RA[10,11] emphasise the importance of a "treat-to-target" strategy (T2T) which advocates monitoring disease activity using composite disease activity scores such as Disease Activity Score-28 (DAS28)[12] and escalating treatment from conventional disease modifying agents such as methotrexate to biological agents until low disease activity or clinical remission is achieved. Similar approaches to that established for RA are now being applied to spondyloarthritis[5] and psoriatic arthritis.[13]

Clinical Relevance of Musculoskeletal Ultrasound (MSUS)

Establishing a Diagnosis

There are many potential diagnoses in a patient with polyarticular joint pain. Whilst clinical examination is considered the method of choice for detecting joint inflammation,[14] ultrasound is more sensitive, especially in early disease, when patients may have fewer symptoms to meet the clinical criteria (otherwise termed subclinical).[4]

Diagnostic ultrasound has therefore become another tool in routine rheumatology practice and is performed by a range of clinicians including sonographers, nurses, rheumatologists, and radiologists.

Positive ultrasound findings (e.g., the presence of moderate or severe inflammation and bone erosion) are good predictors of IA.[11] Although these are not specific to a single disease,[15] the distribution of changes can help to make a diagnosis. These are discussed later in the chapter.

Monitoring Response to Treatment

The role of MSUS in monitoring treatment response is best studied in relation to RA, although is developing for other conditions such as psoriatic arthritis.[16]

Assessing response to treatment is usually made based on clinical assessment for joint inflammation using disease activity scores such as DAS28.[10] The systematic addition of MSUS has been investigated[17,18] but studies concluded that the systematic addition of MSUS was not superior to tight clinical management alone in either clinical or imaging outcomes.

In view of this, whilst UK RA guidelines highlight that ultrasound should not be used routinely in monitoring disease activity in patients with RA,[5] it can be helpful where there is clinical uncertainty, for example, where there are elevations in inflammatory markers but little joint tenderness or swelling and the detection of active inflammation may necessitate an increase in drug therapy. Conversely, in patients with significant joint damage where clinical joint tenderness may not relate to active inflammation but to mechanical issues, surgical intervention may be more appropriate.

Determining Clinical Remission and Likelihood of Successful Treatment Discontinuation

The ultimate aim of T2T regimens for RA is disease remission. Usually this is determined clinically with no tender or swollen joints and established DAS28 cut offs.

However, it has been shown that approximately 44% of patients in clinical remission have evidence of persistent inflammation on Doppler MSUS,[19] which is important as it can predict both radiographic progression[20] and the likelihood of disease flare if biologics treatments are withdrawn.[21] Given the costs of biologics and the impact of disease flares on patients, Doppler MSUS provides a potential method for more accurately predicting which patients are suitable for treatment tapering and which patients, who have ultrasound evidence of disease activity despite clinical remission, risk disease progression if treatment is tapered.

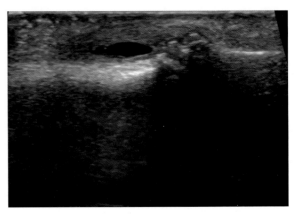

Fig. 10.1 Effusion Within the Proximal Interphalangeal Joint Capsule.

ULTRASOUND APPEARANCES OF PATHOLOGY RELATED TO RHEUMATOLOGICAL CONDITIONS

In this section, there are definitions of pathologies seen on ultrasound, written by Outcome Measures in Rheumatology (OMERACT),[22] which is an international committee that stimulates development of consensus in the context of MSK and autoimmune diseases.

As IA is a chronic, autoimmune disease in which the synovium is the primary site of the inflammatory process, it is important for the practitioner to understand the anatomical location of the synovium in relation to the joint, tendon, and bursal structures and the ultrasound appearances of inflammatory pathologies relating to those structures.

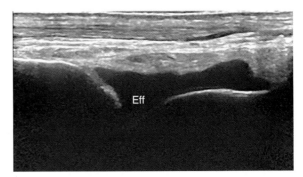

Fig. 10.2 Large Tibiotalar Joint Effusion *(Eff).*

Effusion

Effusion (Fig. 10.1) is an abnormal amount of fluid within an anatomical structure such as a joint, bursa, or tendon sheath and is defined on ultrasound as:

"Abnormal hypoechoic or anechoic (relative to subdermal fat, but sometimes may be isoechoic or hyperechoic) intraarticular material that is displaceable and compressible but does not exhibit Doppler signal."[22]

Small, asymptomatic joint effusions can occur in healthy individuals and are commonly seen on ultrasound. Even when larger amounts of joint fluid are identified (Fig. 10.2), in isolation their presence is relatively nonspecific and little conclusion can be drawn about particular potential pathologies.[23] Differential diagnoses would include overuse, trauma, or infection, in addition to all kinds of arthritis.

Synovial Hypertrophy

Various pathologies can cause oedema, proliferation, and hypertrophy of the synovium lining a joint or soft tissue structure (e.g., inflammation, infection, degeneration, trauma, haemorrhage, and neoplasm). These all have the potential to damage adjacent cartilage or tendon and may lead to irreversible joint destruction[24] or tendon rupture. Fig. 10.3A shows a normal metacarpophalangeal joint (MCPj) and Fig. 10.3B shows an MCPj with synovial hypertrophy.

The recognised definition of synovial hypertrophy/proliferation on ultrasound is:

"Abnormal hypoechoic (relative to subdermal fat, but sometimes may be isoechoic or hyperechoic) intraarticular tissue that is non-displaceable and poorly compressible, and which may exhibit Doppler signal."[22]

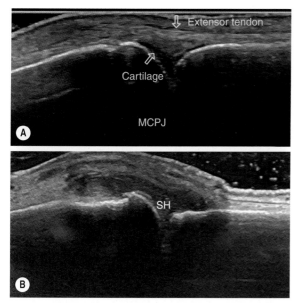

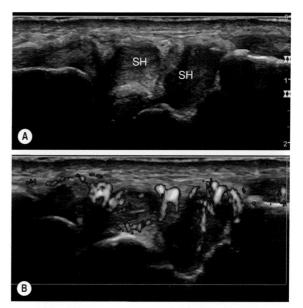

Fig. 10.3 **(A)** Normal longitudinal image of metacarpophalangeal joint *(MCPJ)*. **(B)** Synovial hypertrophy *(SH)* within an MCPJ.

Fig. 10.4 **(A)** Synovial hypertrophy *(SH)* arising from a wrist. **(B)** The same wrist with Doppler activity.

However, the significance of the presence of synovial hypertrophy alone is uncertain. In studies, low grade synovial hypertrophy is seen in the joints of healthy controls,[25] especially those joints with heavy mechanical demand such as the thumb and great toe. Even a moderate grade of synovial hypertrophy is not specific as it may be present in both inflammatory and degenerative pathologies.

It is also important to consider that, as the OMERACT definition states, hypertrophic synovium may be hypoechoic relative to surrounding tissues, but may also be hyperechoic or isoechoic, both of which would be extremely difficult to define during grey scale scanning alone which is important to understand when attempting a diagnosis of active inflammation ("synovitis").

Synovitis

The term "synovitis" is generally reserved for the active inflammatory state of synovial hypertrophy and hence suggests developing/ongoing active inflammatory disease which may lead to destructive changes.[26]

On ultrasound, active synovitis is determined by the presence of neovascularity on colour or power Doppler within synovial tissue (Fig. 10.4).

As previously stated, whilst synovial hypertrophy is usually obvious on ultrasound (as in Fig. 10.4A), there are

cases where it is isoechoic and difficult to define separate from normal tissue and in these cases, increased Doppler signal within the joint capsule can be key (Fig. 10.5).

In view of this and in order to carry out a thorough examination to diagnose or exclude active synovitis, it is vital that all relevant joints are scanned using both grey scale and colour or power Doppler.

> ◎ **TOP TIP**
>
> Synovial hypertrophy/active synovitis is not always obvious on grey scale imaging. It is important to use colour/power Doppler with sensitive settings to capture low velocity blood flow on all joints.

Tenosynovitis

The definition and physiology of tenosynovitis are described in Chapter 3 and can be associated with IA but causes also include infection, overuse, or injury. For whatever cause, if left untreated, it may result in tendon rupture causing considerable hardship to patients.

In its normal state, the tendon sheath can barely be detected on ultrasound and is seen as a thin, hypoechoic band around the tendon. Once inflamed, the sheath becomes increasingly hypoechoic, thickened and may

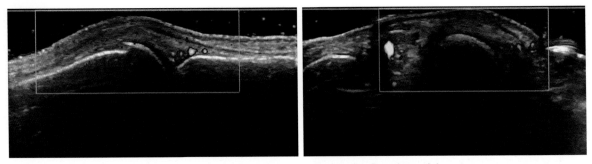

Fig. 10.5 Isoechoic synovial hypertrophy with Doppler activity.

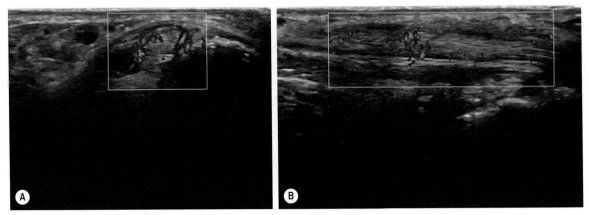

Fig. 10.6 Tenosynovitis of the extensor carpi ulnaris tendon and sheath in **(A)** transverse and **(B)** longitudinal section.

display internal vascularity on Doppler (Fig. 10.6). The recognised definition of tenosynovitis on ultrasound is:

> *"Hypoechoic or anechoic thickened tissue with or without fluid within the tendon sheath, which is seen in two perpendicular planes and which may exhibit a Doppler signal."*[22]

It is worth noting that not all tendons are surrounded by a sheath and that the ultrasound appearance of inflammation varies—for example, the extensor tendons of the fingers, over the MCPjs which have only a paratenon that does not completely surround the tendon but sits on its dorsal surface. Inflamed tendons without sheaths have more diffuse peripheral oedema inflammatory appearances because inflammatory fluid is not contained (Fig. 10.7). Instead of "tenosynovitis", these appearances are described as "paratendinitis" or "paratenonitis."[27]

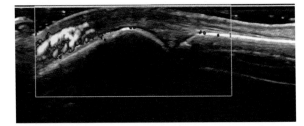

Fig. 10.7 Extensor paratenonitis of the extensor tendon over the proximal metacarpophalangeal joint.

Enthesitis

Enthesitis is a feature of certain IA conditions which are often seronegative, for example psoriatic arthritis, and may result in joint and tendon damage. Entheses—sites where tendons or ligaments insert into bone—are complex areas involving not only ligament/tendon and cartilage tissue but also sometimes bursal tissue and it is

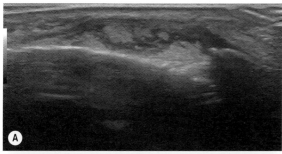

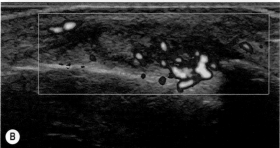

Fig. 10.8 Active enthesitis of the extensor tendon slip at the proximal interphalangeal joint without **(A)** and with **(B)** power Doppler.

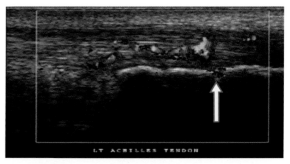

Fig. 10.9 Active enthesitis of the Achilles insertion with bone erosion *(white arrow)*. Doppler activity is relatively common in Achilles tendon disease but the presence of erosion and lack of an obvious biomechanical cause aids the diagnosis.

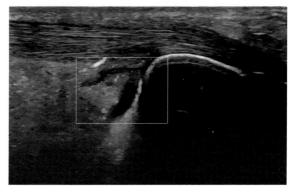

Fig. 10.10 Hyperemia and effusion in retrocalcaneal bursitis in Spondyloarthropathy.

thought to be inflammation of the bursal element of the enthesis which may cause the inflammatory appearances on ultrasound.[28] Enthesitis remains difficult to assess clinically and can also occur in repetitive strain injuries, so correlation between ultrasound appearances, symptoms, and clinical history is vital.

The recognised definition of enthesitis on ultrasound is:

"Abnormally hypoechoic (loss of normal fibrillar architecture) and/or thickened tendon or ligament at its bony attachment (may occasionally contain hyperechoic foci consistent with calcification), seen in 2 perpendicular planes that may exhibit Doppler signal and/or bony changes including enthesophytes, erosions, or irregularity."[22]

Common sites include the extensor tendon enthesis at the base of the middle phalanx of the fingers (Fig. 10.8) where it may be mistaken for PIPj synovitis or degenerative change, and the Achilles insertion at the posterior ankle (Fig. 10.9).

Bursitis

The term "bursitis" refers to abnormal distension of the bursa with thickened synovium and/or effusion, with or without hyperemia of the bursal wall. Bursitis may occur in degenerative or biomechanical conditions such as Haglund's syndrome (see Chapter 9) or subacromial pain syndrome (see Chapter 3), as well as spondyloarthropathy so again, clinical correlation with imaging findings is essential. Fig. 10.10 shows a retrocalcaneal bursitis in a patient with spondyloarthropathy.

Bone Erosions

As stated previously, IA is characterised by a chronic inflammatory process that targets the synovial lining of joints and as the disease advances, may attack articular cartilage and bone at the joint margins, causing erosive change (Fig. 10.11).

The recognised definition of an erosion on ultrasound is:

"An intra-articular discontinuity of the bone surface that is visible in two perpendicular planes."[22]

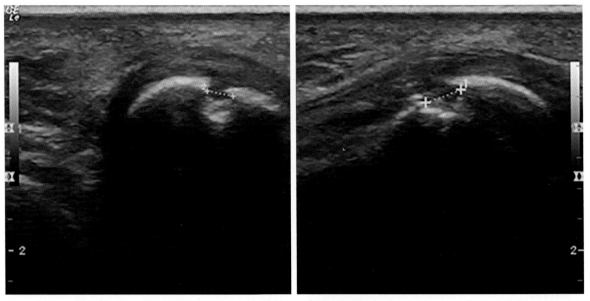

Fig. 10.11 Erosion on a metacarpal head seen in two planes.

Erosions are considered to be features of a poor prognosis of IA and suggestive of more severe disease.[26] Treatment strategies previously mentioned are aimed at halting soft tissue inflammation and preventing or arresting the development of adjacent bone erosions and joint damage, so detection and monitoring of erosions is important. Historically, radiographs have been used to detect and monitor erosions, but ultrasound is now proven to detect them before they are visible on plain radiographs[29] which may help in early diagnosis. However, there are areas of most joints that are difficult to access with the transducer, making erosions difficult to exclude; therefore plain film radiography is still widely used to track bony disease progression.

Research studies suggest that detection of flow within erosions on Doppler (Fig. 10.12) is suggestive of ongoing active bone destruction,[30] which is important when assessing the efficacy of current treatment and prompt reporting of this to the referrer is important.

Osteophytes

Osteophytes are bony projections that form around joint lines, often associated with cartilage damage. In addition to joint space narrowing and subchondral sclerosis, they are one of the main criteria for the diagnosis of OA.

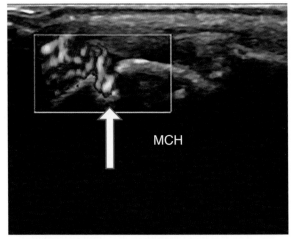

Fig. 10.12 Active erosion on Doppler (white arrow) on a metacarpal head (MCH).

Although historically the diagnosis and monitoring of OA has been predominantly the realm of plain film radiography, degenerative bony changes are often visible on ultrasound (Fig. 10.13) and may form part of a differential diagnosis. It is therefore important to recognise bony appearances but also to appreciate soft tissue changes that may occur in some stages of the disease.

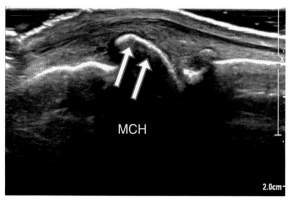

Fig. 10.13 Large osteophyte *(white arrows)* on a metacarpal head *(MCH)*.

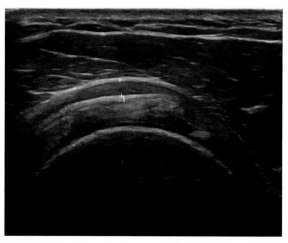

Fig. 10.14 Symptomatic subacromial/subdeltoid bursa *(yellow calipers)* measuring 2.5 mm reported as "bursitis."

It is now understood that synovitis plays an important role at a cellular level in some stages of OA[31] as the synovial membrane of joints hypertrophies and may show increased Doppler signal and effusion in a similar way to IA. This is most evident in specific joints such as the wrist, thumb CMCj, dorsal surfaces of the tarsal joints, and the first MTPj and it is important that degenerative change with evidence of active synovitis on Doppler in patients with symptomatic OA is not mistaken for a more inflammatory arthritis such as RA.

Large Joint Involvement

As a first-line tool, ultrasound can be useful in larger joints which can be difficult to assess clinically. However, limitations include the inability to access structures deep to bone which is of particular relevance when looking for inflammatory appearances in the shoulder, elbow, hip, and knee.

Whilst the presence of synovial hypertrophy or effusion may aid diagnosis of arthritis, it is not specific to inflammatory disease and its absence does not exclude joint disease. Whilst bursitis is often seen in IA, it is commonly reported around the shoulder in patients with subacromial pain syndrome (Fig. 10.14) and differentiating between the two diagnoses on ultrasound alone can be difficult.

In that respect, it is therefore often prudent to consider alternative imaging to ultrasound of large joints either primarily to reduce the number of investigations, or when an ultrasound scan is negative for IA or does not provide sufficient information.

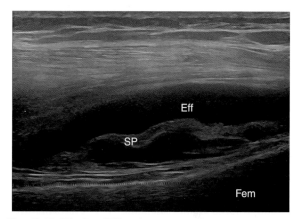

Fig. 10.15 Effusion *(Eff)* and synovial proliferation *(SP)* in the suprapatellar bursa of a patient with osteoarthritis on x-ray. *Fem*, femur.

Fig. 10.15 shows effusion and synovial proliferation in the suprapatellar bursa of the knee but the differential diagnoses for these appearances is wide and access to the joint with ultrasound is limited, meaning that alternative primary imaging such as MRI may be more appropriate.

Whilst the use of colour or power Doppler has been proven to reliably detect active synovitis in small, superficial joints, its use in large deeper joints is more problematic and relies on the ability of the equipment to detect Doppler signal at depth and in the operator to use the machine controls effectively. Fig. 10.16 shows obvious synovial hypertrophy in the glenohumeral joint of a patient with known active RA. Flow could not be detected

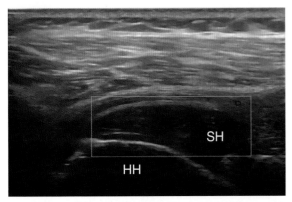

Fig. 10.16 Severe glenohumeral joint synovial hypertrophy *(SH)* with no obvious vascularity on Doppler in a patient with known, active rheumatoid arthritis. *HH,* Humeral head.

on power Doppler despite extensive manipulation of controls such as colour frequency, gain, and pulsed repetition frequency (PRF). One reason for this may be the obvious fatty atrophy of overlying muscle attenuating the ultrasound beam and reducing penetration.

ULTRASOUND TECHNIQUE AND SYSTEM SETTINGS FOR SMALL JOINTS OF THE HANDS AND FEET

The specific technique for scanning hands and feet is well covered in Chapters 5 and 9 but it may be useful to adopt some minor adaptations to protocol when scanning a patient following rheumatology referral.

The expectations of the referrer should be focused on the diagnosis or exclusion of an IA and whilst it is often useful to visualise an alternative cause of symptoms, this may not be practical in terms of scan times and expertise of the operator. In view of this, specific scanning and reporting protocols should be developed, discussed with referrers, and used as a standard for scanning these patients.

Patient Position

Patient comfort is of paramount importance during any ultrasound examination and is vital if they are to comply with the procedure. Scanning multiple joints can be time consuming and may involve several areas of the body in order to aid a diagnosis, requiring adaptation of scanning techniques to accommodate patient needs. One simple adaptation is to alter the position of the patient from the position noted in Fig. 10.17A to the one highlighted in Fig. 10.17B.

This ensures that both patient and sonographer are in a more ergonomically correct position.

The patient's hands may be placed on a pillow on their lap in a relaxed position so as not to compromise blood flow within joints and soft tissues. The feet are usually scanned with the knees flexed and soles of the feet flat on the couch for stability.

> ### ◎ TOP TIP
>
> Make sure that you and your patient are comfortable. Scanning may take some time and require a variety of joints to be scanned. Seating your patient on the examination couch gives access to multiple joints without tiring the patient.

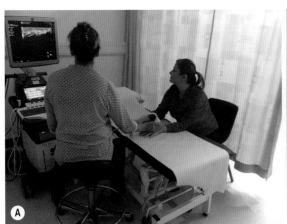
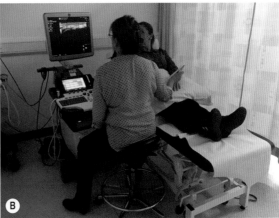

Fig. 10.17 Altering patient position from **(A)** to **(B)** can aid patient comfort.

Scanning Technique

As with all ultrasound examinations, a systematic approach to assessing each structure should be adopted, particularly when screening for signs of early disease when only small changes may be visible. Each joint and tendon should be scanned in longitudinal and transverse planes (Fig. 10.18), from one aspect to the other.

System Settings

Ultrasound system set-up must be appropriate and allow differentiation between tissues of similar densities in order to produce images of good resolution. High frequency (in the range of 10–18 MHz) linear transducers are required for the high-resolution imaging and a small footprint transducer such as a "hockey stick" can be useful for assessing small joints of the hands and feet.

Grey scale controls such as frequency, dynamic range, and overall gain (see Chapter 1) must be used appropriately.

Examination presets may be useful to ensure standardisation of settings between patients but should be constructed with the help of company applications specialists if necessary. Some of these settings may need to be altered to allow for specific joints, patient body habitus,

or the detection of ultrasound features, so the operator must have the skills and knowledge to do this.

Split-screen

The split screen function may be useful to compare two planes of the same joint or soft tissue structure in order to confirm the presence of activity within the structure (Fig. 10.19) or to compare one joint with the contralateral side when changes in structure are subtle.

There are two modes of Doppler ultrasound currently in use to detect active synovitis, colour and power Doppler. Either can be used and in modern equipment, there is often no discernible difference in their sensitivity to detect low flow.

Specific Doppler Functions

The most important aspect of Doppler use is the setting of correct parameters within the system (i.e., low PRF, appropriate gain, and wall filters). This can be difficult without specialist knowledge of ultrasound and appropriate training is essential. There are several Doppler functions to consider which may affect the sensitivity in detecting blood flow within the synovium. Some

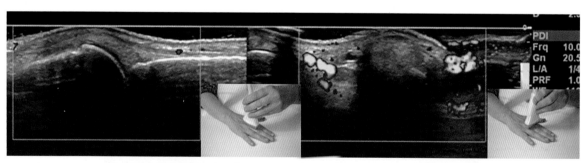

Fig. 10.18 Longitudinal and transverse views of a metacarpophalangeal joint.

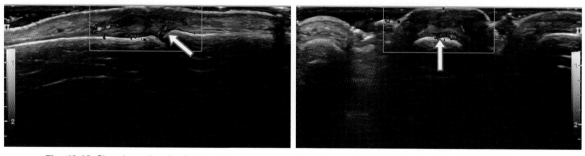

Fig. 10.19 Showing a longitudinal and transverse section of a proximal interphalangeal joint demonstrating the presence of Doppler signal at the enthesis *(white arrow)* in two planes.

functions are set during examination preset construction and then rarely altered but others are used constantly throughout each examination to ensure accurate detection of flow.

Doppler Box Size

General recommendations state that the Doppler box should cover from the deepest area of interest, extending up to the skin surface to show any superficial vessels that may cause artefactual colour signal in the structures below.[32] However, if by doing this, large, fast-flowing vessels sit within the large Doppler box, the system will use a high degree of processing power which, in a mid-low-end system, may compromise the detection of small, deeper vessels. Reducing the box size to the area of interest alone may in fact increase the sensitivity of the system to detect low flow within that area. Also, the visualisation of spurious large, fast-flowing vessels may detract the operator's eye from the region of interest, making subtle flow there difficult to see.

Pulsed Repetition Frequency (PRF)/Wall Filter

These controls are often linked and altering one will automatically alter the other. They affect the sensitivity of colour and power Doppler by filtering out unnecessary signal. A high PRF should be used for high velocity vessels in order to filter out artefact, for example in cardiac examinations. Similarly, low PRF will use less filters and detect vessels of low velocity such as those in synovitis, tenosynovitis, or bursitis. Machine manufacturers may use different numerical thresholds for low flow presets, so it is important to have in-depth knowledge of your system.

Doppler Gain

In a similar way to the grey scale gain, increasing the Doppler gain amplifies the signal seen on the screen and decreasing it may reduce the signal to a level not seen by the operator. Standard practice is to increase the Doppler gain to such a level that the box is flooded with colour, then reduce it slowly until only true flow is seen. This ensures detection of low velocity blood flow despite changes in the depth of the structure from the skin surface (Fig. 10.20).

Doppler Frequency

In grey scale imaging, the frequency of the beam is one of the most important factors, especially when imaging deeper structures where the frequency must be lowered in order to penetrate deep tissues. This is similar when using the Doppler function in deep joints where the colour frequency should be reduced in a similar way; however, it should be remembered that reducing frequency allows more penetration at the expense of resolution and although flow may be detected, image quality of the vessels may be reduced.

◎ **TOP TIP**

When scanning small joints, position the transducer to get a good image of the joint, select the power/colour Doppler function with the appropriate box size. Reduce the transducer pressure, then increase the colour/power Doppler gain until you have artefactual colour on the screen. Then reduce the gain slowly, until the artefact has disappeared. Then move the transducer across the joint to cover all areas.

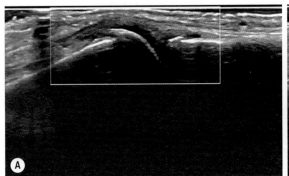 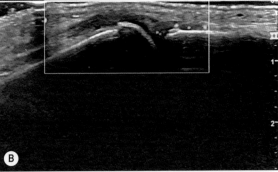

Fig. 10.20 (A) Shows a metacarpophalangeal joint with power Doppler box positioned over the joint. The pulsed repetition frequency is set to detect low flow, the Doppler box is covering the joint and the Doppler gain is set at 22.5. No Doppler signal is seen on the image. **(B)** Shows the same image and parameters except the Doppler gain, which has been increased to 29.5. In this image, flow is seen within the joint.

PITFALLS

Pitfalls in ultrasound scanning for IA include poor scanning technique, the use of incorrect equipment settings, and lack of appreciation of the effects of current treatments.

Pitfalls in Technique and Equipment Settings

Good technique for scanning is vital in accurately assessing joints for synovitis. Of particular importance is the lack of transducer pressure on the skin surface. Too much pressure may compress the small blood vessels present in joint synovitis or tenosynovitis and obliterate Doppler signal. Firm transducer grip and use of thick coupling gel as stand-off can also help eliminate compression.

As Doppler is used frequently to detect the presence of active inflammation, it is vital that the ultrasound system used is sensitive enough to detect low flow and the settings are optimised to avoid missing synovitis (see earlier).

Synovial hypertrophy may appear relatively hypoechoic to the adjacent joint tissue on the grey scale images, so it is important to manipulate the transducer in order to eradicate any anisotropy (see Chapter 1) as this may mimic pathological changes within the joint. Fig. 10.21 presents views of the same joint showing the effect of slight angulation of the transducer. Fig. 10.21A shows the joint with the transducer angled appropriately. Fig. 10.21B shows the same joint with angulation of the transducer causing anisotropy.

> ◎ **TOP TIP**
>
> Make sure the settings on your ultrasound system are appropriate to detect low flow within the synovium. If you are not sure, approach the applications specialist from the relevant company to help you. You will need a patient with active synovitis when setting your system up.

Pitfalls in Interpretation of Current Treatments

Steroids—oral, intramuscular, or infusion—either for the treatment of inflammatory disease or concurrent problems such as asthma, bronchiectasis, and chronic obstructive pulmonary disease, will temporarily reduce synovial inflammation.[33] Rheumatology clinicians may use steroids as a temporary measure to relieve symptoms whilst patients are undergoing investigations and these clinicians may not be aware of their effect on imaging. It is therefore important to take steroid use into account when reporting on ultrasound studies to detect or grade active synovitis. Fig. 10.22 shows the effects of steroid use on Doppler flow in a case of RA.

It is therefore suggested that ultrasound examinations should be scheduled at least 6 weeks after any steroid intervention. If that is not possible, the sonographer should add a comment in the report to ensure that the referrer is aware, for example, "The patient reports that they are taking oral steroids/has had a recent intraarticular or intramuscular steroid. This may reduce the ultrasound features of IA seen on today's scan. If there is ongoing clinical concern, a rescan 6 weeks after any steroid use is suggested."

There has been some research suggesting a similar problem with the long-term use of nonsteroidal antiinflammatory drugs (NSAIDs) and this may be more difficult to manage as they are widely used and required for pain relief. It may not be practical to limit their use, but care should be taken when questioning the patient to ensure the practitioner is aware of any long-term NSAID use. In these cases, areas of synovial proliferation with no Doppler signal and no obvious cause should be taken into consideration when reporting and may require rescan.[34]

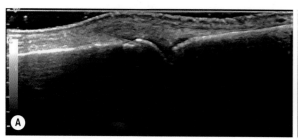
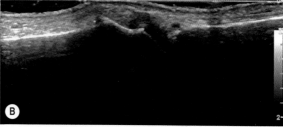

Fig. 10.21 (A) Normal metacarpophalangeal joint. **(B)** With the transducer angled in such a way to cause anisotropy, thus giving the appearances of hypoechoic synovial hypertrophy.

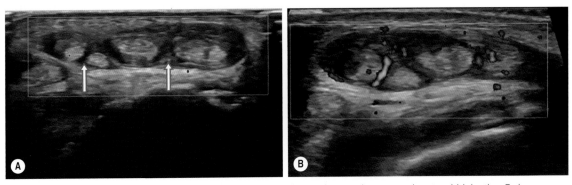

Fig. 10.22 (A) Extensor tendons of a patient who has been given an intramuscular steroid injection 5 days previously. There is evidence of synovial hypertrophy around the tendons *(white arrows)*, but no Doppler signal seen. **(B)** The same tendon sheath 6 weeks after intramuscular steroid showing the return of Doppler signal.

◎ TOP TIP

Steroids will have an effect on active inflammation for around 6 weeks after administration—maybe longer with long-term oral steroids. This will affect Doppler signal and may reduce the true grading of active synovitis, or make the scan appear "normal."
This should be mentioned in the report.

ULTRASOUND APPEARANCES RELATED TO SPECIFIC INFLAMMATORY ARTHRITIDES

Whilst it is difficult to apportion certain ultrasound appearances to specific inflammatory arthritides, there are some which, when seen in addition to clinical information, may help in determining a diagnosis.

Rheumatoid Arthritis

RA is known to commonly affect the wrists, MCP, and PIPjs of the hands as well as tendon sheaths and is often symmetrical.[4] Early ultrasound appearances may include effusion and synovial hypertrophy but as these appearances are common in age- or use-related changes, it is the site-specific presence of significant active synovitis or tenosynovitis seen with Doppler ultrasound, or erosive bony changes in these joints, that often supports the diagnosis. Fig. 10.23 shows active synovitis on power Doppler in an index finger MCPj.

Grading/Scoring of Disease

There have been several grading/scoring systems devised for the quantification of active joint synovitis in an attempt to aid the clinician in the use of appropriate treatment options and to provide data for research.

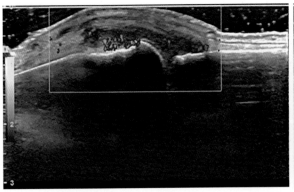
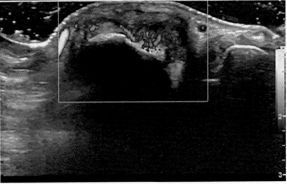

Fig. 10.23 Active synovitis on Power Doppler in an index finger metacarpophalangeal joint.

These grading systems attach a numerical value (usually 0 to 3) to either grey scale or Doppler changes or may use descriptive terms such as "normal, mild, moderate, severe" in a similar way. Whilst numbered grading systems are useful for repeat scanning in research clinics, their interpretation must be understood by referrer and reporter alike and as most reports are now electronic and accessed by multiple health care professionals, a more descriptive system may be safer.

Grey Scale Grading of Synovial Hypertrophy

In some circumstances, it may be clinically appropriate to grade synovial hypertrophy independently as a response to treatment, but because its presence is common in healthy subjects,[35] grey scale grading alone may lead to difficulties with interpretation and is often confined to research studies. However, the presence of high-grade synovial hypertrophy without an obvious cause may alert the sonographer to specific joints for particular interrogation with colour Doppler. Examples of grey scale synovial hypertrophy are shown in Fig. 10.24A–D.

Colour/Power Doppler Grading of Active Synovitis

There has been much research into both quantitive and semiquantitive scoring systems to grade active synovitis using Doppler ultrasound with a view to reduce operator dependence[36,37] and aid sequential scanning to monitor response to treatment. There are many good texts around this but as this chapter is aimed at practitioners providing clinical rheumatology services rather than research, a pragmatic approach has been taken around the work of Szkudlarek and colleagues[36] which is widely-used in the field.

Fig. 10.25 shows examples of a semiquantitive scoring system between 0 (normal) to 3 (severe) using both longitudinal and transverse images of the joint. Theoretically, any Doppler signal within the joint is detected by scanning in a longitudinal plane across the full width of the joint, confirmed as being inside the joint in the transverse plane, then graded/scored. This gives the referrer an indication of the severity of activity which may aid diagnosis or track response to treatment.

Spondyloarthropathy

One of the most common spondyloarthropathies is PsA, which may be difficult to detect in primary care due to relatively random symptoms and lack of understanding of the links between psoriasis and PsA. In addition to joint synovitis, spondyloarthropathies such as PsA commonly affect the tendons and entheses around joints. Common presentations on ultrasound include Achilles

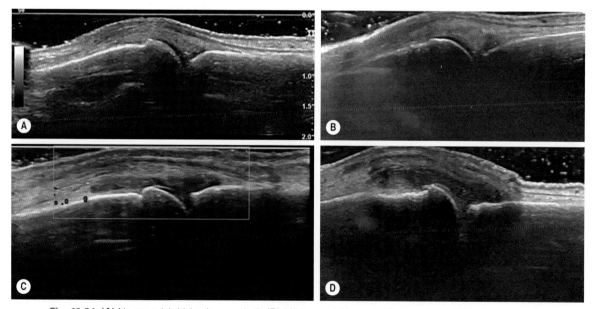

Fig. 10.24 **(A)** No synovial thickening: grade 0. **(B)** Mild synovial hypertrophy: grade 1. **(C)** Moderate synovial hypertrophy: grade 2. **(D)** Severe synovial hypertrophy: grade 3.

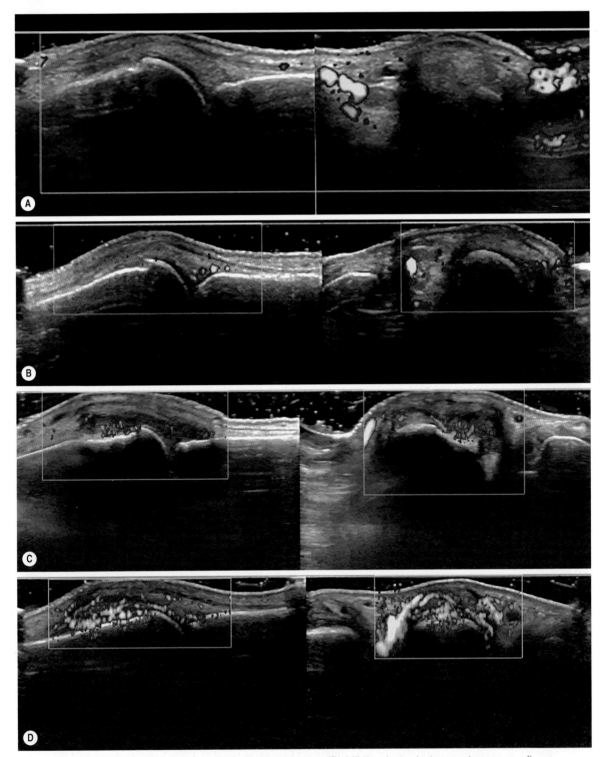

Fig. 10.25 (A) Normal/Grade 0: no flow in the synovium. **(B)** Mild/grade 1: single vessel or one confluent vessel in the synovium. **(C)** Moderate/grade 2: vessels in less than 50% of the synovium. **(D)** Severe/grade 3: vessels in 50% or more of the synovium.

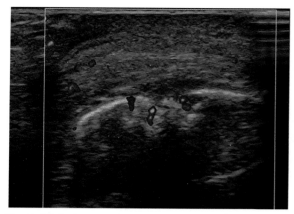

Fig. 10.26 Active, erosive enthesitis at the Achilles insertion on a 21-year-old patient.

tendinopathy/enthesopathy (in particular erosive), plantar fasciitis and dactylitis[38] without obvious biomechanical cause. Fig. 10.26 shows active erosive enthesitis at the Achilles insertion on a 21-year-old patient.

As these pathologies are not specific to PsA, the association between ultrasound appearances and a history (or family history) of psoriasis may be made during scanning and suggested in the report.

More specific ultrasound appearances include paratendinitis/paratenonitis which may be seen where tendons are devoid of a continuous sheath but have a paratenon, for example, around the superficial surface of the Achilles tendon or where the extensor tendons run over the MCPjs of the hand (Fig. 10.27). Appearances include hypoechoic widening and diffuse hyperemia of the soft tissues around the tendon. This is easy to miss when scanning the hand if the Doppler box does not extend proximal to the MCPjs.

Active synovitis at a PIPj with symptomatic OA is common but if there are no osteophytes and Doppler flow is seen within the enthesis, a seronegative inflammatory arthritis such as PsA is likely.[39] Fig. 10.28 shows the extensor enthesitis at the PIPj of a patient with PsA.

A classic site for PsA enthesitis is at the DIPjs of the fingers but this area is difficult to interpret with ultrasound due to its relatively small size and the common presence of osteophytosis from OA. In addition, some patients with psoriatic onychopathy (nail involvement) have very vascular nail beds which can confound the detection of active enthesitis.[38] Because of these difficulties, it is common to exclude DIPjs from a scan protocol to try and avoid increasing false positive results.

In the feet, a common site for SpA is the fifth MTPj which may show evidence of synovitis and erosion (Fig. 10.29). Whilst it is relatively common to see active synovitis in the first MTPj due to symptomatic OA, it is not common to see degenerative changes at the fifth MTPj, making synovitis here a likely result of SpA.

◎ TOP TIP

If there is ultrasound evidence of active enthesitis with no obvious biomechanical cause and the request mentions negative rheumatoid factor, questioning the patient about a history or family history of psoriasis may help the diagnosis. It may not be appropriate to conclude a report with a diagnosis of PsA but the addition of a phrase such as "The patient reports a history of psoriasis and ultrasound appearances would support a diagnosis of a seronegative IA" may help.

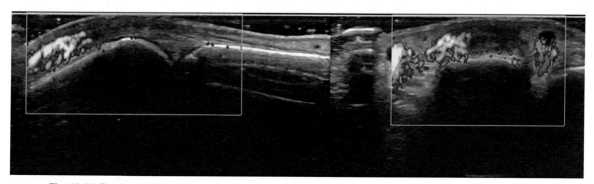

Fig. 10.27 Paratenonitis proximal to metacarpophalangeal joint in a patient with Psoriatic arthritis.

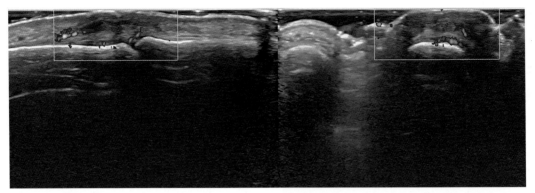

Fig. 10.28 Extensor enthesitis at the proximal interphalangeal joint of a patent with psoriatic arthritis.

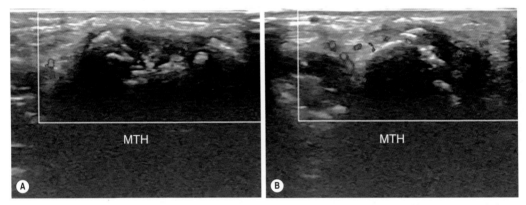

Fig. 10.29 Longitudinal **(A)** and transverse **(B)** images of active erosive change at the fifth metacarpophalangeal joint of a patient with psoriatic arthritis (PsA). *MTH,* Metatarsal head.

Gout

A common ultrasound appearance of gout is that of a "double contour" sign. This appearance occurs as a result of deposition of a layer of hyperechoic MSU crystals on the surface of the hypoechoic cartilage of a joint and is seen most commonly on the head of the first metatarsal and the femoral condyles of the knee[40] (Fig. 10.30).

Care must be taken not to confuse a true double contour sign, which is not dependent on beam angle, from the cartilage interface artefact which is only visible when the beam is perpendicular to the surface of the cartilage as seen in Fig. 10.31. This sign is much more obvious in the presence of a joint effusion.

MSU crystals may also aggregate within soft tissues to form tophus which, in poorly controlled disease,

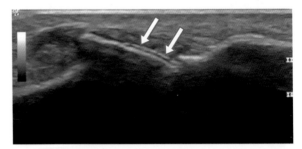

Fig. 10.30 A "double contour" sign *(white arrows)* seen on the first metatarsal head of a patient diagnosed with gout.

may form within joint capsules and tendons, as seen in Fig. 10.32.

Tophi may be asymptomatic but may trigger an inflammatory reaction within the soft tissue causing an episode of acute pain such as tenosynovitis (Fig. 10.33).

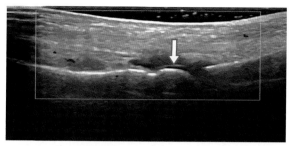

Fig. 10.31 A cartilage interface artefact *(white arrow)* on a metatarsal head.

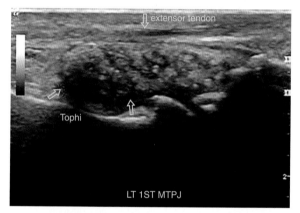

Fig. 10.32 Tophi distending a left *(Lt)* first metatarsophalangeal joint *(MTPJ)* capsule.

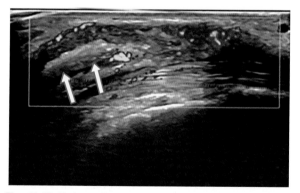

Fig. 10.33 Tophus within a peroneal tendon *(white arrows)* causing an episode of tenosynovitis – hyperemia of the tendon and sheath.

Calcium Pyrophosphate Arthritis - Pseudogout

As with gout, it is often the site of symptoms that indicates the specific crystal arthropathy of pseudogout and a common appearance is that of CPPD within the triangular fibrocartilage of the wrist (Fig. 10.34) and menisci

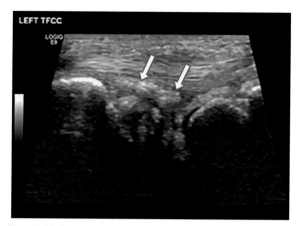

Fig. 10.34 Pseudogout. CPPD within the triangular fibrocartilage complex of the wrist.

of the knee, often seen on X-ray. These deposits may be denser than tophi on ultrasound but equally may cause episodes of adjacent synovitis as they irritate the adjacent structures.

As a double contour sign may be seen in both arthropathies, with a subtle difference in the actual location of crystals, it can be difficult to distinguish between the two, especially around the small joints of the hand with mid-to-low end ultrasound systems, as in Fig. 10.35.

This lack of specificity of the double contour sign may be due to operator, patient, or equipment issues and if there is doubt, a suggestion of a more general "crystal arthropathy" in the report is appropriate, leaving the referrer to correlate with clinical findings and blood results to give a more definitive diagnosis.

> ### ◎ TOP TIP
> Ultrasound appearances may be similar for gout and CPPD—the site of pathology may aid diagnosis—so it may be safer to use the general term "crystal arthropathy" in a report so the referrer will correlate clinically.

PROTOCOLS

Which Patients?

National Institute for Health and Clinical Excellence (NICE) has published specific criteria to assist in the early referral of primary care patients suspected to have

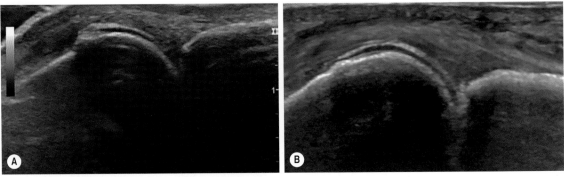

Fig. 10.35 (A) Shows proven CPPD on a MC head. **(B)** Shows proven MSU on an MC head.

inflammatory disease for specialised rheumatology assessment.[10] Any diagnostic test such as ultrasound or MRI requested by the general practitioner (GP) to look for signs of IA should never delay symptomatic patients from being referred to a rheumatologist.

In view of this, it would seem appropriate for radiology departments to discourage GPs and other nonspecialised services from referring symptomatic patients for ultrasound scanning without prior rheumatology assessment. However, it is important that practitioners accepting referrals for MSK scans from GPs are aware of the common ultrasound appearances of inflammatory disease so that they may be able to alert referrers to the possibility of an unexpected underlying IA as a cause for symptoms.

Rheumatologists may or may not need to refer for any imaging in order to appropriately manage their patients. In general, it is the more clinically equivocal cases that require MSUS as those more obviously clinically positive or negative for the disease are relatively straightforward to manage.

Which Joints?

In view of the often-limited time given for diagnostic scans and the ever-increasing demands on imaging departments, it is important to balance the need to detect small, subtle changes on imaging with the time taken to scan the appropriate joints on each patient.

There have been attempts to determine the joints most likely to reflect the stage/degree of inflammatory activity and to limit the joints scanned to those most symptomatic in an attempt to make examination times shorter and scans more focused.[41] However, as yet, there

has been little agreement and scanning protocols are developed locally and may vary. It is therefore vital that ultrasound operators and rheumatology staff have close links and dialogue in order that expectations are agreed and reached.

The number of joints scanned may be determined by the clinical history and disease status of the patient. If ultrasound is being used to aid diagnosis of IA where clinical signs are equivocal, more time may be required in order to look for small subtle changes. However, if the patient has known disease and the scan is being used to stage current activity and efficacy of treatment, the examination may be limited to a few joints, especially if those first few joints show significant disease activity.

Studies have shown that ultrasound can detect more single joint synovitis than clinical examination and frequently changes the diagnosis from oligoarthritis to polyarticular, which may have important implications for disease management.[42] In view of this research, the scanning of purely symptomatic joints would seem likely to frequently miss cases of IA. In addition to small joints, studies have proved the importance of extensor (in particular extensor carpi ulnaris [ECU]) and flexor tenosynovitis as predictors for progression of RA in early disease[43]; therefore it would seem logical to include tendons in the routine scan.

The aspect of the joint scanned has also been discussed, with most studies showing that Doppler signal is more readily detected when imaged from the dorsal aspect of the small joints of the hand.[44] In most centres, the dorsal aspect of the joints is routinely imaged as the palmer aspects will be seen when scanning the flexor tendons.

Foot involvement in IA is common, but symptoms may be confounded by pathologies that are not necessarily inflammatory—Morton's neuroma, plantar fasciopathy, and Haglund's syndrome being relatively common. Whilst it is often helpful to identify these pathologies if they are likely to be the cause of current symptoms, this will depend on the training and experience of the operator and the time allowed for scanning. A pragmatic and standardised approach is outlined in the following section.

Example of a Scanning Protocol for Rheumatology Patients

Hands/Wrists:
- Dorsal wrist to include radioulnar, radiocarpal, ulnocarpal and carpal joints
- Extensor tendons—in particular ECU
- Dorsal aspect of MCP and PIPjs,
- Volar wrist/carpal tunnel
- Flexor tendons

Feet/Ankles:
- Dorsal tibiotalar joint
- Medial and lateral ankle tendons
- Achilles and plantar fascia insertions if seronegative disease is suspected
- MTPjs—dorsal for synovitis, plantar surface for erosions

Scan the joint in longitudinal from the medial to the lateral border and in transverse, to cover the width of the joints.
Look for:
- Synovial hypertrophy
- Effusion
- Bone erosions
- Degenerative change

Repeat the scan using colour/power Doppler
Look for:
- Active synovitis-if present, grade using local guidelines

Stored Images

As with all ultrasound examinations, storing of images is highly recommended and local arrangements based on national guidelines should be followed.[45]

A standard hand and wrist series may include the following minimum images for a normal rheumatology scan:
- Dorsal wrist and carpal joints in longitudinal with colour box

- ECU tendon with colour box
- All MCPjs in longitudinal with colour box
- All PIPjs in longitudinal with colour box
- Flexor tendons with colour box

As with all diagnostic ultrasound scans, any pathology should be imaged in addition to the standard protocol if possible, shown in two planes. All images should be correctly annotated.

REFERENCES

1. O'Neill TW, McCabe PS, McBeth J. Update on the epidemiology, risk factors and disease outcomes of osteoarthritis. Best Pract Res Clin Rheumatol. 2018;32(2):312–326.
2. Hunter DJ, Bierma-Zeinstra S. Osteoarthritis. Lancet. 2019;393(10182):1745–1759.
3. Abhishek A, Doherty M, Kuo CF, Mallen CD, Zhang W, Grainge MJ. Rheumatoid arthritis is getting less frequent-results of a nationwide population-based cohort study. Rheumatology (Oxford). 2017;56(5):736–744.
4. Aletaha D, Neogi T, Silman AJ, et al. Rheumatoid arthritis classification criteria: an American College of Rheumatology/European League Against Rheumatism collaborative initiative. Arthritis Rheum. 2010;62(9):2569–2581.
5. National Institute for Health and Clinical Excellence (NICE) guidelines. Spondyloarthritis. 2018. Available at: https://www.nice.org.uk/guidance/qs170.
6. Solmaz D, Eder L, Aydin SZ. Update on the epidemiology, risk factors, and disease outcomes of psoriatic arthritis. Best Pract Res Clin Rheumatol. 2018;32(2):295–311.
7. Dehlin M, Jacobsson L, Roddy E. Global epidemiology of gout: prevalence, incidence, treatment patterns and risk factors. Nat Rev Rheumatol. 2020;16(7):380–390.
8. Versus Arthritis. What is acute CPP crystal arthritis? Available at: https://www.versusarthritis.org/about-arthritis/conditions/acute-cpp-crystal-arthritis/.
9. Mathsson Alm L, Fountain DL, Cadwell KK, Madrigal AM, Gallo G, Poorafshar M. The performance of anti-cyclic citrullinated peptide assays in diagnosing rheumatoid arthritis: a systematic review and meta-analysis. Clin Exp Rheumatol. 2018;36(1):144–152.
10. National Institute for Health and Clinical Excellence. Rheumatoid arthritis in adults: management. [NG100]. 2018. Available at: https://www.nice.org.uk/guidance/ng100. Accessed November 25, 2019.
11. Combe B, Landewe R, Daien CI, et al. 2016 update of the EULAR recommendations for the management of early arthritis. Ann Rheum Dis. 2017;76(6):948–959.
12. Prevoo ML, van't Hof MA, Kuper HH, van Leeuwen MA, van de Putte LB, van Riel PL. Modified disease activity

scores that include twenty-eight-joint counts. Development and validation in a prospective longitudinal study of patients with rheumatoid arthritis. Arthritis Rheum. 1995;38(1):44–48.

13. Gossec L, Smolen JS, Ramiro S, et al. European League Against Rheumatism (EULAR) recommendations for the management of psoriatic arthritis with pharmacological therapies: 2015 update. Ann Rheum Dis. 2016;75(3): 499–510.

14. Rubin DA. MR and ultrasound of the hands and wrists in rheumatoid arthritis. Part II. Added clinical value. Skeletal Radiol. 2019;48(6):837–857.

15. Kawashiri SY, Suzuki T, Okada A, et al. Musculoskeletal ultrasonography assists the diagnostic performance of the 2010 classification criteria for rheumatoid arthritis. Mod Rheumatol. 2013;23(1):36–43.

16. Mandl P, Aletaha D. The role of ultrasound and magnetic resonance imaging for treat to target in rheumatoid arthritis and psoriatic arthritis. Rheumatology (Oxford). 2019;58(12):2091–2098.

17. Haavardsholm EA, Aga AB, Olsen IC, et al. Ultrasound in management of rheumatoid arthritis: ARCTIC randomised controlled strategy trial. BMJ. 2016;354:i4205.

18. Dale J, Stirling A, Zhang R, et al. Targeting ultrasound remission in early rheumatoid arthritis: the results of the TaSER study, a randomised clinical trial. Ann Rheum Dis. 2016;75(6):1043–1050.

19. Nguyen H, Ruyssen-Witrand A, Gandjbakhch F, Constantin A, Foltz V, Cantagrel A. Prevalence of ultrasound-detected residual synovitis and risk of relapse and structural progression in rheumatoid arthritis patients in clinical remission: a systematic review and meta-analysis. Rheumatology (Oxford). 2014;53(11): 2110–2118.

20. Foltz V, Gandjbakhch F, Etchepare F, et al. Power Doppler ultrasound, but not low-field magnetic resonance imaging, predicts relapse and radiographic disease progression in rheumatoid arthritis patients with low levels of disease activity. Arthritis Rheum. 2012; 64(1):67–76.

21. Naredo E, Valor L, De la Torre I, et al. Predictive value of Doppler ultrasound-detected synovitis in relation to failed tapering of biologic therapy in patients with rheumatoid arthritis. Rheumatology (Oxford). 2015; 54(8):1408–1414.

22. Brown A, Machold KP, Conaghan PG, et al. Musculoskeletal ultrasound including definitions for ultrasonographic pathology. J Rheumatol. 2005;32;2485–2487.

23. Wang L, Xiang X, Tang Y, Yang Y, Qiu L. Sonographic appearance of fluid in peripheral joints and bursae of healthy asymptomatic Chinese population. Quant Imaging Med Surg. 2018;8(8):781–787.

24. Turan A, Çeltikçi P, Tufan A, Öztürk MA. Basic radiological assessment of synovial diseases: a pictorial essay. Eur J Rheumatol. 2017;4(2):166–174.

25. Witt M, Mueller F, Nigg A, et al. Relevance of grade 1 gray-scale ultrasound findings in wrists and small joints to the assessment of subclinical synovitis in rheumatoid arthritis. Arthritis Rheum. 2013;65(7):1694–1701.

26. Brown A, Conaghan P, Karim Z, et al. An explanation for the apparent dissociation between clinical remission and continued structural deterioration in rheumatoid arthritis. Arthritis Rheum. 2008;58:2958–2967.

27. Ramrattan LA, Kaeley GS. Sonographic characteristics of extensor tendon abnormalities and relationship with joint disease activity in rheumatoid arthritis. J Ultrasound Med. 2017;36:985–992.

28. Watad A, Cuthbert RJ, Amital H, McGonagle D. Enthesitis: much more than focal insertion point inflammation. Curr Rheumatol Rep. 2018;20(7):41.

29. Wakefield RJ, Gibbon WW, Conaghan PG, et al. The value of sonography in the detection of bone erosions in patients with rheumatoid arthritis: a comparison with conventional radiography. Arthritis Rheum. 2000; 43(12):2762–2770.

30. Hau M, Schultz H, Tony HP, et al. Evaluation of pannus and vascularization of the metacarpophalangeal and proximal interphalangeal joints in rheumatoid arthritis by high-resolution ultrasound. Arthritis Rheumatism 1999;42(11):2303–2308.

31. Pelletier JP, Martel-Pelletier J, Abramson SB. Osteoarthritis, an inflammatory disease. Arthritis Rheum. 2001;44: 1237–1247.

32. Wakefield RJ, D'Agostino MA. Essential Applications of Musculoskeletal Ultrasound in Rheumatology. Expert Consult Premium Edition. Philadelphia: Saunders; 2010.

33. Teh J, Stevens K, Williamson L, Leung J, McNally EG. Power Doppler ultrasound of rheumatoid synovitis: quantification of therapeutic response. Br J Radiol. 2003;76(912):875–879.

34. Zayat AS, Conaghan PG, Sharif M. Do non-steroidal anti-inflammatory drugs have a significant effect on detection and grading of ultrasound-detected synovitis in patients with rheumatoid arthritis? Ann Rheum Dis. 2011;70:1746–1751.

35. Ellegaard K, Torp-Pedersen S, Holm C, Danneskiold-Samsøe B, Bliddal H. Ultrasound in finger joints: findings in normal subjects and pitfalls in the diagnosis of synovial disease. Ultraschall Med. 2007;28(4):401–408.

36. Szkudlarek M, Court-Payen M, Jacobsen S, Klarlund M, Thomen HS, Østergaard M. Interobserver agreement in ultrasonography of the finger and toe joints in rheumatoid arthritis. Arthritis Rheum. 2003;48:955–962.

37. Qvistgaard E, Torp-Pedersen S, Christensen R, Bliddal H. Reproducibility and inter-reader agreement of a scoring system for ultrasound evaluation of hip osteoarthritis. Ann Rheum Dis. 2006;65(12):1613–1619.

38. Gutierrez M, Filippucci E, De Angelis R, Filosa G, Kane D, Grassi W. A sonographic spectrum of psoriatic arthritis: "the five targets." Clin Rheumatol. 2010; 29(2):133–142.

39. Filippou G, Di Sabatino V, Adinolfi A, et al. Enthesitis of the extensor digitorum tendons. J Rheumatol. 2013; 40(3):335.

40. Checa A. Consistency of the sonographic image (double contour sign) in patients with gout after ambulation. J Med Ultrasound. 2019;27(1):40–42.

41. Ohrndorf S, Halbauer B, Martus P, et al. Detailed joint region analysis of the 7-joint ultrasound score: evaluation of an arthritis patient cohort over one year. Int J Rheumatol. 2013;2013:493848.

42. Wakefield R, Green M, Marzo-Ortega H, et al. Should oligoarthritis be reclassified? Ann Rheum Dis. 2011; 70(3):500–507.

43. Sahbudin I, Pickup L, Nightingale P, et al. The role of ultrasound-defined tenosynovitis and synovitis in the prediction of rheumatoid arthritis development. Rheumatology. 2018;57(7):1243–1252.

44. Witt MN, Mueller F, Weinert P, et al. Ultrasound of synovitis in rheumatoid arthritis: advantages of the dorsal over the palmar approach to finger joints. J Rheumatol. 2014;41(3):422–428.

45. SCoR and BMUS. Guidelines for Professional Ultrasound Practice. 4th ed. London: Society and College of Radiographers and British Medical Ultrasound Society; 2019. https://www.bmus.org/static/uploads/resources/Guidelines_for_Professional_Ultrasound_Practice_v3_OHoz76r.pdf.

Soft Tissue Masses

Katie Simm and Sylvia Connolly

CHAPTER OUTLINE

LEARNING OBJECTIVES

The aim of this chapter is to enable the reader to:
- Employ a methodical approach to ultrasound examination of a STM
- Describe the ultrasound features of commonly encountered STM
- Be confident in utilising the most appropriate local and national guidance for managing the patient dependent on the specific ultrasound features encountered

INTRODUCTION

The use of ultrasound for the initial triage of the patient presenting with a new or changing soft tissue mass (STM) is becoming increasingly common and now makes up a large proportion of the referrals for musculoskeletal (MSK) ultrasound.

The ultrasound evaluation of soft tissue lesions is complex, due to the myriad of possible imaging features and the number of different tumours that can originate from various locations.[1] Operators should gain as much exposure as possible and be fully aware of their local guidelines for investigation and management of STMs.

There are national guidelines for the management of soft tissue sarcomas that can inform departments and enable them to draw up local protocols for clinical and imaging assessment of STM to enable appropriate management.[2] Most soft tissue masses are benign; however, it is clearly important to recognise and provide rapid diagnosis of malignant tumours, and imaging is often used in an attempt to classify lesions.

It is recommended that patients with STMs with the following clinical features should be referred directly to the soft tissue sarcoma (STS) multidisciplinary team (MDT) for further investigation and management[2]:
- Rapid growth
- Deep location
- Pain
- Size greater than 5 to 7 cm
- Recurrent following previous excision

However, in practice, clinical assessment may be challenging with a considerable overlap in the presentation of benign and malignant masses.

It is advisable, in any one clinical setting, to restrict imaging of STM to a select group of operators to allow a level of expertise to be acquired. In many instances, STM can be attributed to a specific diagnosis, for example, a muscle hernia, accessory tendon, or palpable lump post trauma from retracted muscle/tendon complex. As such, operators adept at performing MSK ultrasound examinations are best equipped to carry out imaging of STMs.

ULTRASOUND TRIAGE OF SOFT TISSUE MASSES

Ultrasound is well suited for triage of STM, aiding clinical management of nonspecific masses and confirmation of benign features, providing reassurance to the patient.[3] Rigorous triage of referrals is important to facilitate urgent scanning of patients with suspicious symptoms via a FastTrack, 2-week wait service (2ww).[4] Routine, non-urgent ultrasound assessment is acceptable for patients with low clinical suspicion of malignancy.

Ultrasound and magnetic resonance imaging (MRI) are the principal imaging modalities employed for the diagnosis and management of patients presenting with a new or changing palpable STM. It is important for the operator to have a good understanding of the relative merits and limitations of each.[5]

Ultrasound is effective at differentiating solid from cystic lesions and can readily identify a variety of benign STMs that require no further investigation. In the main, for most peripheral and superficial masses, ultrasound provides all the information required.

Some STM exhibit nonspecific features or may be deep or large and may require further evaluation by MRI. Often in small lesions less than 2 cm, MRI may offer little extra information and, in these circumstances, a wide excision biopsy by an appropriately trained physician should be considered.[5]

It is important to remember other imaging modalities, such as radiographs and computed tomography (CT). These offer information regarding the presence or pattern of ossification and calcification within a STM or its involvement with or effect on the underlying bone.

ULTRASOUND EXAMINATION

The following section describes a strategy of how to approach the ultrasound examination of STM to help with interpretation of appearances.

Equipment

Superficial masses should be examined with a high frequency 6 to 15 MHz linear transducer. Ensure the highest frequency possible is utilised but for deeper, larger lesions the operator may need to employ the use of a lower frequency transducer (9 MHz) to aid depth penetration. For the examination of smaller superficial lesions, or those that are difficult to access, the use of a hockey stick transducer should be considered. The vascularity of a mass should be evaluated with colour or power Doppler in all examinations. The operator should maintain minimal probe pressure during examination of superficial lumps to ensure that vascularity in small lesions can be detected, and use of copious amounts of gel can aid in this. Careful use of compression can be useful in some deeper lesions as this reduces the thickness of the tissues between the lesion and the probe and thereby improves visualisation. A minimum of two grey scale images in orthogonal planes should be obtained to allow measurement of the lesion in three planes, and these images, as well as the accompanying Doppler images should be securely stored and made available for future review if necessary.

Clinical History

As already discussed, it can be difficult to interpret clinical or imaging findings to accurately detect malignancy in a STM and misdiagnosis can have serious consequences to the patient and potentially to clinicians, medico legally. However, there are pointers from the patient's clinical history which may help the sonographer interpret the ultrasound findings.

Questions to ask the patient:
- How long has the lesion been present?
- Is it rapidly changing in size?
- Is it painful to touch?
- Is it mobile?
- Is there a history of injury?
- Does it discharge?
- Has there been previous resection of a lesion at this site? Is this a recurrence?

Lesions that have been present and unchanging for long periods of time are generally benign; however, a long-standing lesion that suddenly changes in size or becomes painful should raise suspicion. New, recurrent, or rapidly growing lesions should raise the concern for malignancy.[4] However, a benign lesion with associated haemorrhage, inflammation, or infection may also increase in size. Untreated malignant lesions do not reduce in size unless there is associated resolving haemorrhage. The patient presenting with a history of trauma and subsequent soft tissue swelling is common; however, the diagnosis of benign haematoma following injury should be exercised with caution. A preexisting malignant lesion, with disorganised internal vasculature, that is aggravated by trauma may haemorrhage. A benign haematoma will resolve at subsequent follow up scan, although this may take several months depending on the size of the haematoma.[6]

It is common for ganglia to fluctuate in size and this, combined with common locations around the hand, wrist, and foot, can steer the operator to a specific diagnosis even before scanning.

In general, lesions that are mobile are more commonly benign, whilst a greater number of malignant lesions, due to their infiltrative nature, tend to be fixed to the surrounding tissues. Nerve sheath tumours tend to be mobile in the axis perpendicular to the nerve but fixed in their long axis.

Location

Ultrasound has good spatial resolution and can identify the origin of many lesions, especially when they are located superficially. Palpation of the lesion prior to scan is helpful as it can guide the operator to the location and depth of the lesion. It also allows visual inspection of potential overlying skin changes or the presence of a punctum. Careful considerations include:

- Does the lesion lie within the subcutaneous soft tissues?
- Is it intramuscular?
- Is it associated with or in close proximity to a vessel or nerve?
- Does it arise from a joint or tendon sheath?
- Is it associated with or arising from a fascial structure?

A larger proportion of benign lesions are located within the subcutaneous soft tissues; however, these should still be assessed with care. Any subcutaneous lesion that has indeterminate or concerning features on examination will still require further investigation and the operator should be aware of locally agreed investigation and management pathways. All lesions deep to the fascia warrant further investigation and appropriate onward referral.[6]

Certain pathologies are diagnostic by their location and will be discussed in the next section.

It is good practice in any situation to describe the location of a soft tissue lesion by its proximity to other vessels and the neurovascular bundle for planning should surgical excision be required.[6]

Grey Scale Appearance

The operator should consider the following:

- Is the STM completely cystic?
- Is it homogenous or heterogeneous?
- Does it have characteristic appearances?
- Are there any artefacts present confusing the diagnosis (near field artefacts in cysts) or useful artefacts such as dirty shadowing (indicating the presence of air)?

In isolation, the grey scale appearance of some soft tissue lesions can cause diagnostic uncertainty. Some benign lesions of mixed echogenicity may demonstrate the same characteristics as their malignant counterparts. In these situations, it is important for the operator to take into account other presenting characteristics of the lesion during examination. If the lesion demonstrates other indeterminate features, then the operator should consider recommending further imaging or referral for consideration of biopsy in a specialist centre. Suspicious solid lesions should always be treated with caution and require further imaging or specialist assessment for consideration of biopsy. Not all malignant soft tissue masses are sarcomas and lymph node masses, for example, will have a different investigative pathway.

Purely cystic lesions that can be seen to arise from a joint or tendon sheath that do not demonstrate any other indeterminate features are rarely malignant. In these instances, the operator can make a positive diagnosis and no further imaging is required. Caution should, however, be exercised as some small malignant cystic sarcomas can present with benign features.[6]

Margins

The operator should consider the following:

- Does the lesion have a well-defined smooth border?
- Is the lesion irregular and ill-defined?
- Does the lesion cross tissue planes?

Most benign soft tissue lesions have clear, well-defined borders; however, many sarcomas, when confined by the fascia, can also appear well-defined and this should not be used as a discriminator alone. Likewise, some benign conditions, such as fibromatosis, endometriosis, fatty necrosis and certain inflammatory masses, are ill-defined and can present diagnostic uncertainty. These should be examined with caution in conjunction with good clinical history from the patient.

Any lesion which is seen to cross tissue planes should immediately raise the suspicion of malignancy and requires further assessment.[5]

Calcification and Ossification

The operator should consider the following

- Is this a site of previous trauma?
- Does the patient regularly inject into this area?
- Where is the calcification located?[7]

Calcification within soft tissues can occur for a number of reasons, including previous injury, post injection, as part of a generalised medical condition, or at the site of a previous invasive procedure.[8] The operator should take this into consideration when performing the ultrasound examination. Some benign soft tissue lesions, such as pilomatricoma, commonly demonstrate characteristic internal calcification.

Calcification associated with a lump or swelling can be seen within tendons or bursae associated with hydroxy-apatite deposition disease (e.g., calcific tendinopathy). Some collagen diseases cause calcification to be laid down in the soft tissues of the fingers. Dystrophic calcification occurs following tissue damage, for example, phleboliths in thrombus within a benign vascular malformation.

Ossification appears bonelike with cortication and can occur with connective tissue disorders and following trauma. Malignant osteosarcoma can also cause ossification within the soft tissues. These features can only be characterised with radiographs and these are mandatory when ossification or calcification is suspected on the ultrasound examination (Fig. 11.1).

Occasionally an apparent soft tissue mass is related to the underlying bone (e.g. osteochondroma). Although ultrasound may be able to identify a cartilage cap which is diagnostic, radiographs are still required to visualise the entire lesion.

Vascularity

The operator should consider the following:
- Is there vascularity associated with the lesion?
- Is the vascular pattern florid, branching, or disorganised?
- Does the lesion abut a vessel?
- Has the lesion been adequately assessed for low-flow vascularity, which can be easy to miss?

The use of colour and power Doppler with appropriate flow settings enables detection of internal vascularity and this is important to assess on all STMs. However, it should be taken in context as alone it is not a predictor of malignancy. The presence of blood vessels in some lesions can help with characterisation (e.g., hemangioma, vascular malformation, aneurysm). The operator should apply minimal compression during examination to avoid obliterating the blood flow; the use of copious amounts of gel should help.[8]

Malignant lesions can demonstrate disorganised internal vascularity. Vascularity within a lesion can, however, be misleading. Some STSs may have little demonstrable blood flow or may be necrotic centrally. Some benign lesions such as hemangiomas and schwannomas can be highly vascular.[7]

Lesions abutting vessels should be described for the purposes of surgical planning due to the risk of bleeding.

Dynamic Evaluation

The operator should consider the movement of a lesion relative to the surrounding structures, for example, a mass related to a tendon should move when the joint is flexed or extended.

Compression of cystic masses close to joints can distinguish ganglia from simple joint effusions. Ganglia will not compress, whereas a simple joint effusion will disperse when pressure is applied or when the joint is moved during examination.

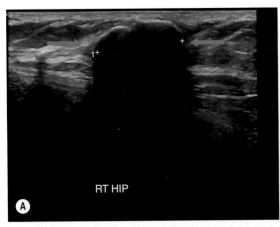
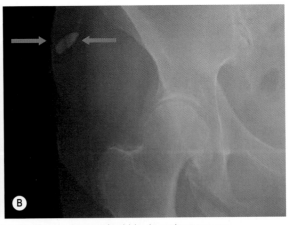

Fig. 11.1 **(A)** Dystrophic calcification on ultrasound: Calcified lesion **(arrows)** within the subcutaneous tissues demonstrating strong posterior acoustic shadowing. **(B)** Dystrophic calcification X-ray: Xray image of the same patient confirms benign dystrophic calcification within the soft tissues **(arrows)**

As previously discussed careful use of compression can improve visualisation of some deeper lesions by minimising tissue thickness between the lesion and the probe, but this compression must be withdrawn whilst Doppler is being used to assess for vascularity.

Hernias are a common cause for a lump in the abdominal wall or groin (see Chapter 6) and these arise from defects in the muscle fascia. Compression/release techniques should be used to encourage contents of the hernia to emerge from the confines of the fascia and gentle compression will assess reduction of the hernia.

Post Examination

Once the ultrasound examination has been performed, it is important for the operator to have a good understanding of the most appropriate onward management of the patient. Ultrasound features of soft tissue masses generally fall into one of three categories after examination:

A. Completely benign.

These require no further action and can be discharged back to the referring clinician.

Examples include: (some of these will be discussed later)

- Simple cyst, bursa synovial/ganglion cyst
- Superficial lipoma
- Vascular malformation
- Foreign body
- Superficial fibromatosis, e.g., plantar and palmer fibromatosis (discussed in appropriate chapters)
- Muscle hernia
- Morton's neuroma (discussed in Chapter 9)
- Normal lymph nodes[1]

In some instances, an interval ultrasound scan may be employed. Many centres employ an 8- to 10-week follow up scan to check that posttraumatic haematoma is resolving.[6] The operator should be aware of locally agreed guidelines to manage these patients. Haematoma and potential pitfalls of scanning haematoma will be fully discussed later in the chapter.

B. Indeterminate.

These STMs have features that require further evaluation with either MRI or excision biopsy. Indeterminate features include:

- Associated calcification
- Size greater than 5 to 7 cm
- Deep to the superficial muscle fascia
- Crossing tissue planes

- Lack of internal uniformity or internal haematoma without history of trauma
- Branching internal vascularity[1]

C. Malignant.

These STMs have positive features of malignancy that require further imaging for staging purposes.[1,6] These features are described later in the chapter.

NORMAL ANATOMY AND ULTRASOUND APPEARANCES OF THE SUBCUTANEOUS TISSUES

As with all areas of ultrasound scanning it is importance to have an appreciation of the anatomy and normal ultrasound appearances of the tissues under examination. The skin or cutaneous layer comprises the epidermis—the thinner outer layer of skin—along with the dermis, which is the deeper element comprising the connective tissue layer. The two layers cannot be differentiated on ultrasound and appear together as a thin hyperechoic layer.

Deep to this is the subcutaneous tissue consisting of hypoechoic adipose tissue interposed by linear striations of bright connective tissue that in the main run parallel to the skin. Veins and nerves can often be visualised within the subcutaneous tissues.

The muscle fascia can be seen deep to the subcutaneous tissues that surrounds the underlying muscle and is seen on ultrasound as a thin, uninterrupted hyperechoic covering (Fig. 11.2).

Fatty Tumours

Fatty tumours are the most commonly encountered soft tissue lesions referred for ultrasound examination. They can be found in any part of the body; however, a large

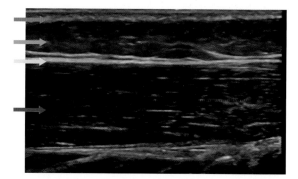

Fig. 11.2 Normal Soft Tissue Anatomy. The epidermis and dermis **(blue arrow)**, subcutaneous soft tissues **(green arrow)**, muscle fascia **(yellow arrow)** and muscle belly **(red arrow)**.

proportion occur within the subcutaneous soft tissues of the abdomen, back, and shoulders. Most subcutaneous fatty tumours are benign: it is rare for a subcutaneous fatty tumour to be malignant and when this is the case, the features on ultrasound are normally concerning.[9]

Clinically the majority of benign lipomas present as nonpainful, slow-growing, mobile lumps that are soft when palpated. In many instances the patient may have more than one. Malignant fatty tumours (liposarcoma) are more likely to be deep and fixed in comparison.

Ultrasound features of benign lipomas are variable. On grey scale they may appear hyperechoic, hypoechoic, or isoechoic to the surrounding soft tissues (Fig. 11.3). In most instances, lipomas are well-defined elliptical lesions sitting within the subcutaneous tissues or within the inter-fascial planes (Fig. 11.3B), containing thin septations (less than 2 mm) and demonstrating no or minimal internal septal vascularity on colour or power Doppler. These lesions are not concerning and can be reported as benign. Larger, multilobulated lipomas may be more ill-defined, and superficial lipomata larger than 5 to 7 cm with benign features should still be referred to the sarcoma unit for nonurgent review (not usually via the 2-week rule referral pathway) as the malignant potential is increased. They will often be managed in the long-term with follow-up ultrasound in the local department to ensure stability.

More concerning features include thick septations greater than 2 mm or nodules, increased number of internal and peripheral blood vessels, disorganised neovascularity, and peripheral oedema. These lesions may require further imaging with MR and/or the opinion of the sarcoma MDT.[2] In a primary care or triage setting, specialist advice is advisable even in superficial lesions.[5] It is important to understand how to correlate the appearances on ultrasound with the local guidelines to ensure that the correct pathway is followed for management of lipomatous lesions.

Less commonly, fatty tumours are found deep to the fascial layer. These can represent intermuscular or intramuscular lipomas or atypical lipomatous tumours. These can take on the shape and echotexture of the infiltrated muscle and can be difficult to distinguish from the muscle itself, especially when large, and comparison with the asymptomatic side may help with location. Sometimes, only the most superficial lobulation is seen and examined. All intramuscular fatty tumours of any size should be considered for referral to the sarcoma unit for further investigation and MRI may be requested to evaluate the true extent[9] (Fig. 11.4).

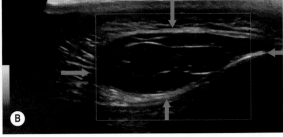

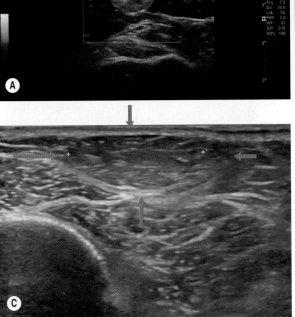

Fig. 11.3 Simple Subcutaneous lipomata (**blue arrows**). (**A**) Hyperechoic. (**B**) Hypoechoic. (**C**) Isoechoic.

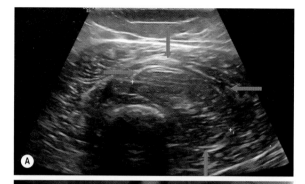

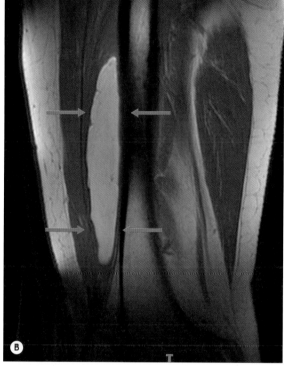

Fig. 11.4 (A) Deep intramuscular lipoma of the vastus intermedialis (**blue arrows**) **(B)** MRI scan of the same intramuscular lipoma *(arrows)*.

Soft tissue sarcomas (STS) are a rare type of cancer that originate in the tissues that connect, support, and surround other body structures. Tissues that can be affected by STS include fat, muscle, blood vessels, deep skin tissues, tendons, ligaments, and the lining of joints. They can occur anywhere in the body and more than 50 subtypes of STS exist. The role of ultrasound in the diagnosis and management of these tumours has been discussed earlier in the chapter and although ultrasound is not able to determine the exact subtype, by determining the location of the lesion, in some cases the

origin can be established. One of the most common types is liposarcoma.

Features concerning for liposarcoma include:
- Disorganised Doppler signal within a fatty mass
- Nodular area of non-fatty tissue within a deep fatty tumour
- Invasive margins
- Heterogeneous deep mass[4] (Fig. 11.5)

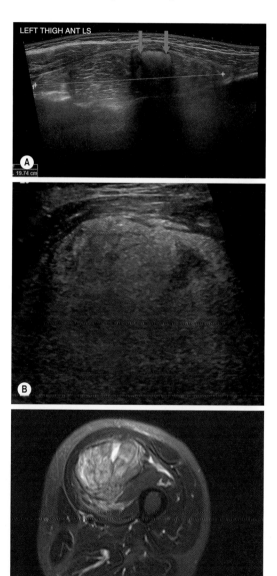

Fig. 11.5 (A–C) Liposarcoma The **blue arrows** demonstrate a nodular area of non-fatty tissue and the full extent of the lesion can be appreciated on MRI.

Synovial Sarcoma

Synovial sarcoma is also one of the most common subtypes of STS and it can present imaging challenges.

Often affecting the extremities, particularly the popliteal fossa of young adults, synovial sarcoma is an intermediate to high-grade malignancy and the fourth most common type of soft tissue sarcoma. They account for 2.5% to 10.5% of all primary soft tissue malignancies worldwide. The lesion is not usually intraarticular but commonly near joints. Compared with other masses, it has a high recurrence rate following surgical resection. Although many are detected early, diagnosis is often delayed as the vast majority of periarticular lesions are benign. Synovial sarcomas in many instances can mimic Baker's cyst or parameniscal cysts, therefore a high index of suspicion should be applied if there is no demonstrable joint communication.[10]

Ultrasound features include cystic or solid and cystic appearance, a lobulated outline, septae, and haemorrhage may be present (Fig. 11.6). It is every sonographer's nightmare and can be easily mistaken for a ganglion or fluid-filled bursa especially in the early stages when it is small. The presence of the more complex features described and neovascularity within the lesion makes it more suspicious. Further imaging with MRI is required although it can also be misdiagnosed on MRI.[10] It is therefore prudent to have a cautious approach when imaging and reporting lesions which are adjacent to the joints.

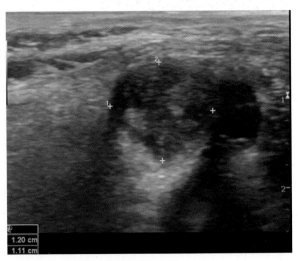

Fig. 11.6 Synovial Sarcoma.

Osteosarcoma (Comparison with Benign Osteochondroma)

Some STMs arise from the bone as seen in the case of a malignant osteosarcoma (Fig. 11.7); sarcoma arising in bone are the second most common type after STS. The destructive nature of the lesion causes disruption of the normal smooth bony/periosteal contour and an often palpable soft tissue component is also present. Two terms commonly used to describe the slightly differing ultrasound features of associated periosteal new bone formation bone growth are "sun-burst," where radiating bone spicules arise from a narrow surface of bone destruction, or "hair-on-end," describing bone spicules from a broad-based lesion. Doppler ultrasound shows increased vascularity of the lesion. Patients with osseous malignancy are referred to a specialist tertiary bone centre for management.[11]

Osteosarcoma should not be confused with a benign osteochondroma, a developmental lesion arising from the separation of a fragment of epiphyseal growth plate cartilage which herniates through the periosteal bone cuff that normally surrounds the growth plate. This cartilage ossifies with the end result of a bony exostosis and distinctive cartilage cap covering (Fig. 11.8). These lesions are often discovered whilst the patient is young but may be a later presentation due to trauma or inflammation to the area resulting in a fracture of the bone protrusion or bursitis of the adjacent tissues (Fig. 11.9). Thickened cartilage caps in adults (greater than 1.5–2 cm diameter) are more concerning and may reflect malignant transformation requiring further imaging. Patients may have solitary or multiple osteochondroma which may be broad-based or pedunculated in appearance.[12,13]

X-ray is helpful in both of these scenarios to confirm findings. Patients with osteosarcoma will normally undergo MRI and biopsy.

Other malignant manifestations can present as STMs as well as STS and bone tumours, including metastases and lymphoma.

Soft Tissue Metastases

As with many soft tissue lesions, it is often not possible for the operator to positively diagnose soft tissue metastases in the absence of other clinical features; however, the operator should have an awareness of the possible presenting ultrasound characteristics. Again, good clinical history should be sought and soft tissue

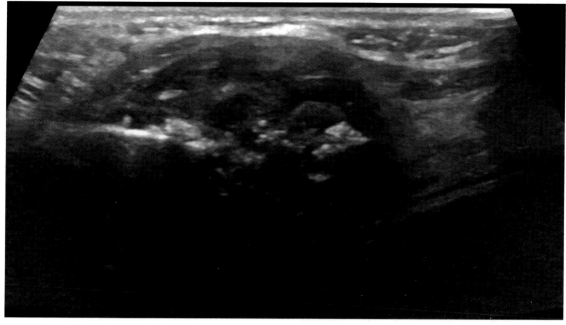

Fig. 11.7 Osteosarcoma.

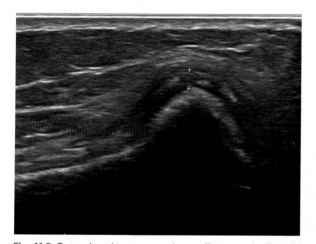

Fig. 11.8 Osteochondroma, note the cartilage cap (**callipers**).

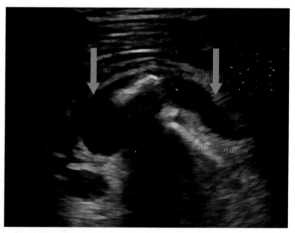

Fig. 11.9 Osteochondroma with Bursitis (**blue arrows**).

metastasis should be considered with a patient presenting with known malignancy. It is important for the operator to be aware that a soft tissue metastasis may be the initial finding in a patient with no history of malignancy. Often patients with soft tissue metastases have the same clinical features as those with STS and as with all lesions with indeterminate features, they should be

considered for assessment at the appropriate diagnostic centres as for patients with suspicious lumps.[3]

Clinically the patient often presents with a new painful lump. Lesions can have variable appearances on ultrasound and most occur within the subcutaneous soft tissues; however, they can be found deep to the muscle fascia. They can be multiple or occur in isolation and can vary in size. Typically, lesions are echo poor, with ill-defined margins and branching disorganised internal vascularity. The operator should, however, appreciate that lesions can demonstrate benign features including well-defined margins and homogenous appearances (Fig. 11.10).

Lymphoma

Lymphoma within the lymph nodes or extra-nodal, in the soft tissue structures, may be the cause of a STM. The case shown in Fig. 11.11 is of a patient with HIV presenting

with a year-long history of a soft swelling in the axilla. Ultrasound shows classic features of huge pathological lymph nodes with rounded shape and loss of the normal hilar architecture. These normally require a staging CT scan of the chest abdomen and pelvis to see the extent of the disease and biopsy of the mass/pathological node. In this case, the patient was diagnosed with non-Hodgkin's lymphoma, which is associated with HIV infection. It is important to note that patients with suspected lymphoma with pathological lymph nodes on ultrasound are referred to hematology for management rather than the sarcoma team.

OTHER COMMONLY ENCOUNTERED STMS

Epidermal Cyst

These are common cutaneous lesions that, in most cases, can be readily identified with ultrasound. They are derived from stratified squamous epithelium of the follicular infundibulum. Commonly referred to as "sebaceous" cyst, this term is misleading and should be avoided as internal contents are not of sebaceous nature. Imaging characteristics vary according to their contents.[14]

Clinically, they present as hard palpable, freely movable lesions and in many cases demonstrate a central punctum. Lesions may remain stable or grow steadily and patients may present for ultrasound examination due to spontaneous inflammation that is slow to resolve.

Ultrasound features vary according to their internal contents. Epidermal cysts are generally well defined and echo poor to the surrounding soft tissues with good through transmission of sound and posterior enhancement. Their most distinguishing feature is a demonstrable punctum that communicates with the skin surface. Internal contents such as fat, mucoid, or pus can give a variable grey scale appearance. (Fig. 11.12) If a lesion becomes inflamed or ruptures, this may affect the surrounding soft tissues and borders may become lobulated or ill-defined. The operator must combine imaging features with a good clinical history. Epidermal cysts do not demonstrate internal vascularity. However, a recently ruptured or infected cyst does often demonstrate peripheral vascularity.[14]

Peripheral Nerve Sheath Tumour (PNST)

These can arise from any peripheral nerve throughout the body and are most commonly identified within the

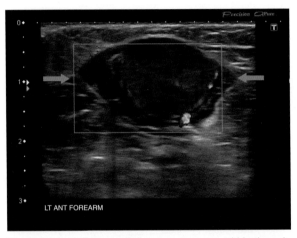

Fig. 11.10 A confirmed soft tissue metastases within the subcutaneous soft tissues of the anterior forearm in a patient with metastatic cervical cancer. The lesion has well-defined margins and a homogenous grey scale appearance with some associated vascularity.

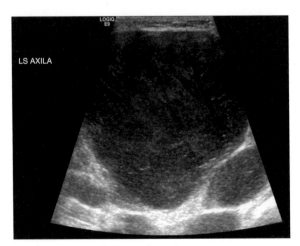

Fig. 11.11 Lymphoma.

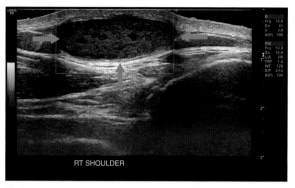

Fig. 11.12 Epidermal Cyst Within the Subcutaneous Tissues (**blue arrows**). Note the posterior acoustic enhancement.

extremities. Whilst ultrasound will readily identify these lesions due to the typical appearance of the nerve root entering and exiting the lesion, ultrasound cannot readily differentiate benign from malignant lesions.[15] The exception is a large lesion with ill-defined margins, rapid growth, and central necrosis (fluid) which is highly suspicious for a malignant lesion.

The most commonly identified PNST include schwannoma, neurofibroma, and much less often, malignant PNST can present. Clinically the patient presents with a palpable lump and may also report loss of nerve function, and/or pain. PNST are usually solitary but can be multiple in inherited conditions such as neurofibromatosis.

Ultrasonically it is often challenging to differentiate schwannoma from neurofibroma; however with careful scanning an appreciation of some key features can help to distinguish the two, the most common of which is the position of the entering and exiting nerve root (Fig. 11.13A). In a higher proportion of schwannomas, the nerve root will enter and exit in an eccentric position (specific feature but not sensitive); however, the operator must remain alert to the fact that in a small percentage of schwannomas, the nerve can be observed entering and exiting the lesion in a central position. In contrast, in all neurofibromas, the nerve root can be seen to enter and exit in a central position.[15]

The shape of the lesion may also help the operator to distinguish neurofibroma from schwannoma. Most schwannomas have an oval appearance, whereas neurofibromas tend to take on a fusiform appearance relative to the nerve.

Both schwannomas and neurofibromas are typically hypoechoic relative to muscle and exhibit through transmission of sound. Both can demonstrate variable degrees of vascularity[15] (see Fig. 11.13B).

Ganglion

Ganglia are cystic lesions that can arise from any joint or tendon sheath throughout the body. They have a fibrous capsule and are filled with thick synovial fluid. Ganglia are most commonly found around the hand, wrist, and dorsal aspect of the foot and can be readily identified with ultrasound due to their typical appearance and location. They are the most common mass in the hand and wrist. Seventy percent arise from the dorsal band of the scapholunate ligament and the next most common site is the radial aspect of the volar wrist. The proximity of the lesion to the radial artery is important to note in the report as this can affect management.[6,8]

Clinically, ganglia present as smooth, firm noncompressible lesions that may fluctuate in size. Symptoms can vary depending on size and location. Some patients may describe pain, or restricted joint movement, whilst others may describe altered sensory/motor function due to compression of an abutting nerve.

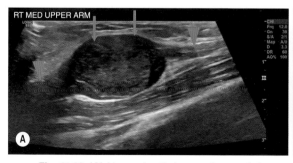
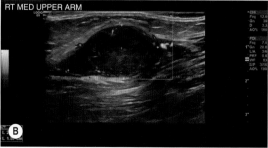

Fig. 11.13 (A) Nerve sheath tumour *(arrows)*. A nerve can clearly be demonstrated in continuity with the lesion **(arrow heads)**. **(B)** Nerve sheath tumour demonstrating internal vascularity.

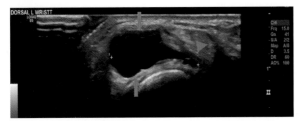

Fig. 11.14 Ganglion Cyst. Note the neck arising from the underlying joint **(arrow head)**.

Traditionally, ultrasound characterisation of a ganglion cyst describes a simple anechoic lesion with a smooth border, good through transmission of sound, and absence of any associated vascularity (Fig. 11.14). In practice, however, the ultrasound characteristics can be variable including internal septa, lobulated irregular shape, and thick walls. The presence of vascularity should alert the operator to a potential suspicious mass or collapsed cyst. Due to their variable appearance, the operator should seek to demonstrate a neck communicating with the associated joint, tendon sheath, or ligament which will define the origin of the lesion to provide a positive diagnosis. The neck of the ganglion can be quite some distance from the palpable abnormality. It is important to trace the neck of the cyst in the event of surgical excision as recurrence is much less likely if the surgeon can reach the origin of the cyst.[6,8]

Pilomatricoma

Pilomatricoma are benign superficial tumours of the hair follicle and can be readily identifiable with ultrasound. Clinically, patients present with a solid palpable mass that is freely movable and can grow slowly over a long period of time.[6]

Ultrasonically, pilomatricomas can present one of two ways:

- Lesions are small, well-defined, and hypoechoic, situated within the subcutaneous tissues, demonstrating echogenic foci within and a hypoechoic halo or rim (Fig. 11.15).
- Lesions can be partially or completely calcified and demonstrate strong posterior acoustic shadowing depending on the degree of internal calcification.

Soft Tissue Venous Malformations

These STMs are more commonly referred to as soft tissue hemangiomas and are benign, vascular lesions. According to the International Society for the Study of

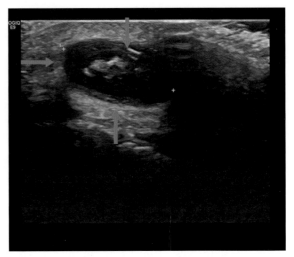

Fig. 11.15 Pilomatricoma (Blue arrows).

Vascular Anomalies (ISSVA) classification, the term "hemangioma" is now considered a misnomer and the more accurate term is slow-flow venous malformation. However, it may be helpful to include the term hemangioma in the imaging report as it is more familiar to many clinicians.[16]

They can arise in various locations throughout the body, including striated muscle, skin, subcutaneous tissue, and synovial tissue, and they are the most common angiomatous lesions, representing up to 7% of all benign soft tissue tumours.[16]

On ultrasound these lesions can have variable grey scale and Doppler appearances, typically seen as an ill- or well-defined hypoechoic mass of heterogeneous echotexture with multiple cystic spaces within. On colour Doppler, there may be florid internal vascularity, no detectable signal, or only weak signal (Fig. 11.16). Theses variable appearances can pose a diagnostic challenge to the operator and appearances must be correlated with clinical presentation. The patient may report a palpable mass with varying degrees of pain.

Bursae

These are fluid-filled sacs or sac-like cavities that can be found throughout the body. They are designed to facilitate movement and reduce friction that may potentially occur between bone and soft tissues, including tendons, muscles, or ligaments. Bursae can often become inflamed or irritated due to repetitive movement and pressure or injury to the affected joint or area. This causes the bursa

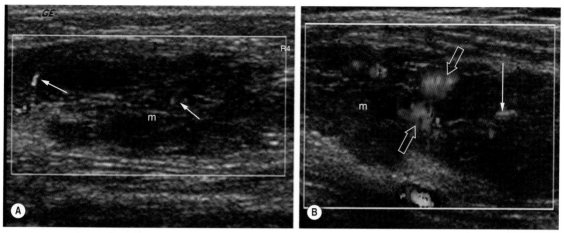

Fig. 11.16 (A and B) Soft Tissue Venous Malformation. (From Keng C-Y, et al. Soft tissue hemangiomas: high-resolution grayscale and color Doppler ultrasonographic features in 43 patients. J Med Ultrasound. 2008;16(3):223-230.)

to fill with fluid, with associated synovial thickening/proliferation, which in turn causes pain and restricted movement. These pathological changes are referred to as bursitis.

They can appear variably solid/cystic on ultrasound and can frequently have swirling contents. They often have thick vascular walls. Location is often key in making the diagnosis.[17]

Adventitious bursae (described as non-native bursae in Chapter 2) are bursae that are not usually present, that form within soft tissues exposed to repetitive external rubbing, friction, or irritation, commonly found at the knee, elbow, or the plantar aspect of the foot (Fig. 11.17).

Foreign Body

Ultrasound is an excellent tool for the identification of superficial soft tissue foreign bodies. A foreign body can be appreciated as an echo-bright structure within the surrounding reactive hypoechoic subcutaneous soft tissues (granuloma).[3] Often, the surrounding granulomatous soft tissue may demonstrate an inflammatory response, seen as increased vascularity when colour Doppler is applied (Fig. 11.18).

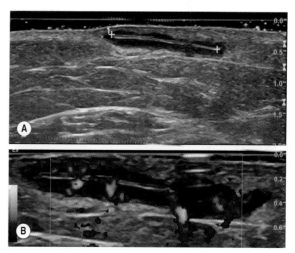

Fig. 11.18 (A) Foreign body with peripheral granulomatous tissue. **(B)** Foreign body with associated inflammatory response of the surrounding soft tissues.

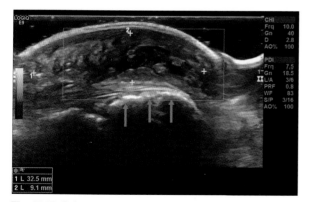

Fig. 11.17 Submetatarsal Bursa within the soft tissues just superficial to the metatarsal head **(arrows)**.

It is useful for the operator to include specific information to the referring clinician when a foreign body is identified, to aid in localisation for its removal. These may include:

- The size of the foreign body, measured in two orthogonal planes if possible
- Its position relative to an adjacent structure
- Depth of the foreign body from the skin surface

The operator should be aware that the patient may often present with no suitable history and should be vigilant to the presence of a foreign body in apparently simple soft tissue infection. If not considered, an undiagnosed foreign body can be an ongoing source of recurrent infection.

Abdominal Wall Endometrioma

Abdominal wall endometriomas occur when endometrial tissue from the uterine cavity becomes embedded within soft tissues of the abdomen after caesarean section (c-section). The patient will present with a palpable lesion in the area of the scar that is tender to the touch. Abdominal wall endometriomas can cause diagnostic uncertainty as they can often demonstrate many of the clinical and ultrasound features of malignant neoplasms, such as STS or soft tissue metastases. Ultrasound features can include irregular margins, disruption of fascia, heterogeneous echotexture, and echo poor grey scale appearance. Lesions can demonstrate branching internal vascularity or be avascular.[18]

Fig. 11.19 demonstrates an echo-poor, solid-looking lesion with irregular margins within the soft tissues of the abdomen. The lesion appears to disrupt the underlying fascia. On first consideration the lesion has several features that would alert the operator to malignant potential. In this instance, it is the clinical history that is pivotal to making an informed decision as to the nature of the lesion. A history of previous c-section with the lesion located at the site of the c-section scar, should alert the operator to the potential diagnosis of abdominal wall endometrioma.[18] It is, however, important for the operator to be aware that if there is still diagnostic uncertainty after the ultrasound examination, then the patient should be managed appropriately, according to locally agreed pathways.

Another soft tissue lesion of the abdominal wall musculature is a desmoid tumour. This is a rare benign, noninflammatory fibroblastic tumour, most frequently occurring in females between the age of 20 and 40 years. It has a hypoechoic appearance on ultrasound and may demonstrate neovascularity. It can have similar appearances to an endometrioma, and MRI is usually required for further assessment. Recurrence is high following surgical resection. Radiotherapy and hormone therapy are also used to limit tumour growth.[19]

Trauma and Infection

Patients presenting with soft tissue complaints relating to trauma or infection are commonplace within both primary care and also accident and emergency settings. Traditionally, when imaging is required in these patients CT and MRI are the modalities of choice. However, due to its accessibility and better resolution of the superficial structures, ultrasound is increasingly becoming the preferred imaging modality for the initial investigation of these patients. Some of these conditions are discussed below.

Fat Necrosis

Fat necrosis is a common condition caused by damage to the subcutaneous fatty tissue following injury and can occur anywhere in the body, but is most prevalent in the shins, buttocks, thighs, arms, and breasts. The trauma may be significant such as a fall or blunt force trauma, but often it is relatively innocuous, and the patient may not recall the injury at all.

The patient may present with any combination of the following:

- Palpable lump
- Localised depression of the soft tissues

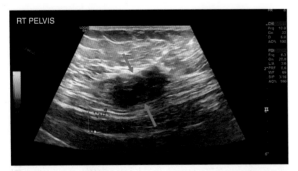

Fig. 11.19 Abdominal wall endometrioma (**blue arrows**) within the subcutaneous soft tissues of the abdominal wall post caesarean section. Power Doppler box has been placed over the lesion to assess for internal vascularity.

- Discolouration of the skin
- Localised area of pain[20]

Often the time interval between the injury and discovery of a lesion can be significant and the patient cannot recall injury when questioned.

Ultrasound features are variable. Common findings include a diffusely echo-bright area of subcutaneous fatty tissue when compared to that of the surrounding soft tissues. In other instances, the area of necrosis may be encapsulated and demonstrate an echo-poor halo. Oil cysts can commonly be seen as central small cystic areas within the area of increased echogenicity. The subcutaneous tissues are often thinned at the site of injury and the perceived lump may in fact be the normal thickness adjacent tissue.[20] If in a limb, it can be useful to use the contralateral limb to compare.

Usually, the patient does not present acutely, and internal vascularity is not commonly seen. The main differential diagnosis in the subcutaneous fat layer would be a lipoma with atypical features (Fig. 11.20). The location and subcutaneous tissue involvement near a bony prominence are usually sufficient to confirm the diagnosis. If there is any clinical or diagnostic doubt, then the patient may require further investigation, either by MRI or by follow-up scan. This is best performed under the guidance of a specialist.

Cellulitis

Initially, ultrasound imaging features include diffuse increased echogenicity of subcutaneous soft tissues;

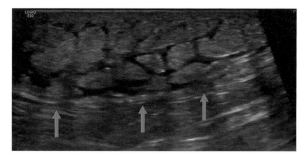

Fig. 11.21 Cellulitis (**blue arrows**).

however, as the condition progresses the amount of subcutaneous soft tissue fluid increases, causing a lobulated effect that can be described as "cobblestone"[21] (Fig. 11.21). It is, however, important for the operator to appreciate that these are nonspecific features of cellulitis and may also be present with generalised subcutaneous soft tissue oedema, often present in conditions such as heart failure. Cellulitis can be treated with antibiotics.

Abscess

The patient will typically present with focal swelling or a lump that is often painful, with accompanying cellulitis of the surrounding soft tissues.

Ultrasound features are wide ranging and can include anechoic or hypoechoic collections of fluid with internal debris.[21] Gas may also be present within the abscess, typically seen as echo-bright foci. Transducer pressure may illicit swirling movement if pus is present with the lesion. Often the borders may be ill-defined and the lesion may demonstrate some peripheral vascularity when colour Doppler is applied[21] (Fig. 11.22).

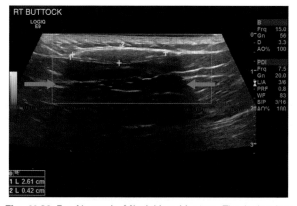

Fig. 11.20 Fat Necrosis Mimicking Lipoma. The lesion has atypical features demonstrating posterior acoustic enhancement (**blue arrows**). The lesion was confirmed at MRI to be an area of fat necrosis from previous injury.

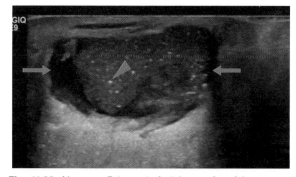

Fig. 11.22 Abscess. Echogenic foci (**arrow heads**) represent gas within the lesion.

No colour flow should be demonstrated within the collection. It is important for the operator to appreciate that these features are, however, nonspecific and can be present in other lesions. The main differential diagnosis is necrotic tumour. The operator must always take into consideration the clinical history of the patient when performing the examination. Identification of occult abscess warrants incision and drainage in the vast majority of cases, so when scanning for potential abscess, the operator should aim to delineate the involved soft tissues and proximity to vessels.[21]

Haematoma

It is relatively easy for the operator to appreciate a haematoma within the soft tissues when accompanied by a strong clinical history, which may include previous trauma, surgery, or use of anticoagulation therapy. Ultrasound features vary depending on the time frame in which the lesion is scanned. Acute haematoma will generally present as a well-defined ovoid or lentiform lesion, often with fluid/fluid levels due to settling blood products, or varying degrees of internal echoes (Fig. 11.23). As the internal blood products are broken down, the lesion will become more homogenous and anechoic. Some peripheral vascularity may initially be observed and you may often see a small amount of neovascularity associated with resolving haematoma at the site of a muscle injury as the muscle starts to repair[6].

As previously discussed, the diagnosis of benign haematoma should always be exercised with caution. The disorganised internal vascularity present in some preexisting malignant lesions may spontaneously rupture and bleed after minor trauma and can mimic benign haematoma. It is therefore prudent for the operator to carry out a follow-up scan when haematoma is identified, even if the patient provides a good clinical history

to explain the haematoma. Benign haematoma will resolve at subsequent scan. Occasionally, haematoma may form a chronic collection which is anechoic with a well-defined wall and gelatinous content which can persist long term. The operator should be aware of locally agreed pathways for the follow up of haematoma.

The main differential diagnoses the operator should be aware of are abscess and necrotic tumour.

POTENTIAL PITFALL CASE 1

1. Malignant Lesion with Benign Features

Low-grade myxofibrosarcoma in a 54-year-Old female

Patient presented with a tender firm lump just below the buttock that was not present on the contralateral side. There was no stated history of trauma.

Ultrasound imaging demonstrated a homogenous echo-poor lesion with well-defined borders and an apparent lack of associated vascularity when power Doppler was applied (Fig. 11.24A). Whilst these are, on first consideration benign features, they are not sufficient to reliably characterise the lesion as benign.

However, there are indications from the clinical history and the location of the lesion that should alert the operator to the potential for malignancy. Clinically, the lesion was a new presentation, was tender when palpated and there was no history of trauma. The lesion was intramuscular, and measured over 5 cm.

The patient was referred for MRI scan for further assessment. Fig. 11.24B shows a well-defined ellipsoid lesion lying within the biceps femoris muscle. Following Gadolinium contrast, there was marked irregular enhancement. The patient was referred to the regional sarcoma unit. The lesion was confirmed to be a myxofibrosarcoma.

POTENTIAL PITFALL CASE 2

2. Benign Lesion with Malignant Features

Hemangioneurofibroma in a 35-year-old male

Patient presented with a tender palpable lump at the left lateral thigh that had grown larger over a period of 3 months.

Fig. 11.25A demonstrates a complex, solid-looking lesion with heterogeneous echotexture, irregular borders, and branching disorganised internal vascularity. Ultrasound characteristics along with the associated clinical features of a tender fast-growing lesion also suggest malignant potential.

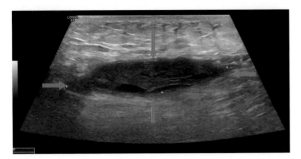

Fig. 11.23 Haematoma seen in the acute phase.

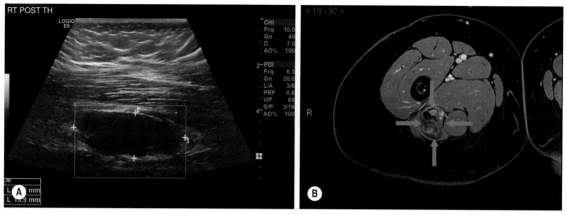

Fig. 11.24 Case 1: **(A)** Myxofibrosarcoma. **(B)** MRI image representing low-grade myxofibrosarcoma *(arrows)*.

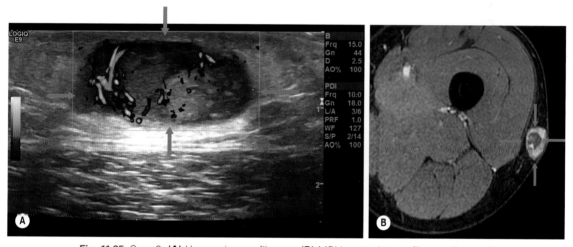

Fig. 11.25 Case 2: **(A)** Hemangioneurofibroma. **(B)** MRI hemangioneurofibroma *(arrows)*.

The patient was urgently referred via the 2-week pathway to the regional sarcoma MDT. The patient also underwent an MRI scan to further characterise the lesion. In Fig. 11.25B the MRI scan shows a lesion within the subcutaneous soft tissue at the left lateral thigh which demonstrates marked heterogeneous enhancement post gadolinium. The lesion was eventually diagnosed at histology as a hemangioneurofibroma, with a potential differential diagnosis of schwannoma.

◎ KEY RECOMMENDATIONS

1. Any patient with a soft tissue mass that is increasing in size, or measures more than 5 cm whether or not it is painful, should either be referred for an urgent ultrasound scan or referred directly to the sarcoma diagnostic centre.
2. If the ultrasound scan does not confidently confirm a benign diagnosis, then the patient should be referred for further investigation on an urgent suspected cancer pathway referral.[1]

MULTIPLE CHOICE QUESTIONS

1. Post examination, which of the following ultrasound features of a STM would prompt the operator to refer the patient for further investigation/management?
   a) Crossing tissue planes
   b) Size greater than 2 to 5 cm
   c) Hypoechogenic compared to surrounding tissues

2. Ganglia can be distinguished from simple joint effusions due to the fact that,
   a) ganglia are often hypoechoic on ultrasound, whereas joint effusions are not.
   b) ganglia will compress, whereas a simple joint effusion will not compress when pressure is applied.
   c) ganglia will not compress, whereas a simple joint effusion will disperse when pressure is applied.

3. A traumatic event can cause the following soft tissue manifestation:
   a) fatty hypertrophy.
   b) fatty infiltration.
   c) fat necrosis.

4. Utilising colour or power Doppler can be useful when assessing STM but when assessing superficial lesions, it is important to apply:
   a) minimal pressure to ensure small vessels are not obliterated.
   b) maximum pressure to ensure small vessels are not excluded from the assessment.
   c) maximum pressure to minimise tissue thickness.

5. Soft tissue sarcomas (STS) are a rare type of cancer that can originate in:
   a) blood.
   b) fat.
   c) omentum.

REFERENCES

1. Fletcher CDM, Bridge JA, Hogendoorn PCW, Mertens F. WHO Classification of tumours of soft tissue and bone. 5th ed, Volume 3. Lyon, France: IARC; 2020. https://publications.iarc.fr/Book-And-Report-Series/Who-Classification-Of-Tumours/Soft-Tissue-And-Bone-Tumours-2020

2. Dangoor A, Seddon B, Gerrand C, Grimer R, Whelan J, Judson I. UK guidelines for the management of soft tissue sarcomas. Clin Sarcoma Res. 2016;6:20.

3. Lakkaraju A, Sinha R, Garikipati R, Edward S, Robinson P. Ultrasound for initial evaluation and triage of clinically suspicious soft-tissue masses. Clin Radiol. 2009;64:615–621. doi:10.1016/j.crad.2009.01.012.

4. Rowbotham E, Bhuva S, Gupta H, Robinson P. Assessment of referrals into the soft tissue sarcoma service: evaluation of imaging early in the pathway process. Sarcoma. 2012; 2012:781723. doi:10.1155/2012/781723.

5. Chung HW, Cho KH. Ultrasonography of soft tissue "oops lesions". Ultrasonography. 2015;34(3):217–225.

6. Hwang S, Adler RS. Sonographic evaluation of the musculoskeletal soft tissue masses. Ultrasound Q. 2005; 21(4):259–270.

7. O'Sullivan P, Harri AC, Munk P. Radiological features of synovial cell Sarcoma. Br J Radiol. 2008;81:346–356.

8. Toprak H, Kiliç E, Serter A, Kocakoç E, Ozgocmen S. Ultrasound and Doppler US in evaluation of superficial soft-tissue lesions. J Clin Imaging Sci. 2014;4:12.

9. Al-ani Z, Fernando M, Wilkinson V, Kotnis N. The management of deep-seated, low grade lipomatous lesions. Br J Radiol. 2018;91(1086):20170725.

10. Belli P, Costantini M, Mirk P, Maresca G, Priolo F, Marano P. Role of color Doppler sonography in the assessment of musculoskeletal soft tissue masses. J Ultrasound Med. 2000;19:823–830.

11. Jamshidi K, Yahyazadeh H, Bagherifard A. Unusual presentation of synovial sarcoma as meniscal cyst: a case report. Arch Bone Jt Surg. 2015;3(4):296–299.

12. Loberant N. Sonographic hair-on-end sign in osteosarcoma. An Bras Dermatol. 2013;88(4):631–634.

13. Murphey MD, Choi JJ, Kransdorf MJ, Flemming DJ, Gannon FH. Imaging of osteochondroma: variants and complications with radiologic-pathologic correlation. Radiographics. 2000;20:1407–1434.

14. Lee HS, Joo KB, Song HT, et al. Relationship between sonographic and pathologic findings in epidermal inclusion cysts. J Clin Ultrasound. 2001;29(7):374–383.

15. Tsai WC, Chiou HJ, Chou YH, Wang HK, Chiou SY, Chang CY. Differentiation between schwannomas and neurofibromas in the extremities and superficial body. J Ultrasound Med. 2008;27:161–166.

16. Keng CY, Lan HHC, Chen CCC, Gueng MK, Su YG, Lee SK. Soft tissue hemangiomas: high-resolution grayscale and color Doppler ultrasonographic features in 43 patients. J Med Ultrasound. 2008;16(3):223–230.

17. Ruangchaijatuporn T, Gaetke-Udager K, Jacobson JA, Yablon CM, Morag Y. Ultrasound evaluation of bursae: anatomy and pathological appearances. Skeletal Radiol. 2017;46:445–462.

18. Hensen JH, Van Breda Vriesman AC, Puylaert JB. Abdominal wall endometriosis: clinical presentation and imaging features with emphasis on sonography. AJR Am J Roentgenol. 2006;186(3):616–620.

19. Lou L, Teng J, Qi H, Ban Y. Sonographic appearances of desmoid tumors. J Ultrasound Med. 2014;33:1519–1525.

20. Walsh M, Jacobson JA, Kim SM, Lucas DR, Morag Y, Fessell DP. Sonography of fat necrosis involving the extremity and torso with magnetic resonance imaging and histologic correlation. J Ultrasound Med 2008; 27(12):1751–1757.

21. O'Rourke K, Kibbee N, Stubbs A. Ultrasound for the evaluation of skin and soft tissue infections. Mo Med. 2015;112(3):202–205.

ANSWERS

CHAPTER 1

1. **b.** distinguish between two structures in axis or parallel to the beam
2. **a.** Scattering, specular reflection, refraction, and absorption
3. **b.** can cause areas of tendons to appear artefactually echo poor
4. **c.** A low PRF should be set when assessing low velocity flow, which is the aim in most MSK examinations.
5. **a.** minimising scan time and power output

CHAPTER 3

1. **b.** Supraspinatus, infraspinatus, subscapularis, and teres minor
2. **c.** To move the tendon from underneath the coracoid process
3. **c.** Supraspinatus
4. **a.** Scarf test
5. **a.** nonsteroidal antiinflammatory drugs, rehabilitation physiotherapy, pain relieving interventional techniques, and surgery

CHAPTER 4

1. **c.** Long head portion
2. **c.** Olecranon fossa
3. **b.** Resisted flexion
4. **c.** Biceps, artery, median nerve
5. **b.** Brachialis

CHAPTER 5

1. **c.** Extensor carpi radialis brevis. **e.** Extensor carpi radialis longus
2. **a.** Flexor carpi radialis. **b.** Palmaris longus. **e.** Flexor carpi ulnaris
3. **a.** Flexor digitorum superficialis
4. **a.** Median nerve
5. **c.** Associated with a rupture of the ulna collateral ligament of the thumb

CHAPTER 6

1. **c.** Linea alba
2. **a.** Inferior epigastric vessels
3. **b.** Indirect inguinal herniae
4. **a.** An irreducible hernia due to a narrow neck
5. **b.** Potential space medial and adjacent to the femoral vein

CHAPTER 7

1. **c.** Greater trochanteric pain syndrome
2. **a.** Pectineus, adductor brevis, adductor longus, adductor magnus, gracilis
3. **b.** Femoral head and acetabulum
4. **c.** Ischial
5. **b.** Flexor of the hip and an extensor of the knee

CHAPTER 8

1. **b.** Rectus femoris, vastus medialis, vastus lateralis, vastus intermedius
2. **c.** Between the medial head of gastrocnemius and semimembranosus
3. **b.** Patella baja
4. **a.** Medial and lateral gastrocnemius, soleus
5. **c.** Sinding-Larson-Johansson disease

CHAPTER 9

1. **a.** Tibialis anterior
2. **a.** First MTPj. **b.** Second MTPj
3. **d.** Steroid injection
4. **b.** 4 mm
5. **c.** Peroneus brevis, peroneus tertius, lateral cord of the plantar fascia

CHAPTER 11

1. **a.** Crossing tissue planes
2. **c.** Ganglia will not compress, whereas a simple joint effusion will disperse when pressure is applied
3. **c.** Fat necrosis
4. **a.** Minimal pressure to ensure small vessels are not obliterated
5. **b.** fat

INDEX

Page numbers followed by *f* indicates figures and *t* indicates tables.